Mechanical Ventilation in Neonates and Children

Ashok P. Sarnaik · Shekhar T. Venkataraman ·
Bradley A. Kuch

Editors

Mechanical Ventilation in Neonates and Children

A Pathophysiology-Based Management Approach

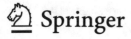

Springer

Editors
Ashok P. Sarnaik
Children's Hospital of Michigan,
Wayne State University
Detroit, MI, USA

Shekhar T. Venkataraman
Children's Hospital of Pittsburgh,
University of Pittsburgh
Pittsburgh, PA, USA

Bradley A. Kuch
Children's Hospital of Pittsburgh
Pittsburgh, PA, USA

ISBN 978-3-030-83740-2   ISBN 978-3-030-83738-9   (eBook)
https://doi.org/10.1007/978-3-030-83738-9

This Springer imprint is published by the registered company Springer Nature Switzerland AG
The registered company address is: Gewerbestrasse 11, 6330 Cham, Switzerland

Preface

With so many books on the subject, a reasonable question may be "why another book"? During our careers as clinicians, investigators and educators, we have observed that the healthcare providers are often intimidated by the ventilators as they focus on the machine rather than the altered pathophysiology that is to be addressed in the least injurious fashion while allowing sufficient time for recovery to occur. The ventilator manufacturers do not make it easier by introducing different terminology for similar interventions adding further confusion. We have also observed that nurses, physicians and respiratory therapists have their own areas of attention. We have attempted to provide a common framework based on growth-dependent pulmonary mechanics and underlying pathophysiologic mechanism necessitating all forms of support of the respiratory system. We hope that this framework is an effective tool to understand the underlying pathophysiologic derangements and the therapeutic rationale behind the supportive measures necessary. We also hope that this book will be useful for readers from different disciplines at varying levels of experience, at the bedside as clinicians, in the classrooms as educators and in the academic settings conducting scholarly activities.

We begin with traditional, age-old principles of pulmonary mechanics and physiology of gas exchange taught by Julius Comroe and simplified by John West. These are important for any student to build his/her understanding the fundamentals of lung dysfunction. The concepts of static and dynamic processes are explained and mechanisms of airflow in health and disease are described. Importance of clinical examination and physical assessment is emphasized followed by description of monitoring techniques. Within this framework, we present both invasive and non-invasive support of respiration. Every attempt is made to not only direct the reader what to do but also the rationale for why a certain approach is superior in some situations but not others. A separate section on special challenges encountered in the neonatal period is presented. Finally, we describe various case-based approaches in managing respiratory failure.

This book is intended for medical students, residents, fellows, attending physicians, nurses and respiratory therapists. We dedicate it to countless parents, who entrusted their most precious possession—the lives of their children, to our care; and to all our patients who taught us so much over the years.

Detroit, USA   Ashok P. Sarnaik, MD
Pittsburgh, USA   Shekhar T. Venkataraman, MD
Pittsburgh, USA   Bradley A. Kuch, MHA, RRT-NPS, FAARC

Contents

Chapter 1
Mechanical Characteristics of the Lung and the Chest Wall

Ashok P. Sarnaik

Mechanical properties of the respiratory system govern the principles of air movement between the alveoli and the atmosphere. For air to move from one end to another, a pressure gradient is required. As long as there is some communication between the alveoli and the atmosphere, gas will flow (volume/time) from a higher pressure to a lower pressure until the pressures at both ends equilibrate resulting in cessation of flow. Pressure equilibration is not instantaneous; it requires time. Insufficient time will prevent pressure equilibration, and therefore the potential change in volume. Resistive properties of the respiratory system oppose generation of flow whereas the elastance characteristics oppose change in volume.

1.1 Lung Volumes and Capacities

Along with pressure, knowledge of lung volumes and capacities is crucial to understanding normal lung function as well as many pathological conditions (Fig. 1.1). *Tidal volume* (VT) is the volume of gas moved with each breath. In health, spontaneous VT is usually between 6-8 ml/kg. This volume refreshes alveolar gas with atmospheric air during inspiration and leads to removal of CO_2 during exhalation. The volume of gas remaining in the lung after tidal exhalation is termed *functional residual capacity* (FRC). FRC is measured either by measurement of

The original version of this chapter was revised with correct labels and text alignment Figures 1.1, 1.2, 1.3 and 1.6. The correction to this chapter can be found at https://doi.org/10.1007/978-3-030-83738-9_14

A. P. Sarnaik (✉)
Professor of Pediatrics, Former Pediatrician in Chief and Interim Chairman Children's Hospital of Michigan, Wayne State University School of Medicine, 3901 Beaubien, Detroit, MI 48201, USA
e-mail: asarnaik@med.wayne.edu

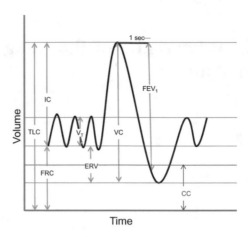

Fig. 1.1 Spirometry showing lung volumes and capacities. Total lung capacity = TLC, IC = Inspiratory capacity, FRC = Functional residual capacity, VT = Tidal volume, ERV = Expiratory reserve volume, VC = Vital capacity, FEV_1 = Forced expiratory volume in 1 s, CC = Closing capacity (measured only by gas dilution techniques). Reprinted with permission from Sarnaik AP, Heidemann S and Clark JA, Nelson Textbook of Pediatrics, 20th Edition, Kliegman, St. Geme et al. Editors, Elsevier 2016

thoracic gas volume by plethysmography or by helium dilution method. FRC acts as a reservoir for gas exchange between the alveoli and the pulmonary capillary blood throughout respiration. Diseases that decrease lung compliance and lower FRC can have profound effects on oxygenation. Positive end-expiratory pressure (PEEP) helps maintain end-expiratory volume and improve oxygenation. *Residual volume* (RV) is the volume of gas remaining in the lung after a maximal forced exhalation. The difference between FRC and RV is the *expiratory reserve volume. Inspiratory capacity* (IC) is the volume that can be inspired from FRC after a maximal inspiration from a normal exhalation and *total lung capacity* is the total volume of gas in the lung at maximum inspiration. Closing capacity (CC) is volume of gas in the lung during exhalation when the dependent airways start to close. Closing capacity can only be measured by specific gas dilution techniques and not by spirometry. In healthy children and adults, CC is well below the FRC, meaning that all the airways remain open during tidal respiration. In intrapulmonary obstructive diseases and even in healthy neonates, dependent airways start to close during tidal exhalation before reaching FRC. When CC is greater than FRC, the alveolar ventilation moves towards the nondependent, less perfused areas, away from dependent and better perfused areas, resulting in V/Q mismatch and a lower PaO_2. This also results in some amount of air trapping.

1.2 Pressure

In regards to pulmonary mechanics, pressure is generally described in relation to atmosphere which is considered to be 0 cm H_2O. During spontaneous breathing, inspiration results from negative pressure in the pleural space and alveoli drawing air from the atmosphere, while during positive pressure breathing air is pushed into the alveoli from a higher pressure source. There is a lack of consistency with terms and symbols used to describe reference pressures and pressure gradients. For the purpose of this discussion, we will use the following terminology (Fig. 1.2).

Proximal airway pressure (P_{AW}) is measured at the mouth during spontaneous breathing, inside the ventilator, at the patient-support device interface during non-invasive breathing support or in the hub of the endotracheal tube during invasive mechanical ventilation. When measured at the mouth during spontaneous respiration, it is same as the atmospheric pressure (P_{ATM}) or body surface pressure (P_B) which is referred to as 0 cm H_2O. During mechanical ventilation, P_{AW} is usually measured in the ventilator via a pressure transducer in various phases of respiratory cycle. Alveolar pressure (P_{ALV}) is inferred by inspiratory and expiratory occlusion techniques, allowing the P_{ALV} to equilibrate with the P_{AW} by accomplishing a "no flow" state and measuring pressure at the proximal airway. A no flow state assumes equalization of pressure at both ends of the system. Intrapleural pressure (P_{PL}) is not directly measured in clinical practice. Instead, it is inferred by measuring esophageal pressure (P_{ES}) by a balloon placed in distal esophagus.

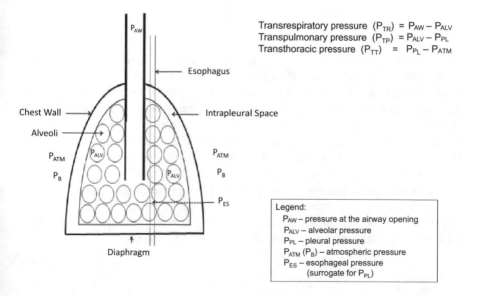

Transrespiratory pressure $(P_{TR}) = P_{AW} - P_{ALV}$
Transpulmonary pressure $(P_{TP}) = P_{ALV} - P_{PL}$
Transthoracic pressure $(P_{TT}) = P_{PL} - P_{ATM}$

Legend:
P_{AW} – pressure at the airway opening
P_{ALV} – alveolar pressure
P_{PL} – pleural pressure
P_{ATM} (P_B) – atmospheric pressure
P_{ES} – esophageal pressure
(surrogate for P_{PL})

Fig. 1.2 Schematic presentation of various sites at which reference pressures are measured. P_{ATM} or P_B = atmospheric or body surface pressure, P_{AW} = proximal airway pressure, P_{ALV} = alveolar pressure, P_{PL} = intrapleural pressure, P_{ES} = esophageal pressure (used as a surrogate for P_{PL})

1.3   Pressure Gradients

Transrespiratory pressure is the pressure difference between P_{AW} and P_{ALV}. Transthoracic pressure ($P_{ATM} - P_{PL}$) is the pressure difference that thoracic cage is subjected to throughout the respiratory cycle. P_{ES} is used as a surrogate measure of P_{PL}. Transpulmonary pressure ($P_{ALV} - P_{PL}$) is the pressure difference between the alveolar pressure and the pleural pressure and is indicative of the pressure responsible for maintaining alveolar inflation. It reflects the stress the alveoli are exposed to during inflation and deflation with mechanical ventilation. Measurement of transpulmonary and transthoracic pressures allow the partitioning of the combined lung-thorax mechanics into separate chest wall and alveolar components. Trans-airway pressure ($P_{AW} - P_{ALV}$) denotes the pressure difference that influences air movement (flow) across the airways. It is used to calculate airway resistance (pressure/flow).

1.4   Surface Tension

Alveolar surface is lined with a liquid film creating an air-fluid interface for gas exchange. Alveoli are connected to each other and the atmosphere via airways. The pressure required to keep an alveolus open is governed by Laplace's law which is expressed as:

$$P = \frac{2T}{r}$$

where P is the pressure required to inflate the alveolus, T is the surface tension at the air-fluid interface, and r is the radius. Pressure needed to keep the alveolus open is greater, with higher surface tension and smaller radius. If surface tension remains the same, smaller alveoli will tend to collapse and empty into larger alveoli resulting in atelectasis. Pulmonary surfactant is produced by type II alveolar cells and forms the lining of alveolar air interface. There are two major functions of surfactant. Surfactant is necessary to decrease the surface tension thereby requiring less pressure (critical opening pressure) for alveolar inflation. Surfactant also decreases the surface tension of smaller alveoli to a greater extent compared to the larger ones. Because the concentration of surfactant is greater in smaller alveoli compared to larger alveoli, the surface tension is decreased to a greater extent thus equalizing the pressure in alveoli of different sizes (Fig. 1.3).

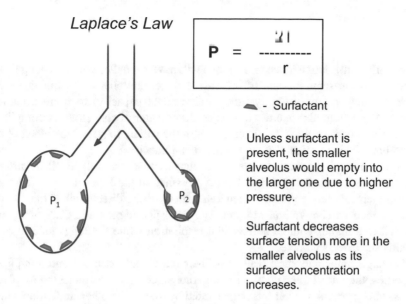

$$P = \frac{2l}{r}$$

- Surfactant

Unless surfactant is present, the smaller alveolus would empty into the larger one due to higher pressure.

Surfactant decreases surface tension more in the smaller alveolus as its surface concentration increases.

Fig. 1.3 Pressure generated in a smaller alveolus (P_2) is greater than that in a larger alveolus (P_1) with a tendency of the smaller alveolus to empty into the larger one. Surfactant, in general, lowers the surface tension. Being more concentrated in a smaller alveolus, surfactant lowers the surface tension to a greater extent allowing alveoli of different sizes to remain open and in communication with each other.

1.5   Elastance and Compliance

Elastance is the property of a substance to return to its original state when the deforming stress (e.g. pressure) is removed. Pulmonary elastance is determined by two factors: elastin in elastic fibers in the connective tissue of the lungs including the airways and surface tension in the alveoli. Elastance is decreased with loss of elastin and increased with increased surface tension or accumulation of fluid and inflammatory material. Elastance of the chest wall is determined by the stiffness and the integrity of its skeletal components and, strength and tone of the musculature.

$$E = \frac{\Delta P}{\Delta V}$$

where E = Elastance, P = Pressure, and V = Volume. Elastic recoil refers to the rapidity and force (pressure) with which a substance returns to its original state when the deforming stress is removed. Compliance, which is the inverse of elastance, refers to the distensibility or stretch-ability of a substance when subjected to a deforming stress.

$$C = \frac{1}{E} = \frac{\Delta V}{\Delta P}$$

Specific compliance Since small lungs will have a smaller volume change when subjected to the same amount of pressure change, compliance is sometimes corrected to lung volume (usually functional residual capacity) to more accurately describe the structural properties of tissues. As a matter of convenience, compliance is sometimes corrected for weight or height of the patient to reflect the effect of size of the lung. This is referred to as specific compliance.

During normal spontaneous breathing, lungs and chest wall recoil in different directions during tidal respiration. Recoil pressures of the lungs and the chest wall refer to their respective pressures generated (in opposite directions) as they tend to return to their passive volume at 0 cm H_2O atmospheric pressure. Chest wall tends to recoil to a higher volume during tidal respiration while the lungs tend to recoil towards the lowest volume.

Although lungs and chest wall have their individual elastance and compliance properties, they need to be considered together since they are connected by pleural space which transmits recoil forces generated by one to the other. Individual elastic recoil pressures of chest wall and lung are represented schematically at various lung volumes corresponding to a percentage of total lung capacity (Fig. 1.4). At any

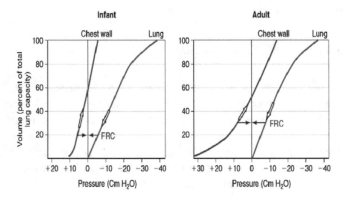

Fig. 1.4 Interaction between chest wall and lung recoil pressures in infants compared to adults. The lower recoil pressure of the chest wall in infants favors a lower FRC in infants. **FRC** – Functional Residual Capacity (Reprinted with permission from Sarnaik AP, Heidemann S and Clark JA, *Nelson Textbook of Pediatrics*, 20th Edition, Kliegman, St. Geme et al. Editors, Elsevier 2016)

volume, both the lung and the chest wall recoil to their passive volumes where their recoil pressure will be 0 cm H_2O. When corrected for volume, an infant's lungs exhibit remarkably similar elastance (and compliance) for an equivalent % change in volume compared to a healthy adult. The major difference between a neonate and an adult lies in the elastance of the chest wall. Neonatal chest wall has much less elastic recoil compared to an adult chest wall. It generates/requires less pressure (i.e. is more compliant) for a given change in volume. It can be easily understood that the elastic recoil pressure generated by the lung will bring about a greater change in the neonatal chest wall compared to the adult chest wall. The amount of air left in the lung at the end of tidal exhalation is referred to the functional residual capacity (FRC) which serves an important function as a reservoir for gas exchange during exhalation. At FRC the recoil pressures of the chest wall and the lungs are equal and opposite. FRC is also therefore termed as the "rest volume" which is achieved by equal and opposite recoil forces of the lung and the chest wall with no energy expenditure. The actual FRC determined in a spontaneously breathing neonate is considerably higher than what can be expected on the sole basis of respective lung and chest wall recoils. It is closer to what is observed in older children and adults corrected for lung volume. This is because (1) a neonate holds its chest wall in inspiratory position at the end of expiration by sustained tonic activity of the diaphragm and intercostal muscles, (2) increased respiratory rate (decreased time for exhalation) does not allow for complete lung deflation and (3) higher closing capacity which exceeds the volume at which tidal ventilation is occurring.

There are several implications of the lung-chest wall interaction in infants compared to older children. In newborns, the chest wall compliance is 3 to 6 times greater than the lung compliance. By 1 year of age, the chest wall elastance increases sufficiently to maintain FRC at a higher level solely on the basis the respective elastic recoils of the lung and the thoracic cage. In younger infants however, a marked decrease in FRC can occur in certain states: (1) conditions where inspiratory muscle tone is decreased, the chest wall becomes increasingly compliant such as during REM sleep, or with neuromuscular diseases (e.g. myopathies, neuropathies), use of sedatives/anesthesia and muscle relaxants, and CNS depression; (2) increased lung elastance (decreased lung compliance) such as with ARDS, pneumonia, pulmonary edema; and (3) extrathoracic airway obstruction which worsens during inspiration necessitating higher negative intrapleural pressure. In all these instances, the increasingly deformable chest wall retracts inward to a greater extent with a loss of FRC at end expiration and impeding air entry during inspiration. Under general anesthesia, because of the relaxed chest wall muscles, FRC declines by 10–25% in healthy adults, 35–45% in 6–18 year olds and greater than 50% in younger children. Application of PEEP is necessary in such instances to prevent atelectasis and hypoxemia.

1.5.1   Static and Dynamic Compliance

The pressure needed to overcome elastic recoil and move air, is measured once pressure has equilibrated and airflow has stopped. When compliance ($\Delta V/\Delta P$) is measured in this manner it is termed static compliance (C_{STAT}). Additional pressure is necessary to overcome resistance when air is flowing. The effect of resistance on compliance can be demonstrated using a pressure–volume plot (Fig. 1.5). The static relationship between pressure and volume is represented by the line A. At any given change in pressure, a corresponding change in volume is achieved, once airflow has stopped. The additional pressure necessary to overcome resistance is represented by the curves B and C when flow is occurring. During air flow, the same change in pressure results in less change in volume depending on the amount of resistance.

The $\Delta V/\Delta P$ relationship during flow is termed dynamic compliance (C_{DYN}). The C_{DYN} for curve C is lower than for curve B because of increased resistance. Therefore, the difference between C_{DYN} and C_{STAT} represents the degree of resistance. Clinically, the difference between static and dynamic compliances can be measured during mechanical ventilation. When patients are receiving a set tidal volume using constant flow (volume control mode), the difference between peak

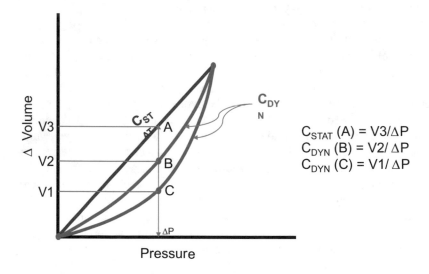

$$C_{STAT} (A) = V3/\Delta P$$
$$C_{DYN} (B) = V2/\Delta P$$
$$C_{DYN} (C) = V1/\Delta P$$

Inspiratory pressure/volume relationship curve
Red line represents the static pressure/volume relationship (C_{STAT})
Blue curves represent dynamic pressure/volume relationship (C_{DYN})

Fig. 1.5 Inspiratory pressure–volume (PV) curves. The red line (A) represents PV relationship during no-flow (static) state. The blue lines (B and C) represent PV curves while flow (dynamic) is occurring. Static compliance (C_{STAT}) and dynamic compliance (C_{DYN}) are calculated at a given ΔP. $C_{STAT} (A) > C_{DYN} (B) > C_{DYN} (C)$

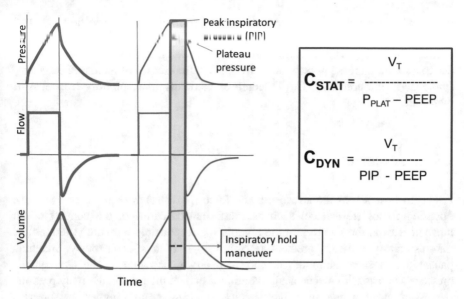

Fig. 1.6 Time relationships are shown for pressure, flow and volume in a volume-controlled ventilation with constant flow. Inspiratory hold is applied after peak pressure (PIP) is reached to allow pressure equilibration to occur between P_{AW} and P_{ALV} resulting in a plateau pressure (P_{PLAT}) which is lower than PIP as resistive forces are overcome

pressure and the plateau pressure obtained using an inspiratory hold maneuver can give an estimate of the airflow resistance (Fig. 1.6).

C_{DYN} can be calculated as the tidal volume divided by the difference between the peak inspiratory pressure and the end-expiratory pressure (Fig. 1.6). C_{STAT} is calculated as the tidal volume divided by the difference between the plateau pressure and end-expiratory pressure (Fig. 1.6). During volume controlled ventilation, P_{PLAT} is always lower than PIP and therefore C_{STAT} is always lower than C_{DYN}, and the degree of difference is dependent of the degree of airway obstruction.

1.5.2 Frequency Dependence of Compliance

Dynamic compliance (C_{DYN}) takes into account both the resistance (when flow is maximum) and the compliance (when flow is zero) of the respiratory system. Unlike C_{STAT}, which is relatively constant and a reflection of structural properties of the lung, C_{DYN} takes into account the flow resistive properties of the airways as well as the structural properties. Since the pressure required is a product of flow and resistance, an increase in either the flow or the resistance will require a greater pressure when considering the dynamic compliance. An increase in respiratory frequency will decrease the amount of time provided for inflation and deflation to occur and necessitate an increase in flow. The resultant increase in flow resistive property will require a greater pressure to deliver the tidal volume and thus a decrease in C_{DYN}. This is termed frequency dependence of compliance; C_{DYN} decreases with increase in respiratory frequency. In diseases of increased resistance (prolonged time constant), C_{DYN} decreases markedly as respiratory frequency is increased.

1.6 Resistance

For air to flow across the airways, some force (pressure) is required to overcome opposing forces (resistance) such as inertia and friction. In the context of air movement from the mouth into the alveoli, the responsible pressure is termed the transrespiratory pressure gradient ($P_{AW} - P_{ALV}$). In a spontaneously breathing patient the pressure at mouth or proximal airway is same as the atmospheric pressure whereas with mechanically ventilated patient the proximal airway pressure is pressure at the patient-machine interface. Air flows from a higher pressure to a lower pressure both during inspiration and expiration. When the pressures at two ends are equal, flow ceases. By the same token, when airway is occluded stopping the flow, pressure is presumed to have equilibrated after a period of time. These airway occlusion techniques are utilized at various phases of respiration to estimate alveolar pressure measured at the proximal airway which is readily available for pressure measurement. Resistance is calculated as transrespiratory pressure gradient required generating a given amount of flow (volume per time) and expressed conventionally as cm $H_2O/L/sec$. Two of the important determinants of resistance to airflow are: (a) airway diameter and (b) nature of the flow, laminar or turbulent.

Laminar versus Turbulent flow: When gas molecules travel in a straight direction, the flow is referred to as being laminar. At higher velocities (distance/time), such as would occur when same amount of flow (volume/time) is pushed through a narrowed airway, the movement of gas molecules becomes chaotic thus resulting in turbulence.

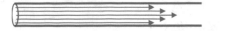   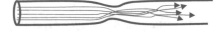

Laminar flow   **Turbulent flow**

Whether the flow is laminar or turbulent depends upon density, viscosity and velocity of gas and the diameter of the airway. When airflow is laminar, resistance is governed by Poiseuille's law:

$$R = \frac{8nL}{\pi r^4}$$

R is resistance, l is length, η is viscosity, and r is the radius. The practical implication of pressure-flow relationship is that airway resistance is inversely proportional to its radius raised to the 4th power. If the airway lumen is decreased in half (1/2), the resistance increases 16-fold. A flow change from laminar to turbulent occurs when Reynold's number exceeds 2000. Reynold's number (Re) is a dimensionless entity represented as:

$$Re = (Diameter \times Velocity \times Density) \div Viscosity$$

Resistance to turbulent flow is much greater than to laminar flow. In clinical situations, the most effective way of decreasing the Reynold's number is to decrease the density of inspired gas. For this purpose, helium is used to replace nitrogen to promote laminar flow. Helium is about 7 times less dense and slightly more (1.1X) viscous than nitrogen. For helium to be effective for this purpose, it needs to be present to a sufficient degree. It is generally believed that for Helium–oxygen mixture (Heliox) to effectively reduce resistance, at least 50–60% of the mixture needs to be comprised of helium. This means patients requiring more than 50% oxygen may not benefit from Heliox.

Resistance to airflow is different during inspiration and expiration. In normal circumstance, expiratory resistance is higher than inspiratory resistance. This is because the intrathoracic airways expand during inspiration as they are subjected to more negative pleural pressure from the outside in spontaneous breathing and positive pressure from the inside in mechanical ventilation. In intrathoracic airway obstruction (asthma, bronchiolitis, vascular ring etc.) this discrepancy increases as expiratory resistance increases exponentially due to airway compression by excessively positive pleural pressure. In extrathoracic airway obstruction (subglottic stenosis, vocal cord paralysis etc.), the inspiratory resistance can exceed the expiratory resistance as the airway outside the thorax collapses because of excessively increased intraluminal negative pressure.

1.7 Flow/Volume Relationships

Flow/volume relationships curves are clinically useful tools for demonstrating the effect changes in pulmonary mechanics have on volumes and gas flow (Fig. 1.7). These curves are generated with spirometry machines and can be used in both the outpatient setting well as the bedside. Typically, a maximal inspiration is followed by maximal forced exhalation, generating a flow/volume loop. Forced vital capacity (FVC) is the total volume exhaled during this maneuver. Forced expiratory volume during the first second of exhalation is termed FEV1. Decreases in FVC and FEV1 result from decreased lung compliance, increased airway resistance and decreased

A normal flow/volume loop. Performed by maximal inspiration followed by maximal forced exhalation to completion.
FEF$_{MAX}$ is synonymous with peak expiratory flow rate (PEFR) and represents the maximum expiratory flow rate during exhalation. This occurs soon after the start of forced exhalation.
FEF$_{25\%-75\%}$ represents the mean flow between 25% and 75% total expiratory volume. Also referred to as mid maximum expiratory flow rate (MMEFR).
FEV$_1$ is the volume of expired gas in the first second of expiration.

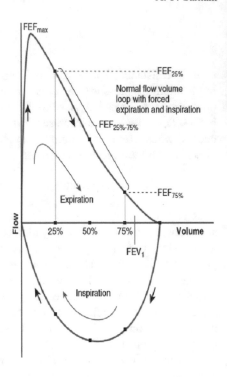

Fig. 1.7 Flow-volume loop created by maximum inhalation followed by forced maximum exhalation

respiratory muscle strength. The maximum flow occurs in the first phase of forced exhalation and is referred to as FEF$_{max}$ (also referred to as peak flow). It is effort dependent but also a marker of airway obstruction. The volume exhaled between 25 and 75% of the expiratory volume (FEF 25–75%) is relatively effort independent. The reason for this is that a higher intrathoracic pressure results in narrowing of intrathoracic airway preventing further increase in flow.

A decrease in FEF$_{25-75\%}$ is indicative of intrathoracic airway obstruction such as in asthma (Fig. 1.8). The shape of the expiratory curve gives clues to disease pathophysiology, as in obstructive disease, where the mid-expiratory curve may be increasingly concave. In restrictive lung and chest wall diseases, all the lung volumes and capacities are decreased without appreciable decreases in flow rates.

Intrapulmonary Airway Obstruction (A): note the decrease in **FEF**~MAX~ and **FEF**~25%-75%~ and the concavity of the mid-expiratory curve.

Restrictive disorder (B): Note the more vertical and narrow shape. **FVC** is decreased but flow rates are relatively less affected.

Reprinted with permission from Sarnaik AP, Heidemann S and Clark JA, *Nelson Textbook of Pediatrics*, 20th Edition, Kliegman, St. Geme et. al. Editors, Elsevier 2016.

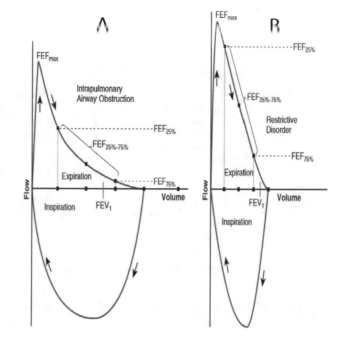

Fig. 1.8 Flow volume loops in intrapulmonary obstructive lung disease (**a**) and restrictive disorders (**b**)

1.8   Equal Pressure Point (EPP)

When intrathoracic airway pressure is increased during exhalation (either by forced voluntary exhalation or in intrathoracic airway obstruction), the pressure must dissipate along the airway to reach the reference atmospheric pressure of 0 cm H_2O or the positive end expiratory pressure set in the mechanical device. The site at which the intraluminal pressure equals pleural pressure is termed the equal pressure point (EPP).

The significance of EPP is that the pressure in the intrathoracic airway proximal to this point (downstream) is less than intrapleural pressure and therefore subject to collapse depending on the magnitude of the pressure difference and stiffness/softness of its wall. With intrathoracic airway obstruction, the EPP is shifted distally towards the alveolus, causing a greater length of airway to collapse above (Fig. 1.9). Softer infantile airways are more susceptible to change in diameter when subjected to increased pressure. Marked dynamic changes in intrathoracic airway diameter during inspiration and exhalation in young infants above EPP are often termed collapsible trachea. Tracheal collapse is often a result of airway obstruction and even contributes to its severity but it is rarely the primary abnormality.

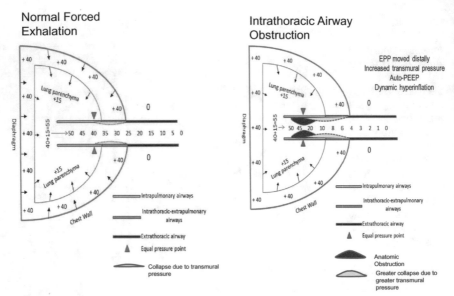

Assume intrapleural pressure of 40 cm H_2O and lung recoil pressure of 15 cm H_2O during forced exhalation

Fig. 1.9 Equal pressure point (EPP) is a site at which intrathoracic and intraluminal pressures during exhalation are equal. Proximal to EPP (downstream), intrathoracic pressure exceeds intraluminal pressure resulting in airway collapse. EPP is displaced distally in intrathoracic airway obstruction, and the magnitude of difference between intrathoracic and intraluminal pressures is increased resulting in greater airway collapse

Suggested Readings

1. Sarnaik AP, Heidemann SM, Clark JA. Respiratory pathophysiology and regulation. In: Kliegman RM, Stanton BF, St Geme JW, Schor NF, editors. Nelson textbook of pediatrics. 20th ed. Philadelphia: Elsevier; 2016. p. 1981–93.
2. Bigeleisen PE. Models of venous admixtures. Adv Physiol Educ. 2001;25:159–66.
3. Sarnaik AP, Clark JA, Heidemann SM. Respiratory distress and failure: In Nelson textbook of pediatrics, 21st Edition. In Kliegman RM, Stanton BF, St Geme JW, Schor NF (eds). Elsevier, Philadelphia 2019
4. Clark J, Chiwane S, Sarnaik, AP. Mechanical dysfunction of respiratory system. In Fuhrman BF, Zimmerman JJ, Rotta A (eds.), Pediatric Critical Care. C.V. Mosby Company, St. Louis, 5th edition, 2020

Chapter 2
Physiology of Inflation and Deflation

Ashok P. Sarnaik and Shekhar T. Venkataraman

The process of breathing, spontaneous or mechanical, involves the physical movement of air in and out of the lungs. Interaction of various physical factors is involved in the way this process occurs physiologically. It is important to understand these factors as they relate to diagnosis and management of lung disease.

2.1 Equation of Motion

A pressure gradient (Δ pressure) is required to move air in and out of the lung. In normal spontaneous respiration, air is drawn from the atmosphere into the alveoli because of negative intrapleural pressure generated by contraction of the diaphragm and intercostal muscles during inspiration and released from alveoli into the atmosphere during expiration by pressure generated from elastic recoil of the lung. During mechanical ventilation, gas flows into the lungs from positive pressure created by the ventilator during inspiration and exhalation results from alveolar pressure generated by elastic recoil of the lung and chest wall.

The original version of this chapter was revised with correct equation at page 17.
The correction to this chapter can be found at https://doi.org/10.1007/978-3-030-83738-9_14

A. P. Sarnaik (✉)
Professor of Pediatrics, Former Pediatrician in Chief and Interim Chairman Children's Hospital of Michigan, Wayne State University School of Medicine, 3901 Beaubien, Detroit, MI 48201, USA
e-mail: asarnaik@med.wayne.edu

S. T. Venkataraman
Professor, Departments of Critical Care Medicine and Pediatrics, University of Pittsburgh School of Medicine, Pittsburgh, PA, USA

Medical Director, Respiratory Care Services, Children's Hospital of Pittsburgh, 4401 Penn Avenue, Faculty Pavilion 2117, Pittsburgh, PA 15224, USA

© Springer Nature Switzerland AG 2022, corrected publication 2022
A. P. Sarnaik et al. (eds.), *Mechanical Ventilation in Neonates and Children*,
https://doi.org/10.1007/978-3-030-83738-9_2

Regardless of the site where it is generated, the pressure necessary to move air is expended for two opposing mechanical factors: (1) *elastance* (inverse of compliance) and (2) *resistance* (Fig. 2.1). Major component of resistance is experienced in generation of airflow across the airways and a minor component is from frictional resistance of tissues. Pressure to overcome elastance is measured by determining the change in volume (Δ volume) after pressure has equilibrated at both ends and flow has ceased. Alveolar pressure is determined in the proximal airway by performing the inspiratory occlusion technique. This means that both the Δ volume and the Δ pressure are determined when pressure has equilibrated throughout and airflow has ceased. Resistance on the other hand is experienced only when airflow is occurring. Thus, the pressure to overcome resistive forces is measured by determining the Δ pressure applied at the source and the flow that results from this. When compliance is measured at a point where there is no flow, it is referred to as static compliance (C_{STAT}). When measured while the flow is occurring, it is referred to as dynamic compliance (C_{DYN}).

2.2   Time Constant

For airflow to occur, a pressure gradient has to be created from one end to the other (proximal airway and the alveoli). Flow will continue as long as the pressure gradient remains between the two ends. When pressure equilibrates at two ends, flow ceases. The equilibration of pressure does not occur instantaneously. It takes some time for pressure to equilibrate at two ends. The time required for pressure

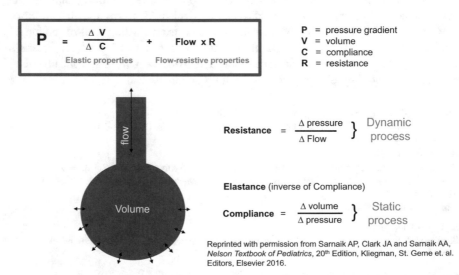

Fig. 2.1 Equation of motion. Pressure required to move air in and out of the lung is to overcome Resistance (dynamic process) and Elastance (static process)

gradient depends on two variables: (1) compliance and (2) resistance. When compliance is low (meaning elastance is high), the elastic recoil pressure of the lung is increased. During inspiration, inflow of air is opposed by high lung recoil (decreased compliance) and during exhalation; outflow of air is aided by it. This results in quicker attainment of pressure and equilibration volume with cessation of flow in a relatively short time. On the other hand, when airway resistance is increased, longer time is required for pressure/volume equilibration and cessation of air flow to occur. Time constant is a reflection of the time necessary for pressure/volume equilibration to occur and airflow to cease. Thus, the required time is directly proportional to both compliance and resistance. Greater the compliance and resistance, longer the time needed and vice versa. Indeed, time constant is calculated as:

$$\tau(Time\ Constant) = Compliance \times Resistance$$

$$\tau = \frac{\Delta V}{\Delta P} \times \frac{\Delta P}{Flow}$$

$$\tau(s) = \frac{mL}{cms} \times \frac{cms}{mL/s}$$

Thus, time constant is appropriately represented as time (Fig. 2.2).

It takes one time constant for 63%, two time constants for 86%, 3 time constants for 95% and 5 time constants for almost complete pressure or volume equilibration to occur. Since time constant is a product of compliance and resistance, patients with increased airway resistance require greater time during inspiration and

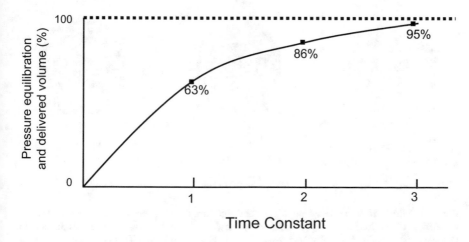

Fig. 2.2 The time required for % of pressure equilibration (and therefore the volume delivery) depends on the time constant of a given system

expiration for pressure and volume equilibration to occur and airflow to cease. Conversely, in patients with diseases of decreased compliance, pressure and volume equilibration occurs quicker. Airways expand during inspiration and narrow during exhalation. Thus, expiratory time constant, because of increased airway resistance is greater than inspiratory time constant. This discrepancy becomes more pronounced in diseases of increased airway resistance (asthma, vascular ring etc.) where expiratory time constant is markedly increased to the point pressure equilibration at the end of expiration does not occur resulting in hyperinflation and auto-PEEP (see below).

The effects of compliance and resistance on time constant are presented in Fig. 2.3. Let's consider that based on compliance and resistance of a normal lung the time constant is X seconds. This would mean that if a pressure of 10 cm H_2O is applied at one end it would take 3X seconds for the other end to receive 9.5 cm H_2O (95% of the driving pressure). The expiratory time constant will be greater than inspiratory time constant because airway resistance is greater in exhalation as they become narrower compared to during inspiration. In diseases with decreased compliance, the time constant will be less than X seconds. Although the volume delivered will be less than in a normal lung, the pressure equilibration is quicker. The inspiratory and expiratory time constants are closer to each other because of greater lung recoil pressure. In diseases of increased airway resistance, the time constant is greater than X seconds as the proximal pressure takes more time to

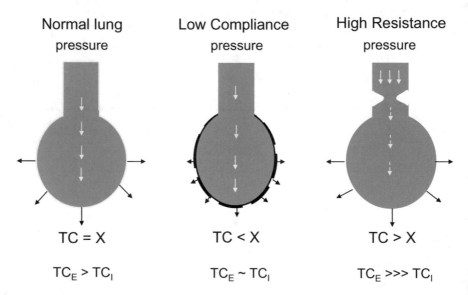

Fig. 2.3 Effect of decreased compliance and increased resistance on time constant (TC). Normally, TC is longer during exhalation as airways get narrower compared to inhalation. Diseases with decreased compliance have decreased TC with expiratory TC (TC_E) getting closer to inspiratory TC (TC_I). Diseases of airway obstruction have prolonged TC with TC_E far exceeding TC_I

overcome airway resistance. In intrathoracic airway obstruction which gets worse during exhalation, the expiratory time constant is much more increased compared to the inspiratory time constant.

Even though a disease can be classified as that of increased resistance (e.g. asthma) or decreased compliance (e.g. ARDS), most lung diseases are often heterogeneous in nature.

Normal lung units are interspersed with units with prolonged time constants (increased resistance) and those with short time constants (decreased compliance). The effect of time on the delivered volume after application of pressure is shown in Fig. 2.4. The units with short time constants fill up (or empty) quickly, with negligible change in volume as time is increased from A to B. The units with increased time constants however fill up (or empty) much slower with greater volume change with time B compared to time A. Consideration of time constant is extremely important when choosing respiratory rate and I:E ratio during mechanical ventilation.

2.2.1 Auto-PEEP and Dynamic Hyperinflation

Auto-PEEP and dynamic hyperinflation exist when exhalation is incomplete and the alveolar pressure has not had sufficient time to equilibrate with atmospheric (or ventilator) pressure during exhalation. As a result, the lung volume is increased above the potential FRC when lung recoil is complete. This occurs in two situations: (1) in patients with airway obstruction such as asthma, time constant is

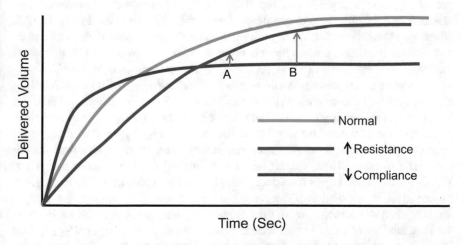

Fig. 2.4 Change in volume delivery in lung units with different time constants. Increasing time from A to B will result in greater volume change in lung units with prolonged time constant (increased resistance) compared to the little change in volume in those units with short time constant (decreased compliance) where pressure equilibration has already occurred

prolonged, much more so during exhalation, preventing complete alveolar empty-ing. Inspiration occurs either spontaneously or is delivered mechanically before alveolar pressure approximates proximal airway pressure at end expiration. This is termed auto-PEEP and (2) at high respiratory rates, the decrease in expiratory time is not sufficient for complete alveolar emptying to occur. This is referred to as dynamic hyperinflation. Neonates, with their high respiratory rates experience dy-namic hyperinflation. Dynamic hyperinflation also results during exercise where both tidal volume and respiratory frequency are increased.

2.3   Work of Breathing

2.3.1   Pressure–Volume Work

In physics, work is defined as the product of force and distance. In the context of respiratory mechanics, work of breathing (WOB) is defined as the product of pressure and volume. It represents the energy required to move air in and out of the lungs. In spontaneous breathing, the work is done by the patient whereas in con-trolled mandatory breaths, the work is done by the ventilator. Except in situations when expiration is active (obstructive lung disease and forced expiration), WOB is performed during inspiration while the exhalation is passive and the work is accomplished by elastic recoil of the lung. In obstructive lung disease, the patient has to perform expiratory work by creating positive intrapleural pressure by diaphragmatic and intercostal contraction. Calculation of WOB requires consider-ation of pressure–volume relationship. As stated in equation of motion, one com-ponent of pressure required to effect a change in lung volume is to overcome its elastance and the other is to overcome its flow-resistance properties. In the Fig. 2.5, where spontaneous respiration is presented, the red line represents the static pres-sure volume relationship when there is no flow. Area covered by ACDA represents the inspiratory elastic work (W_{ELAST}) whereas the area covered by ABCA repre-sents the work that represents the flow-resistive work (W_{RESIST}). The total WOB for a given breath is the sum of W_{ELAST} and W_{RESIST}. Total WOB/min is WOB for each breath X respiratory rate. As tidal volume is increased, W_{ELAST} increases since greater amount of volume is moved at higher pressure. W_{RESIST} on the other hand is greatest at maximum flow. At faster respiratory rates, there is less time for air movement to occur. Therefore, air needs to be moved at a higher flow rate. Thus, W_{RESIST} increases at higher respiratory rates. In health as well as in disease, a given minute alveolar ventilation [(Tidal volume—Dead space) X Respiratory rate] is accomplished at a combination of tidal volume and respiratory rate that necessitates the least amount of energy expenditure. Young infants have a larger W_{ELAST} than W_{RESIST} compared to older children and adults. This is not because their lungs have greater elastic recoil (less compliance), but because their chest wall is more com-pliant and it tends to retract inwards in response to negative intrapleural pressure during inspiration making lung inflation more difficult. The total WOB is lowest at a rate of 35–40/min for neonates and 14–16/min for older children and adults.

W_{ELAST} increases disproportionately in diseases with decreased compliance and W_{RESIST} increases in diseases with increased airway resistance. Respirations are therefore shallow (low VT) and rapid in diseases of low compliance and deep and relatively slow (decreased flow rate) in diseases of increased resistance in order to minimize energy expenditure. In healthy children, the energy cost of WOB is only approximately 2% of total body expenditure. In children with chronic lung disease, WOB may contribute to as much as 40% of total energy expenditure.

2.4 Airway Dynamics in Health and Disease

Airways in infants are much more compliant compared to older children and adults resulting in greater changes in airway diameter when subjected to similar trans-mural pressure changes. To understand the phasic dynamic changes during the respiratory cycle, the airway can be divided into 3 anatomic parts: the extra-thoracic airway from the nose to thoracic inlet, the intrathoracic-extrapulmonary airway from the thoracic inlet to the main stem bronchi, and intrathoracic airway which is embedded in the lung parenchyma. Transrespiratory pressure ($P_{AW} - P_{ALV}$) is responsible for air movement. Please note that P_{AW} refers to proximal airway pressure which is same as mouth or atmospheric pressure during spontaneous ventilation and pressure applied to patient-positive pressure interface (ET tube, face

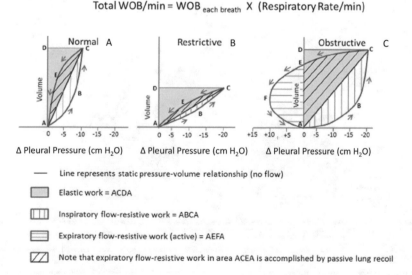

Fig. 2.5 Work of Breathing (WOB) in normal state (**a**), restrictive disease (**b**), and obstructive disease (**c**)

mask, nasal cannula etc.) during mechanical ventilation. P_{ALV} depends on two factors; P_{PL} and recoil pressure of the lung. Lung recoil pressure is greater at higher lung volume and increased elastance (decreased compliance). For the purpose of simplicity, we will assign the value of +5 cm H_2O to lung recoil pressure in order to describe transmural pressures the airways are subjected to during respiration.

During normal spontaneous respirations, intrathoracic airways expand in inspiration because of negative intrapleural pressure, and somewhat narrower during exhalation as they return to the FRC. In diseases characterized by increased airway resistance, a much greater change in intrapleural pressure is required to generate adequate airflow. The transluminal pressure that the walls of the airway are subjected to increase proportionate to the extent the intrapleural pressure is increased. During mechanical ventilation, airways are subjected to positive pressure during inspiration. During exhalation however, it is the positive pressure in the pleural cavity that the alveoli and intrathoracic airways are subjected to. The changes in the size of the airways, which are softer and more compliant, are accentuated in young infants during respiration.

In extra-thoracic (ET) airway obstruction, (retropharyngeal abscess, laryngotracheitis, vocal cord paralysis etc.), most of the increased negative transrespiratory pressure (P_{TR}) during inspiration is transmitted up to the site of obstruction beyond which it is rapidly dissipated. The ET airway below the site of obstruction is subjected to a marked increase in negative intraluminal pressure resulting in collapse. This leads to inspiratory difficulty, prolonged inspiration and inspiratory stridor. Increase in negative intrapleural pressure results in suprasternal, intercostal and subcostal retractions. During exhalation, the increased P_{TR} is again transmitted to the site of obstruction resulting in distension of the ET airway and amelioration of obstruction (Fig. 2.6).

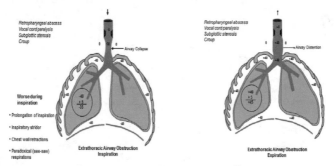

During inspiration, increased negative pleural pressure is transmitted to all airways including the extra-thoracic. This results in collapse of the extra-thoracic airways distal to the site of obstruction. The end result is increased inspiratory resistance and worsening of obstruction.
During exhalation, positive pleural pressure is transmitted to all airways including the extra-thoracic. This results in distention of the airway below the site of obstruction and improvement of symptoms.
Pressures are presented relative to atmospheric pressure (0 cm H_2O). Distal airway pressures are taken as pleural pressure plus lung recoil pressure (arbitrarily taken as +5 cm H_2O for simplicity).

Fig. 2.6 Airways dynamics in extra-thoracic airway obstruction

These symptoms are especially pronounced in newborns and infants with their compliant chest wall and airways. One may observe paradoxical or see-saw respiration as the chest wall retracts inwards and abdomen bulges out due to diaphragmatic descent during inspiration and the converse occurring during exhalation. In obstruction of intrathoracic-extrapulmonary (IT-EP) airways such as vascular ring, pulmonary sling, mediastinal mass etc. the equal pressure point (EPP) is displaced distally and the intrathoracic airway above the obstruction is subjected to an excessive positive intrathoracic pressure (Fig. 2.7).

This results in intrathoracic airway collapse above the EPP, worsening the obstruction leading to the signs and symptoms of expiratory difficulty and wheezing, prolongation of expiration and hyperinflation. During inspiration, there is relatively less obstruction as the IT airway above the obstruction is surrounded by much more negative extraluminal pressure than intraluminal and thus tends to distend with improvement in symptoms. The classic findings of expiratory wheezing in IT-EP obstruction has led to the axiom "all that wheezes is not asthma". In unilateral IT-EP obstruction, such as in foreign body aspiration, the clinical manifestations are predominantly at the site of the lesion. In IP airway obstruction such as with asthma and bronchiolitis, the EPP moves further into the distal airways causing a widespread intrathoracic collapse during expiration resulting in expiratory wheezing, prolonged expiration, air trapping and hyperinflation (Fig. 2.8).

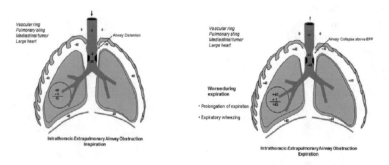

During inspiration, increased negative pleural pressure is transmitted to all structures inside the chest including the airways up to the site of obstruction beyond which it is rapidly dissipated. This results in distension of the intra-thoracic airways proximal to obstruction as it is surrounded by even greater negative intrathoracic pressure.
During exhalation, the increased airway pressure rapidly dissipates above the obstruction. There is a collapse of the intrathoracic airway above the obstruction because of markedly increased positive intrathoracic pressure outside the airway making the obstruction worse during exhalation. Equal pressure point (EPP) is the point at which intra and extra luminal pressures during exhalation are equal.
Pressures are presented relative to atmospheric pressure (0 cm H_2O). Distal airway pressures are taken as pleural pressure plus lung recoil pressure (arbitrarily taken as +5 cm H_2O for simplicity).

Reprinted with permission from Sarnaik AP, Heidemann S and Clark JA, *Nelson Textbook of Pediatrics*, 20th Edition, Kliegman, St. Geme et. al. Editors, Elsevier 2016.

Fig. 2.7 Airway dynamics in intra-thoracic extrapulmonary airway obstruction

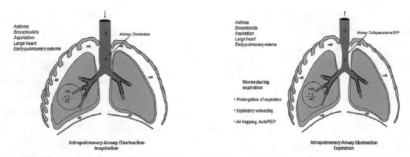

During inspiration, increased negative pleural pressure is transmitted to all structures inside the chest including the airways. The intrathoracic extraluminal airway pressure is more negative especially above the site of obstruction resulting in airway distension. During exhalation, the positive intrathoracic pressure rapidly dissipates above the site of obstruction and the equal pressure point moves distally towards the alveoli. The end result is widespread airway collapse and worsening of symptoms. Pressures are presented relative to atmospheric pressure (0 cm H_2O). Distal airway pressures are taken as pleural pressure plus lung recoil pressure (arbitrarily taken as +5 cm H_2O for simplicity).

Reprinted with permission from Sarnaik AP, Heidemann S and Clark JA, *Nelson Textbook of Pediatrics*, 20th Edition, Kliegman, St. Geme et. al. Editors, Elsevier 2016.

Fig. 2.8 Airway dynamics in intra-thoracic intrapulmonary airway obstruction

Suggested Readings

1. Sarnaik AP, Heidemann SM, Clark JA. Respiratory pathophysiology and regulation. In: liegman RM, Stanton BF, St Geme JW, Schor NF, editors. Nelson textbook of pediatrics. 20th ed. Philadelphia: Elsevier; 2016. p. 1981–93.
2. Bigeleisen PE. Models of venous admixtures. Adv Physiol Educ. 2001;25:159–66.
3. Sarnaik AP, Clark JA, Heidemann SM. Respiratory distress and failure. In: Kliegman RM, Stanton BF, St Geme JW, Schor NF, editors. Nelson textbook of pediatrics, 21st ed. Elsevier, Philadelphia; 2019.
4. Clark J, Chiwane S, Sarnaik AP. Mechanical dysfunction of respiratory system. In: Fuhrman BF, Zimmerman JJ, Rotta A editors. Pediatric critical care, 5th ed. St. Louis: C.V. Mosby Company; 2020.

Chapter 3
Gas Exchange

Ashok P. Sarnaik

The main function of the respiratory system is to remove CO_2 from and add O_2 to systemic venous blood brought to the lung. Tissue demands of O_2 supply and CO_2 removal requires the process of matching perfusion and alveolar ventilation (V_A), diffusion of gases across the alveolar capillary membrane, O_2 delivery (DO_2) and consumption (VO_2). These processes are schematically represented in (Fig. 3.1).

3.1 Alveolar Gas Equation

The total pressure of atmosphere (P_{ATM}) at sea level is 760 torr or mm Hg. P_{ATM} is also sometimes expressed in kilopascal unit. 1 kilopascal is approximately 7.5 torr. P_{ATM} decreases progressively at higher altitude (Table 3.1). The total atmospheric pressure is the sum of pressures exerted by each of its component gases. With increasing altitude, P_{ATM} decreases while the fraction of O_2 (FiO_2) remains constant. At temperature of 37°C (98.6°F), and 100% humidity, water vapor exerts pressure of 47 torr regardless of the altitude. Alveolar air is 100% humidified, therefore the inspired gas is also assumed to be fully saturated with water. To subtract the contribution of water vapor, 47 torr is subtracted from the atmospheric pressure to account for the pressure exerted by gases alone. Our atmosphere contains 20.93% ($\approx$21%) oxygen at any altitude. Thus, the fraction of atmosphere

---

The original version of this chapter was revised with correct equation at Figure 3.6. The correction to this chapter can be found at https://doi.org/10.1007/978-3-030-83738-9_14

A. P. Sarnaik (✉)
Professor of Pediatrics, Former Pediatrician in Chief and Interim Chairman Children's
Hospital of Michigan, Wayne State University School of Medicine, 3901 Beaubien,
Detroit, MI 48201, USA
e-mail: asarnaik@med.wayne.edu

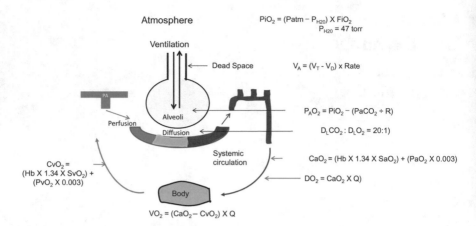

Fig. 3.1 Various factors involved in respiration; Atmospheric composition, Ventilation, Diffusion, Perfusion, Oxygen delivery (DO_2), Oxygen consumption (VO_2), CO_2 production (VCO_2)

Table.3.1 Relationship of barometric pressure and partial pressure of inspired air (PiO_2) when 100% humidified at different altitudes

Altitudes (feet)	P_{ATM}(Torr)	(P_{ATM}-47[P_{H2O}])Torr	O_2%	PiO_2(Torr)
0	760	713	20.93	149
600	747	700	20.93	147
5000	632	585	20.93	123
10,000	523	476	20.93	100
15,000	429	382	20.93	80
18,000[a]	380	333	20.93	70
20,000	349	302	20.93	63
25,000	282	235	20.93	49
30,000	225	178	20.93	37

[a]Highest Village. Modified from Comroe JH. Physiology of Respiration, Year Book Medical Publishers, 2nd ED, Chicago, USA 1974

comprising of oxygen (FiO_2) is 0.21. Partial pressure of oxygen in inspired gas (PiO_2) is calculated as:

$$PiO_2 = (P_{atm} - 47) \times FiO_2$$

At sea level, PiO_2 = (760–47) × 0.21 = 149 torr. When breathing 40% O_2 at sea level, PiO_2 = (760 – 47) × 0.4 = 285 torr. At higher altitudes, breathing the same FiO_2 results in a lower PiO_2. In Denver (altitude 5,000 feet, P_{ATM} = 632 mmHg) for example, breathing FiO_2 of 0.21 will result in PiO_2 = (632 – 47) × 0.21 = 123 torr and at FiO_2 of 0.4, it will be (632 – 47) × 0.4 = 234 torr.

3.2 Oxygenation and Ventilation

The amount of air moved in and out of the lungs every minute (V_T x respiratory rate) is termed minute volume. Part of the inspired V_T occupies conducting airways (anatomic dead space) which does not contribute to gas exchange. Still another part of V_T enters alveoli that are not sufficiently perfused (alveolar dead space). Total dead space ($V_D$tot) is the sum of anatomic dead space ($V_D$anat) and alveolar dead space ($V_D$alv). Alveolar ventilation (VA) is calculated as:

$$\dot{V}_A = [V_T - (Vd_{anat} + Vd_{alv})] \times RR$$

where RR is the respiratory rate (Fig. 3.2).

Although dead space is often looked at as moving in bulk, in reality the gas moves at a higher velocity in the center compared to the periphery where frictional resistance slows it down. Thus, alveolar ventilation may be higher than expected because of asymmetric velocity of the inspired gas compared to uniform velocity in a bulk flow model. The relationship of V_T and $V_D$tot is calculated as:

$$\frac{V_D}{V_T} = \frac{\left(P_{A_{CO2}} - P_{\bar{E}_{CO2}}\right)}{P_{A_{CO2}}}$$

where, $P_E CO_2$ is mixed expired PCO_2. $P_A CO_2$ is assumed to be same as $PaCO_2$ since there is no A-a CO_2 gradient. To calculate $V_D$alv, $P_{ET}CO_2$ is used to replace mixed $P_E CO_2$.

$V_D$alv/V_T = ($PaCO_2$ − $P_{ET}CO_2$) ÷ $PaCO_2$.

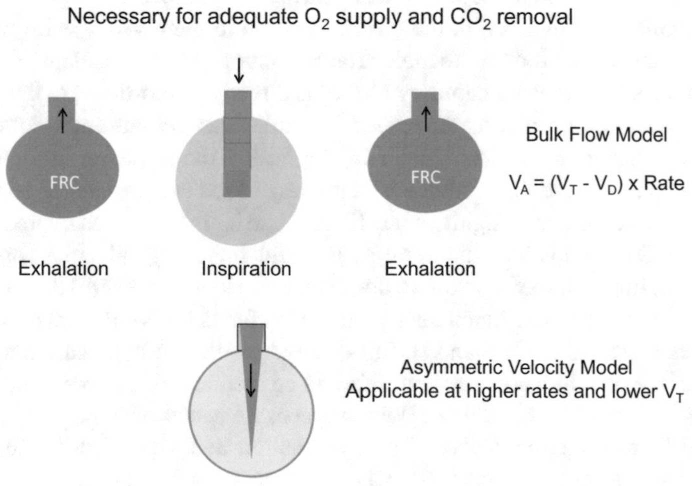

Fig. 3.2 Alveolar ventilation with bulk flow model and asymmetric velocity model

In normal lungs, $P_{ET}CO_2$ should be close to $PaCO_2$ and thus V_Dalv should be negligible. Increasing difference in $PaCO_2$ and $P_{ET}CO_2$ is indicative of increasing V_Dalv. Increased V_Dalv is encountered when pulmonary perfusion is insufficient to match ventilation such as in decreased cardiac output, pulmonary embolism, hypovolemia and excessive PEEP. V_A is inversely proportional to $PaCO_2$. The relationship between V_A and $PaCO_2$ is hyperbolic but at the bedside, in the ranges of $PaCO_2$ commonly seen, it can be assumed to be linear. Therefore, when V_A is doubled, $PaCO_2$ is halved. Conversely when V_A is halved, $PaCO_2$ is doubled. With minor changes during the respiratory cycle the total pressure of all gases in alveoli is very similar to the total pressure of inspired gas. Alveolar gas composition depends on partial pressure of gases in the inspired gas, $PaCO_2$ (assumed to be same as alveolar PCO_2) and respiratory quotient (R). The simplified alveolar air equation is used to calculate the alveolar PO_2 (P_AO_2) as follows:

$$P_AO_2 = PiO_2 - (\frac{P_aCO_2}{R})$$

For practical purposes, R is assumed to be 0.8. According to the alveolar air equation, for a given PiO_2, a rise in $PaCO_2$ of 10 torr will result in a decrease in P_AO_2 by $10 \div 0.8 = 10 \times 1.25 = 12.5$ torr. Thus, pure hypoventilation will decrease P_AO_2 with increase in $PaCO_2$ by a factor of 1.25. In a normal person, PiO_2 is about 150 torr. With a $PaCO_2$ of 40 torr, the P_AO_2 will be $150 - (40 \times 1.25)$ torr or $150 - 50 = 100$ torr. An increase in FiO_2 and therefore the PiO_2 will raise P_AO_2 without affecting $PaCO_2$. Dangerous level of hypercarbia may coexist without hypoxia in hypoventilating patients who are breathing supplemental O_2.

The alveolar gas is is exchanged with the systemic venous (pulmonary arterial) blood through the process of diffusion which is influenced by the alveolar capillary barrier and the time available for equilibration. The "arterialized" blood is returned via pulmonary venous circulation to the heart to be pumped through the systemic arterial circulation. Diffusion in the gas phase (within the alveoli) is inversely proportional to the square root of the molecular weight of a gas molecule. Diffusion into the liquid phase (pulmonary capillary blood) is directly proportional to the solubility of a gas molecule. Considering the respective molecular weights and solubility, CO_2 is about 20 times more diffusible than O_2. In health, the diffusion for both O_2 and CO_2 is complete by the time pulmonary capillary blood is no longer in contact with the alveolar gas. Clinically significant diffusion barrier manifests as hypoxia without impairing CO_2 elimination. Increasing FiO_2 and increasing alveolar-capillary O_2 gradient will improve oxygenation to some extent. However, even 100% O_2 is only about 5 times more concentrated than room air (as far as O_2 is concerned) while CO_2 is 20 times more diffusible than O_2. In other words, before hypercarbia to develop solely because of a diffusion gradient, life will be incompatible in presence of severe hypoxemia even while breathing 100% oxygen. Presence of hypercarbia suggests additional factors such as alveolar hypoventilation and ventilation/perfusion mismatch. Alveolar-arterial oxygen (A-aO_2) gradient is often utilized to monitor for oxygenation defects in impairment of diffusion and V/Q mismatch.

3.3 Distribution of Ventilation

Alveoli are perfused with systemic venous (pulmonary arterial) blood which gets arterialized after diffusion is complete. Pulmonary venous (systemic arterial) blood should have the same PO_2 and PCO_2 as in the alveolar gas. However, the arterial blood gas composition is different from alveolar gases even in normal individuals because alveolar ventilation (V) and perfusion (Q) are not matched uniformly. Some alveoli receive more ventilation compared to perfusion (high V/Q ratio, dead space ventilation units) while some receive perfusion in excess of ventilation (low V/Q ratio, shunt perfusion units). Ventilation perfusion (V/Q) relationships in a normal lung are easily understood by consideration of West Zones (Fig. 3.5)

Because of the lung recoil and gravitational force, the intrapleural pressure is more negative in non-dependent parts (upper lobes in upright position) of the lung compared to the dependent parts (lower lobes in upright position). At FRC, the alveoli in non-dependent areas of the lung are therefore at a more horizontal part of the pressure volume curve (more distended or aerated but less compliant) whereas the alveoli in the dependent areas are at a more vertical portion of the lung (less distended or aerated but more compliant). For the same change in intrapleural

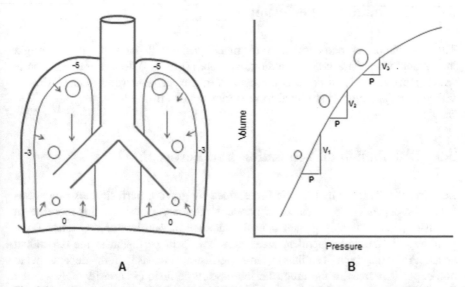

A   B

Fig. 3.3 a Illustrative representation of intrapleural pressures at FRC. Because of the lung recoil pressure and gravitational force, the intrapleural pressure is more negative in the non-dependent (upper lobes in upright position) portions of the lung compared to the dependent (lower lobes in upright position) portions. **b** Alveoli subjected to greater intrapleural pressure are therefore more distended (aerated) but less compliant. Alveoli that are surrounded by less negative pressure are less aerated but more compliant. For an identical change in inflation pressure, the change in volume is greater in dependent regions of the lung compared to non-dependent regions

Fig. 3.4 Distribution of pulmonary perfusion is gravity dependent with dependent areas of the lung getting a larger share of the blood flow

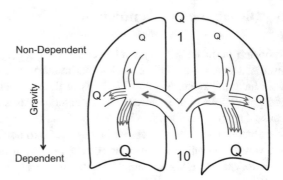

Q increases in the dependent parts of the lung because of greater hydrostatic pressure

pressure during inspiration, the dependent alveoli will receive greater portion of ventilation. At FRC, ventilation increases from non-dependent to dependent areas of the lung (Fig. 3.3).

3.4 Distribution of Perfusion

The distribution of perfusion is very much position dependent. In an upright individual, perfusion is greatest in the lower lobes (Fig. 3.4). In a supine position in which most critically ill patients are cared for, greater proportion of perfusion as well as ventilation are distributed to posterior regions of the lung.

3.5 Distribution of Ventilation and Perfusion

Because of the higher hydrostatic force aided by gravity, perfusion also increases from non-dependent portions to dependent portions. However, the increase in perfusion is considerably greater than the increase in ventilation. V/Q ratios favor ventilation in the non-dependent areas and they favor perfusion in the dependent areas. Although both ventilation and perfusion increase from dependent to non-dependent areas of the lung, the increase in perfusion is considerably greater than the increase in ventilation. While ventilation increases a little over 3 folds, the increase in perfusion may be as much as tenfold. The V:Q ratio is about 3:1 in the non-dependent and about 0.6:1 in the dependent parts of the lung. Thus, the V/Q ratios favor dead space ventilation in non-dependent parts and venous admixture in the dependent parts (Fig. 3.5). In situations such as ARDS, the dependent areas are more affected with capillary leakage. These areas receive less ventilation while still receiving larger share of perfusion. This leads to marked V:Q mismatch and

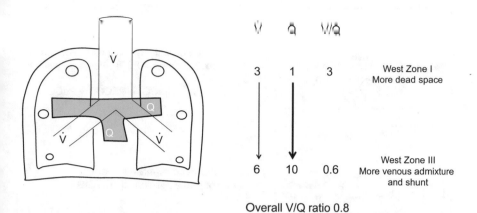

Overall V/Q ratio 0.8

Fig. 3.5 Regional ventilation, perfusion and V/Q Ratios: Both ventilation and perfusion increase from non-dependent to dependent parts of the lung. The increase in perfusion is disproportionately greater than increase in ventilation resulting in V:Q ratios approximately 3:1 in non-dependent areas and 0.6:1 in dependent areas

hypoxemia. Caring such patients in prone position, shifts the perfusion to anterior portions of the lung which are less affected and better ventilated.

3.6   Regional V:Q Relationships (West Zones)

Alveolar pressure (P_A) , pulmonary capillary arterial pressure (Pa) and pulmonary capillary venous pressure (P_V) determine the type of V:Q relationship and they form the basis of West zones described by John West. In West zone I, P_A is > Pa which is > Pv. The alveolar pressure tamponades the pulmonary blood flow in Zone I. Ventilation is in excess of what is required to fully arterialize the pulmonary arterial blood amounting to wasted or dead space ventilation. Zone I is accentuated in hypovolemia, low cardiac output, pulmonary hypertension, excessive PEEP and pulmonary embolism. The overall VD/VT ratio is increased in Zone I. In West zone II, Pa is > P_A which is > P_V. Ventilation and perfusion are better matched in the sense the pulmonary arterial blood is adequately arterialized with appropriate amount of ventilation. In West zone III, both Pa and Pv exceed P_A resulting in a relationship of Pa > Pv > P_A. In these areas ventilation is insufficient to fully arterialize the pulmonary arterial blood thereby leading to venous admixture or right to left shunting. Zone III is increased in pulmonary edema, fluid overload and atelectasis. When using prone positioning in ARDS, the clinician attempts to improve V:Q matching by converting Zone III to Zone II type of V:Q relationship (Fig. 3.6).

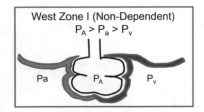

V:Q ratio 3:1   Dead space ventilation
Accentuated with Hypovolemia, Low cardiac
output, Excessive PEEP, Pulmonary HTN

$$V_D/V_T = (PaCO_2 - PECO_2) \div PaCO_2$$

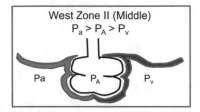

V:Q more evenly matched
Aim of prone positioning in ARDS

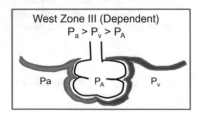

V:Q ratio 6:10 (0.6)   Venous admixture
Accentuated with High closing capacity,
Atelectasis, ARDS, Pulmonary edema

$$Q_S/Q_T = (C_CO_2 - C_aO_2) \div (C_CO_2 - C_{\bar{v}}O_2)$$

Fig. 3.6 Ventilation–Perfusion Relationship (West zones). Zone I is characterized by high V:Q ratios whereas Zone III has lower V:Q ratios

3.7   Ventilation (V) and Perfusion (Q) Mismatch

There are 3 prototypical V:Q relationships (Fig. 3.7). The first one is when venti-lation is inadequate to fully arterialize the blood flowing past the hypoventilating alveolus. The end-result is a part (or all) of pulmonary capillary blood to remain variably deoxygenated and mix with the arterialized blood from other adequately ventilating lung segments. In this situation the arterial PO_2 (PaO_2) will be less than alveolar PO_2 (P_AO_2) as calculated by the alveolar air equation. The blood gas abnormality is referred to as venous admixture or intrapulmonary right to left shunt. The second V:Q relationship is when ventilation is appropriate for the given per-fusion. In this situation, the pulmonary capillary blood is fully arterialized and PaO_2 and P_AO_2 are equal. The third V:Q relationship characterizes areas with decreased perfusion compared to ventilation. The part of the atmospheric air enters and leaves alveoli without contributing to the gas exchange. This type of V/Q mismatch is termed dead-space ventilation. In such situations P_ACO_2 is markedly less than $PaCO_2$.

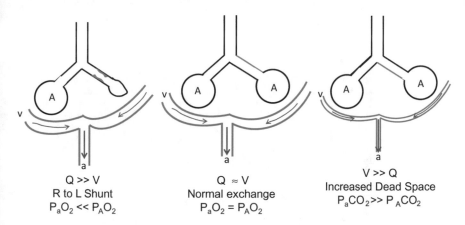

Fig. 3.7 Three types of V:Q relationship may exists: Normal V/Q, Shunt units and Dead space units

3.8 O_2 Transport and Utilization

The amount of oxygen carried by the arterial blood is in two forms: (i) in a dissolved state and (ii) combined with hemoglobin. The amount of dissolved oxygen is linearly related to PO_2. For every 100 torr PO_2, there is 0.3 mL oxygen dissolved in 100 mL of solvent. Dissolved O_2 serves two important functions. In this form O_2 is immediately available for tissue uptake. Dissolved oxygen also determines the extent to which hemoglobin is saturated by O_2. However this amount in and of itself, is hardly sufficient to satisfy tissue O_2 demands (Fig. 3.8).

The O_2 consumption for a healthy adult is approximately 250 mL/min. At a normal PaO_2 of 100 torr, there is 3 mL/L of dissolved O_2 in blood. If all of O_2 in blood was in the state of dissolved oxygen, it would require 83 L/min of cardiac output even if all of it were to be utilized by the body. The way hemoglobin associates and dissociates with O_2 constitutes an efficient means of transporting and utilizing oxygen. Each gram of hemoglobin when 100% saturated with O_2, carries 1.34 ml of oxygen. Thus, 15 G of hemoglobin per 100 mL of blood can carry approximately 20 ml of O_2 when nearly fully saturated with oxygen. This amounts to 200 mL of O_2 in 1000 mL of blood. With cardiac output of 5L per minute, an adult delivers 200 X 5 or 1000 mL of oxygen to the tissues every minute. With a resting O_2 consumption of 250 mL/min, as much as 750 mL (75% HbO_2 saturation) can still be returned back to the heart in mixed venous blood. Normally, arterial blood HbO_2 saturation is nearly complete much before we attain a normal PaO_2 because of the dissociation curve. For example, at PO_2 of 100 torr; hemoglobin-oxygen saturation is 97.5%, an increase of only 3.5% compared to the saturation at PO_2 of 70 torr where it is 94%. Relatively little O_2 can be added at higher PO_2s (Fig. 3.9).

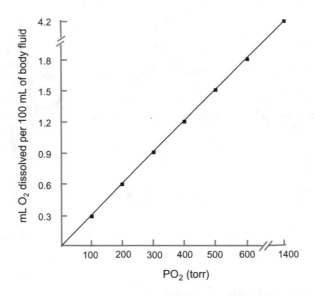

Fig. 3.8 Relationship of dissolved O_2 and PO_2 is linear. For every 100 torr, 0.3 ml of O_2 is in a dissolved state in a solution. Dissolved $O_2 = (PO_2$ in torr $\times$ 0.003)/mL of body fluid

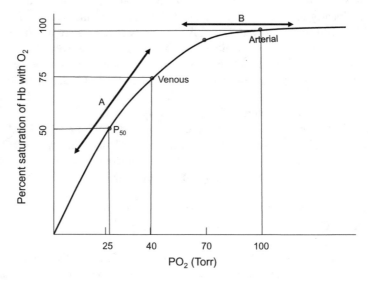

Fig. 3.9 Relationship of Hb-O_2 saturation and PO_2. In part of the curve labeled A, the change in the amount of Hb-O_2 saturation is considerably greater for a given change in PO_2 compared to the part labeled B. P_{50} refers to PO_2 at which Hb is 50% saturated

The hemoglobin molecule contains 4 heme chains each with an iron molecule in a reduced, ferrous ($Fe++$) state, and 4 globin chains. The spatial arrangement of the heme chains, $Fe++$ and globin chains is necessary for O_2 to bind reversibly with the heme part of the hemoglobin molecule. If the iron molecule is in an oxidized to a ferric state ($Fe+ ++$), methemoglobin is formed which is incapable of binding with O_2. Carbon monoxide (CO) reversibly binds with hemoglobin at the same sites as O_2 but with about 210 time greater affinity. Thus presence of mere 0.1% atmospheric CO will result in 50% carboxyhemoglobin (COHb) and 50% HbO_2 in arterial blood when breathing room air (21% O_2)! Both methemoglobinemia and CO poisoning can lead to life-threatening decline in blood O_2 content despite adequate PaO_2. 2,3-DPG, a product of RBC anaerobic glycolysis, plays an important part in association and dissociation of hemoglobin and oxygen. It binds with deoxyhemoglobin much more efficiently than with oxyhemoglobin. At lower PO_2 levels such as would occur in the tissues, 2,3-DPG facilitates O_2 to dissociate from the hemoglobin and make itself available for aerobic metabolism. At higher PO_2 levels such as would occur in the lung, oxygen binds more readily with hemoglobin not allowing 2,3-DPG to bind with hemoglobin. At high altitudes and in patients with anemia and other hypoxic conditions, 2,3-DPG concentration is increased allowing for greater release of O_2 to the tissues. Fetal hemoglobin has less affinity to 2,3-DPG and therefore it binds to O_2 more readily.

Several factors influence the shape of HbO_2 dissociation curve. A shift to the left or a decrease in P_{50} (PO_2 at which HbO_2 saturation is 50%) is a characteristic of fetal hemoglobin, hypothermia, alkalosis and a decrease in 2,3-DPG. On the other hand, a shift to the right or an increase in P_{50} is observed in hyperthermia, acidosis and an increase in 2,3-DPG. A shift to the right facilitates release of O_2 at the tissue level. (Fig. 3.10).

Following equations represent the relationship of arterial O_2 content (CaO_2), venous O_2 content (CvO_2), Cardiac output (CO), Oxygen delivery (DO_2), and Oxygen consumption (VO_2).

$$CaO_2 = [(Hb \times 1.34 \times SaO_2\%) + (PaO_2 \times 0.003)] \times 10$$

where CaO_2 is Oxygen content of blood in mL/L, Hb is Hemoglobin concentration in G/dL, SaO_2 is the Arterial Oxygen Saturation, PaO_2 is the Arterial Oxygen Tension in mmHg. Please note that the multiplication by 10 is to convert O_2 content/100 mL to O_2 content/1000 mL or 1 L.

Similarly, the oxygen content of mixed venous blood can be calculated as follows:

$$CvO_2 = [(Hgb \times 1.34 \times SvO_2\%) + (PvO_2 \times 0.003)] \times 10$$

Delivery of oxygen to the tissues by the circulatory system is estimated using the formula:

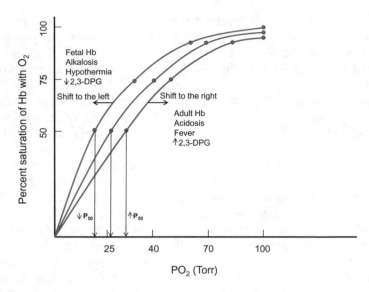

Fig. 3.10 HbO$_2$ dissociation curves shift to the left (increased O$_2$ affinity) or to the right (decreased O$_2$ affinity) under certain clinically encountered situations

$$\dot{D}O_2 = CaO_2 \times C.O.$$

where DO$_2$ is the delivery of oxygen in mL/min, CaO$_2$ is the arterial oxygen content in mL/L, and C.O. is the cardiac output in L/min.

Oxygen consumption by the tissues is measured in mL of oxygen per minute and is expressed as:

$$\dot{V}O_2 = (CaO_2 - C\bar{v}O_2) \times C.O.$$

where VO$_2$ is oxygen consumption per minute, CaO$_2$ is the arterial oxygen content, CvO$_2$ is the mixed venous oxygen content, and C.O. is the cardiac output.

The ratio of oxygen consumption to oxygen deliver is called Oxygen Extraction. It is the fraction of the oxygen delivery that is consumed by the tissues. It is calculated as follows:

$$Oxygen\ Extraction(O_{2Extr}) = \frac{\dot{V}O_2}{\dot{D}O_2}$$

Since Cardiac Output is in both the numerator and the denominator, oxygen extraction can be simplified as follows (Fig. 3.11):

$$Oxygen\ Extraction(O_{2Extr}) = \frac{(CaO_2 - C\bar{v}O_2)}{CaO_2}$$

Fig. 3.11 As DO$_2$ decreases, VO$_2$ remains constant over a wide range by increasing O$_2$ extraction to maintain aerobic metabolism. Fall in DO$_2$ beyond a certain point (critical O$_2$ delivery) results in anerobic metabolism and lactic acidosis despite continued increase in O$_2$ extraction

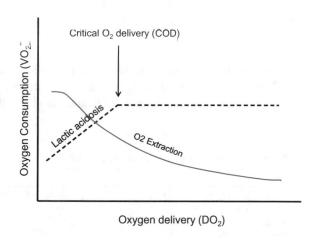

Normal resting adult has DO$_2$ of approximately 1 L/min and VO$_2$ of 250 mL/min. Thus 75% of delivered O$_2$ is returned back to heart in the mixed venous blood. CvO$_2$ is a reflection of the DO$_2$-VO$_2$ relationship. For sake of convenience, SvO$_2$ is substituted for CvO$_2$ since most of the oxygen content is accounted for by hemoglobin saturated with O$_2$. The relationship between VO$_2$, DO$_2$ and O$_2$ extraction is shown in Fig. 3.11. When DO$_2$ is decreased, VO$_2$ is initially kept constant to maintain aerobic metabolism by increasing O$_2$ extraction. A decrease in DO$_2$ below a certain level results in a decreased VO$_2$ despite increased O$_2$ extraction. DO$_2$ below which increased O$_2$ extraction does not satisfy aerobic metabolic demand of the tissues is termed critical O$_2$ delivery (COD). When DO$_2$ falls below COD, anaerobic metabolism begins with accumulation of lactic acid. Provided VO$_2$ and CaO$_2$ remain unchanged, SvO$_2$ is an indication of adequacy of CO to maintain aerobic metabolism. Declining SVO$_2$ is suggestive of decreasing cardiac output.

3.9 Abnormalities of Gas Exchange

As outlined in the preceding discussion, several factors determine gas exchange at the alveolar capillary junction. Analysis of arterial blood gases provides both diagnostic clues as well as therapeutic approach in management of respiratory disorders. The challenge to the clinician is that arterial sample is often not available and a capillary blood sample has to be relied on in many circumstances. Also, a precise FiO$_2$ is usually not available in many patients. The clinician has to rely on many assumptions and clinical experience.

There are four main types of abnormalities in gas exchange. These are (a) alveolar hypoventilation (b) ventilation-perfusion (V-Q) mismatch (c) diffusion defects and (d) absolute right to left shunt (Table 3.2). In many patients more than one disorder may be present. For example, a patient with alveolar hypoventilation may also have a component of V-Q mismatch and a patient with a diffusion defect may become exhausted and develop hypoventilation. In such a situation, the clinician must determine the major component of gas exchange abnormality to plan a targeted intervention.

Alveolar hypoventilation results when sufficient air is not moved in and out of the alveoli. There are 3 major types of clinical situations which manifest as alveolar hypoventilation. These are: airway obstruction above the carina (choanal atresia,

Table.3.2 Interpretation of arterial blood gas (ABG) values

Lesion	Effect	Typical ABG
* Central (above the carina) airway obstruction * Depressed respiratory center * Ineffective neuromuscular function	Uniform alveolar hypoventilation	* Early increase in $PaCO_2$ * Proportionate decrease in PO_2 depending on alveolar air equation * Response to supplemental oxygen: Excellent
Intrapulmonary airway obstruction	Venous admixture V/Q mismatch	* Mild: $\downarrow PCO_2$, $\downarrow PO_2$ * Moderate: "Normal PCO_2 $\downarrow\downarrow PO_2$ * Severe: $\uparrow\uparrow PCO_2$ $\downarrow\downarrow\downarrow PO_2$ * Response to supplemental oxygen: Good
Alveolar-Interstitial pathology	V/Q mismatch, venous admixture, R to L shunt Diffusion defect	* Early decrease in PO_2 depending on severity * Normal or low PCO_2 * $\uparrow PCO_2$ if fatigue occurs * Response to supplemental oxygen: Fair to poor
Extrapulmonary right to left shunt	Systemic venous blood bypasses alveoli, absolute R to L shunt	* Hypoxemia depending on magnitude of the shunt * Response to supplemental oxygen: Very poor

subglottic stenosis, vascular ring etc.), weakness of muscles of respiration (Guillain Barre syndrome, myasthenia gravis, diaphragmatic paralysis etc.) and depressed respiratory center (CNS depressants, congenital central hypoventilation syndrome, brain stem dysfunction etc.). Airway obstruction below the carina may also manifest with predominant alveolar ventilation if the obstruction is relatively uniform such as in bronchiolitis obliterans. Alveolar ventilation is inversely proportional to $PaCO_2$; a certain percentage decline in alveolar ventilation [(Vt − Vd) x rate] will lead to an increase in $PaCO_2$ by a similar percentage. The hallmark of alveolar hypoventilation is elevated $PaCO_2$ and a proportionate decline in PAO_2 as determined by alveolar air equation;

For $FiO_2 < 1$, the equation can be simplified to:

$$PAO_2 = PiO_2 - \frac{PACO_2}{R}$$

For bedside calculations, $PACO_2$ is substituted for $PaCO_2$. Thus for a given PiO_2, PAO_2 will fall only by the rise in $PaCO_2 \div R$. Since R is assumed to be 0.8, the fall in PAO_2 will be approximately by rise in $PaCO_2 \times 1.25$. In the absence of significant parenchymal disease and intrapulmonary shunting, administration of supplemental O_2 will increase PiO_2 and readily reverse hypoxemia despite persistent hypercarbia.

In intrapulmonary airway obstruction (asthma, bronchiolitis, aspiration), the obstruction is not uniform in nature. Some areas are more obstructed than others while some still are relatively unaffected resulting in multiple areas having different extent of ventilation; some are hypoventilated while others are hyperventilated. Pulmonary capillary blood coming from hypoventilated areas has higher $PaCO_2$ and a lower PaO_2, whereas that coming from hyperventilated areas has lower $PaCO_2$ and higher PaO_2. A lower $PaCO_2$ can compensate for the higher $PaCO_2$ because the $Hb-CO_2$ dissociation curve is relatively linear. An equal amount of blood with $PaCO_2$ of 30 torr mixing with $PaCO_2$ of 50 torr will result in a $PaCO_2$ of 40 torr. A higher PaO_2 however cannot compensate for a lower PaO_2 in the presence of desaturated hemoglobin because of the shape of the HBO_2 dissociation curve. It is the % HbO_2 saturation that averages out since far more O_2 is responsible for combing with Hb than the dissolved O_2 reflecting the PO_2. For example, an equal amount of blood with PaO_2 of 25 torr and HBO_2 saturation of 50% mixing with PaO_2 of 110 torr and HbO_2 saturation of near 100% will result in HbO_2 saturation of 75% and PaO_2 of 40 torr. The blood gas abnormality in such situations is referred to as V-Q mismatch, venous admixture or partial right to left intrapulmonary shunting. In mild disease, the hyperventilated areas predominate outnumbering the hypoventilated ones. The end result is hypocarbia and respiratory alkalosis. An elevated PaO_2 in the hyperventilated areas however cannot compensate for the low PaO_2 in hyperventilated area resulting in mild hypoxemia. With increasing severity, more areas become hypoventilated resulting in normalization of $PaCO_2$ (crossover point) with a further progressive decline in PaO_2. A normal or slightly elevated $PaCO_2$ in intrapulmonary airway obstruction raises concern for impending respiratory failure. As the disease severity increases, more and more lung units are hypoventilated, resulting in hypercarbia, respiratory acidosis and hypoxemia. Supplemental O_2 is effective if it is able to reach the hypoventilated alveoli.

In alveolar and interstitial pathology (ARDS, interstitial pneumonia, pulmonary edema), arterial blood gas values reflect intrapulmonary right to left shunting and diffusion barrier. Systemic venous blood flows across unventilated alveoli without getting oxygenated. The diffusion impediment is 20 times greater for O_2 than for CO_2. Hypoxemia developing early and getting progressively severe is a hall mark of such diseases. Most patients develop hyperventilation manifesting hypocarbia. An increase in $PaCO_2$ is observed only after muscle fatigue and exhaustion ensue. Response to supplemental O_2, while life-saving, may not be as robust as in other respiratory pathophysiologic alterations. In severe situations, hypoxemia may become resistant to O_2 therapy.

In conditions where systemic venous blood completely bypasses the alveolar-capillary bed (cyanotic heart disease, pulmonary arteriovenous fistula etc.), hypoxemia is the predominant feature as a fixed amount of deoxygenated blood mixes with oxygenated blood. Supplemental oxygen does not increase PaO_2 since the deoxygenated shunted blood has no chance of getting in contact with alveolar gas.

3.10   Regulation of Respiration

Blood gas homeostasis to suit the body's requirements is maintained by a complex interaction of controllers, sensors and effectors (Fig. 3.12). The central respiratory controller is represented by a group of neurons in the CNS that receives information from sensors and sends motor impulses to muscles of respiration which serve the function of the effectors. The most important effector is the diaphragm which is aided by the intercostal, abdominal and neck muscles as accessories when needed. The effectors target the lungs to adjust alveolar ventilation and control pH, $PaCO_2$ and PaO_2. The entire respiratory regulatory mechanism undergoes maturational changes from the neonatal to adult life. It is also subject to modifications by the sleep states, disease processes, pharmacologic agents and acclimatization to the environment.

3.10.1   Central Respiratory Controller

Two functionally and anatomically distinct group of neurons located in the CNS control the process of respiration: voluntary and automatic.

Voluntary control of respiration resides in the cerebral cortex and limbic forebrain areas. Major sensory inputs consist of smell, vision, emotions, pain, touch

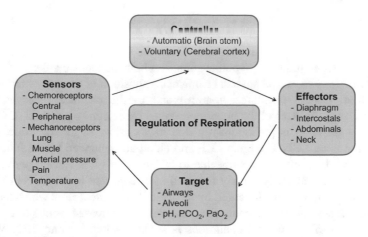

Fig. 3.12 Control of respiration

etc., and motor impulses are sent to the effectors through corticobulbar and corticospinal tracts. Voluntary control of respiration requires a certain level of consciousness, and is important for protection against aspiration and inhalation of noxious gases. Patient with toxic/metabolic/infectious/traumatic encephalopathies and pharmacologic sedation may lose voluntary control of respiration depending on the extent of CNS dysfunction.

Automatic control of respiration is located in the brainstem. Neuronal circuits, referred to as central pattern generators (CPGs) spontaneously generate rhythmic motor output without requiring conscious input, and are responsible for breathing, swallowing and chewing. CPGs responsible for breathing are located in pons and medulla. A group of neurons located in lower pons constitutes the apneustic center which is responsible for pronged inspiratory effort interrupted by brief periods of expiratory activity. Another group of neurons in the upper pons termed pneumotaxic center, is involved in inhibiting the activity of CPGs. The role of apneustic and pneumotaxic centers is to fine-tune the rhythmic respiratory activity of CPGs. Global CNS depression from any cause can manifest as slow and shallow respirations, hypoventilation and respiratory acidosis. Similarly, localized CNS lesions are manifested by specific patterns of abnormal ventilation.

3.10.2   Sensors

Multiple mechanisms exist that can sense abnormalities of gas exchange, acid–base imbalance and respiratory system dysfunction, and send that information to the central respiratory controller to modify the breathing pattern. These mechanisms exist in the form of sensory nerve endings termed chemoreceptors and mechanoreceptors depending on the type of stimulus that is being sensed.

Chemoreceptors are further classified as central or peripheral depending on their location.

Central chemoreceptors are located within the CNS. They reside over a wide area that includes posterior hypothalamus, cerebellum, locus ceruleus, raphe and brain stem. They sense a change in chemical composition of the body fluid they are exposed to. Central chemoreceptors respond to the chemical changes in the extracellular fluid (ECF) of the brain represented by cerebrospinal fluid (CSF). The ventilatory response is predominantly due to a change in the H^+ concentration (pH) of the brain ECF. The brain ECF and blood are separated by the blood brain barrier which is relatively impermeable to H^+ and HCO_3^- but freely permeable to PCO_2. A rise in $PaCO_2$ is quickly reflected in a rapid rise in the CSF PCO_2. The consequent fall in CSF pH is sensed by the central chemoreceptors which then send excitatory impulses to the controller resulting in increased ventilation via the effectors. CSF pH in normal conditions is slightly acidic, around 7.32. With its lower protein level and absence of hemoglobin, CSF also has much less buffering capacity compared to that of the blood. Consequently, for an equivalent change in $PaCO_2$, the change in CSF pH is much more pronounced than that in the blood. In disease states characterized by chronically elevated $PaCO_2$, the CSF pH tends to normalize as HCO_3^- eventually equilibrates across the BBB. Patients with chronically elevated $PaCO_2$ therefore have a relatively normal CSF pH and they do not have the same ventilatory response that is observed with acute hypercarbia.

Peripheral chemoreceptors are clusters of cells referred to as carotid bodies just above the bifurcation of the common carotid and external carotid arteries, and aortic bodies above and below the aortic arch. Carotid bodies are far more powerful sensors than aortic bodies. The cells comprising carotid and aortic bodies have a very high metabolic rate as well as blood flow to meet their metabolic demands. The main stimulus for peripheral chemoreceptors is hypoxia. Decrease in PaO_2 (SaO_2), blood flow (low cardiac output), and impaired O_2 utilization (cyanide poisoning) classically described as hypoxemic hypoxia, stagnant hypoxia and histotoxic hypoxia respectively, are potent stimulators of peripheral chemoreceptors. Anemia and dyshemoglobinemias do not stimulate peripheral chemoreceptors as long as PaO_2 and cardiac output are adequate. This is because the dissolved oxygen in the blood in form of PaO_2 and high blood flow easily satisfy the exceptionally high O_2 requirement of the chemoreceptors. Relationship of PaO_2 and stimulation of peripheral chemoreceptors is non-linear. Chemoreceptor stimulation begins at PaO_2 below 500 torr and a small increase in ventilation occurs incrementally until PaO_2 reaches 100 torr. The response time for peripheral chemoreceptor is much faster than central chemoreceptor stimulation. Even during normal respiration, carotid bodies response rate is fast enough to alter their discharges sensing small cyclic changes in PaO_2 during inspiration and exhalation. At PaO_2 less than ~ 50 torr, carotid body stimulation increases exponentially. Subjective feeling of dyspnea from pure hypoxia alone does not occur until PaO_2 falls below ~ 50 torr (SaO_2 below $\sim 85\%$). Peripheral chemoreceptors account for almost all the hyperventilation response to hypoxia. They also respond to PCO_2 but the increase in alveolar ventilation per torr PCO_2 is much less than that from central

Table.3.3 Characteristics of central and peripheral chemoreceptor stimulation

	Central chemoreception	Peripheral chemoreception
Site	Central Nervous System	Carotid and Aortic bodies
Primary Stimulus	CSF pH (PaCO$_2$)	Hypoxia
Response to hypoxia	None or depressed	Marked stimulation
Response to acutely PaCO$_2$	+ + +	+
Response time	Slow	Fast
Acclimatization	Readily occurs	Does not occur easily
Sedation/anesthesia	Easily depressed	Not easily depressed

chemoreceptor stimulation. Adaptation to stimulus (Increased PaCO$_2$) occurs in days for central chemoreceptors but hypoxic stimulation of peripheral chemoreceptors persists for a long time, even for life, for people living at high altitudes as reflected by their lower PaCO$_2$ levels. The difference in central and peripheral chemoreception is presented in Table 3.3.

In certain disease states such as asthma a blunted response to hypoxia is well documented. In recent SARS-CoV-2 pandemic, similar observations of "happy hypoxia" have been reported describing patients with minimal respiratory distress in spite of considerable arterial O$_2$ desaturation. Pure peripheral chemoreceptor stimulation results in bradycardia. In most situations with acute hypoxia, tachycardia develops because of action of muscles of respirations causing lung inflation. Two situations where bradycardia is a pronounced effect of sole peripheral chemoreceptor stimulation are: hypoxic patients with neuromuscular blockade and neuromyopathy, and in intrauterine life. In chronic hypercarbic states, the central chemoreceptors have adapted to elevated PaCO$_2$ and the respirations are maintained mainly by the hypoxic drive from the peripheral chemoreceptors. Administration of high concentration of O$_2$ can potentially abolish the hypoxic peripheral chemoreception resulting in hypoventilation, respiratory acidosis and CO$_2$ narcosis. Care must be taken in delivering supplemental O$_2$ to such patients to avoid serious hypoventilation.

Mechanoreceptors

Stretch receptors located within the airway smooth muscles, are stimulated by lung inflation. They are important in adjusting the respiratory rate in health and disease and minimizing work of breathing. In diseases with decreased lung compliance, alveoli fill up quickly thus the transpulmonary pressure is transmitted quickly to the airways stretch receptors resulting in inhibition of inspiration. The breathing pattern is rapid and shallow. In diseases of increased resistance, alveoli take longer time to fill up thus delaying stimulation of the stretch receptors and thus resulting in deeper and slower respiration.

Muscle receptors are located in diaphragm and intercostal muscles. Stretching of these muscles is sensed by the muscle spindle to control the strength of contraction.

Excessive distortion of diaphragm and intercostal muscles inhibits inspiratory activity.

J receptors are located in the alveolar walls close to the pulmonary capillaries. Pulmonary capillary engorgement and interstitial and alveolar fluid collection activate J receptors resulting in rapid, shallow respiration and dyspnea.

Irritant receptors are located in between the epithelial cells in the airway mucous membrane throughout the respiratory tract. They are stimulated by particulate matter and noxious gases as well as cold air. Their stimulation results in bronchoconstriction and cough.

Arterial baroreceptors located in aortic arch and carotid sinus, respond to arterial blood pressure. Hypotension results in tachypnea and hyperpnea.

3.10.3 Effectors

The most important effector of respiration is the diaphragm. Intercostals and abdominal muscles are recruited when additional increase in ventilation is necessary. Sternocleidomastoids and paraspinal muscles may be called upon to additional contribution to the respiratory effort. Developmental changes significantly influence the ability of the diaphragm to sustain large elastic work load and resist fatigue. As compared to the skeletal muscles which contain primarily fast twitch, fatigable type 2 × and 2b fibers, the predominant muscle fiber types in the diaphragm are the fatigue resistant slow twitch type 1 and intermediate fatigue resistant fast twitch type 2a fibers. The type 1 fibers have slower shortening velocities than fast type 2a fibers but are highly fatigue resistant due to their lower ATP consumption and their reliance almost exclusively on aerobic metabolism. Type 2a fibers on the other hand are fast-twitch, less oxidative and are more prone to fatigue. This combination of fiber types allows for good fatigue resistance and increased force generation when necessary. Diaphragms of newborns and infants have a lower muscle mass when indexed for body size. In addition, they have lower percentages of fatigue resistant type I fibers. The diaphragm of preterm infants contains only 10% type I fibers. This increases to 25% in term neonates and 55% in children greater than 2 years of age. These developmental differences predispose neonates and infants to respiratory muscle fatigue and respiratory failure.

Suggested Readings

1. Sarnaik AP, Heidemann SM, Clark JA. Respiratory pathophysiology and regulation. In: Kliegman RM, Stanton BF, St Geme JW, Schor NF, editors. Nelson textbook of pediatrics. 20th ed. Philadelphia: Elsevier; 2016. p. 1981–93.
2. Bigeleisen PE. Models of venous admixtures. Adv Physiol Educ. 2001;25:159–66.

3. Sarnaik AP, Clark JA, Heidemann SM. Respiratory distress and failure. In: Kliegman RM, Stanton BF, St Geme JW, Schor NF, Phillips Nelson textbook of pediatrics, 21st ed. Philadelphia: Elsevier; 2019.
4. Clark J, Chiwane S, Sarnaik, AP. Mechanical dysfunction of respiratory system. In: Fuhrman BF, Zimmerman JJ, Rotta A, editors. Pediatric Critical Care, 5th edn. St. Louis: C. V. Mosby Company; 2020.

Chapter 4
Clinical Examination and Assessment

Shekhar T. Venkataraman and Ashok P. Sarnaik

4.1 Importance of Clinical Examination

Clinical examination is the first step in both establishing a diagnosis and immediate institution of therapies. The first step in establishing the diagnosis of respiratory disease is appropriate interpretation of clinical findings. Respiratory symptoms and signs may occur not only due to respiratory diseases but also other systems that impact on the respiratory system.

Within the first few minutes of an encounter, the patient can be classified into the following categories:

(1) The clinical examination shows that the patient is in extremis and in imminent danger of dying and requires immediate intervention
(2) The clinical examination shows a serious situation that may require some treatments to be administered before a definitive diagnosis can be made
(3) The clinical examination shows a sick child but one has enough time to perform a detailed clinical exam as well as diagnostic assessment before any preliminary treatment is started

S. T. Venkataraman (✉)
Professor, Departments of Critical Care Medicine and Pediatrics, University of Pittsburgh School of Medicine, Pittsburgh, PA, USA
e-mail: venkataramanst@upmc.edu

Medical Director, Respiratory Care Services, Children's Hospital of Pittsburgh, 4401 Penn Avenue, Faculty Pavilion 2117, Pittsburgh, PA 15224, USA

A. P. Sarnaik
Professor of Pediatrics, Former Pediatrician in Chief and Interim Chairman Children's Hospital of Michigan, Wayne State University School of Medicine, 3901 Beaubien, Detroit, MI 48201, USA
e-mail: asarnaik@med.wayne.edu

© Springer Nature Switzerland AG 2022
A. P. Sarnaik et al. (eds.), *Mechanical Ventilation in Neonates and Children*,
https://doi.org/10.1007/978-3-030-83738-9_4

(4) The clinical examination shows a clinically stable patient but with a problem that needs to be investigated without needing any preliminary treatment.

4.2   Respiratory Distress and Respiratory Failure

The term respiratory distress is used to indicate signs and symptoms of abnormal respiratory pattern with an increased work of breathing and discomfort. A child with nasal flaring, increased rate (tachypnea), increased (hyperpnea) or decreased (hypopnea) depth of respiration, chest wall retractions, stridor, grunting, dyspnea, or wheezing has respiratory distress. Taken together, the magnitude of these findings is used to judge clinical severity.

Nasal flaring is a nonspecific, but a relatively sensitive sign of respiratory distress especially in infants and newborns. Although teleologically intended to decrease airway resistance, flaring of ala nasi is relatively ineffective for that purpose. It is however, a very important sign to identify an infant in some form of distress.

Rate and depth of respiration Prominent tachypnea is a hallmark of children with decrease lung compliance observed in alveolar-interstitial disease. Elastic work of breathing (W_{Elast}), determined mainly by V_T is increased disproportionately compared to resistive work of breathing (W_{Resist}) which is determined mainly by the respiratory rate. Thus, rapid and shallow respirations minimize work of breathing in such situations. Diseases of resistance are associated with increased depth of respiration at relatively slower rates. Young infants, because of their softer chest wall, have greater W_{Elast} and therefore they tend to breathe rapidly in all diseases affecting the respiratory system. Tachypnea is also prominent in situations with stimulation as J receptors which are located in the alveolar walls close to pulmonary capillaries. They are activated by distention of pulmonary capillaries, and accumulation of interstitial fluid. Increased in depth of breathing is seen much more commonly in non-respiratory diseases such as a response to metabolic acidosis, anxiety, and abnormal CNS impulses. For reliable interpretation of tachypnea, the child should be observed in a relative position of comfort and an environment that is least anxiety provoking.

Stridor is a high-pitched, coarse sound, characteristically during inspiration. It is indicative of extra thoracic airway obstruction (laryngotracheitis, vocal cord paralysis etc.) which gets worse during inspiration. In such a situation, the high negative intrathoracic pressure created to overcome the obstruction causes the extra thoracic airway to collapse below it. Inspiration is prolonged when this occurs.

Wheezing is a high-pitched, musical sound mostly heard during exhalation (but may also be during inspiration) in intrathoracic airway obstruction. The equal pressure point (EPP) is moved distally causing widespread intrathoracic airway collapse and prolongation of exhalation.

Rhonchi are low-pitched wheezes that are a result of pulmonary secretions in the larger bronchial airways. They are often biphasic in nature. Air flowing past the loose secretions creates a sound of "gurgling or rattling" throughout the lung fields.

Crackles or Rales are discontinuous "faint popping" sounds heard during inspiration. The sound auscultated is a result of opening of air fluid menisci in the late generation bronchi. When crackles are heard earlier in the inspiration phase it is indicative of fluid in the larger airways (congestive heart failure), whereas crackles later in the inspiratory phase that are fine or high-pitched are associated with fluid in the smaller airways (pneumonia). Pathologies associated with crackles/rales often have poor lung compliance secondary to increased lung water, decrease alveoli surface area, and surfactant dysfunction.

Chest wall retractions are a manifestation of increased negative intrathoracic pressure during inspiration. They can also be observed, even in normal conditions, in children with weak chest walls. Excessively high negative intrathoracic pressures are generated in extra thoracic airway obstruction which worsens during inspiration and diseases of poor compliance where higher pressures are needed to maintain V_T. In newborns, especially those born prematurely, a pattern of paradoxical or see-saw respiration is observed where the chest caves in and abdomen bulges out during inspiration and the opposite occurs during exhalation.

Grunting is the child's attempt to maintain lung volumes without alveolar collapse. Grunting creates positive pressure during exhalation by partial closure of the glottis. This to a) maintain FRC in alveolar-interstitial disease to counter hypoxia and b) decrease transmural pressure and displacing the EPP more proximally to minimize airway collapse during exhalation in intrathoracic airway obstruction. Grunting can also be a manifestation of general distress as associated with pain and sepsis.

Other signs are useful in localizing the site of pathology as described below. Respiratory failure is defined conceptually as the inability to maintain adequate oxygenation or ventilation while breathing spontaneously in room air. Inability to adequately oxygenate results in hypoxemia, which is defined as an arterial oxygen tension (PaO_2) less than 60 mmHg or an arterial oxyhemoglobin saturation of < 90%. Hypoxemic respiratory failure refers to hypoxemia resulting from respiratory disease. Hypercarbia is defined as an increase in arterial carbon dioxide greater than 45 mmHg. Hypercarbic respiratory failure refers to hypercarbia and respiratory acidosis due to respiratory disease while breathing spontaneously. Therefore, whereas respiratory distress is a clinical assessment, the diagnosis of respiratory failure requires measurement of indices of gas exchange.

Diseases characterized by CNS excitation, such as encephalitis, and neuroexcitatory drugs are associated with central neurogenic hyperventilation. Similarly, diseases that produce metabolic acidosis, such as diabetic ketoacidosis, salicylism, and shock, result in hyperventilation and hyperpnea. Patients in either group could present clinically with respiratory distress; they are distinguished from patients with respiratory disease by their increased chest expansion per breath (i.e., tidal volume) as well as the respiratory rate. Patients with neuromuscular diseases, such as Guillain-Barré syndrome or myasthenia gravis, and those with an abnormal respiratory drive can develop severe respiratory failure but are not able to mount sufficient effort to appear in respiratory distress. In these patients, respirations are ineffective or can even appear normal in the presence of respiratory acidosis and hypoxemia.

Caveats:

1. Respiratory distress can occur in patients without respiratory disease
2. Respiratory failure can occur in patients without respiratory distress.
3. Hypoxemia can occur due to reasons other than respiratory disease (e.g., cyanotic heart disease)
4. Hypercarbia can occur without respiratory disease (e.g., diuretic use, excess bicarbonate due to acetate administration)

4.3 Characterizing Severity of Disease with Clinical Examination

Clinical examination of the respiratory system includes inspection, palpation, percussion and auscultation. Inspection of the respiratory system requires observation of respiratory rate, rhythm, pattern and effort of breathing. Auscultation of the lungs may reveal rales/crackles, stridor or wheeze. These can also be graded for severity based on the duration and whether they occur during one phase or both phases of breathing. There are scoring systems such as the croup score or the asthma score which offer a way to quantify the severity of the respiratory distress. The Table 4.1 shows a method to quantify the severity based on the respiratory signs and its effect on gas exchange and other systems.

4.4 Using Clinical Signs to Locate Site of Pathophysiology

While breathing rate, depth of respiration, presence of retractions, stridor, wheezing, and grunting are valuable in evaluating the severity of respiratory distress, they are also very useful in localizing the site of respiratory pathology (Table 4.2). Rapid

Table 4.1 Clinical signs with differing degrees of respiratory distress

Clinical sign	Mild	Moderate	Severe
Respiratory rate	+	++	+++
Retractions	Subcostal	Subcostal + Intercostal	Subcostal + intercostal + suprasternal
Asynchrony	None	Mild Asynchrony	Paradoxical Breathing
Stridor	None	Inspiratory	Inspiratory + Expiratory
Wheezing	None	Expiratory	Expiratory + Inspiratory
Gas exchange	SpO2 > 92% in RA	SpO2 > 92% with FiO2 < 0.3	SpO2 < 92% with FiO2 > 0.3 and < 0.5
Mental status	Awake	Restless	Decreased

Table 4.2 Interpreting the clinical signs of respiratory disease

Sign	Extra-thoracic airway obstruction	Intrathoracic extrapulmonary airway obstruction	Intrapulmonary airway obstruction	Parenchymal pathology
Tachypnea	+	+	++	++++
Stridor	++++	++	–	–
Retractions	++++	++	++	+++
Wheezing	±	+++	++++	±
Grunting	±	±	++	++++

Reprinted with permission from Sarnaik AP, Heidemann S and Clark JA, *Nelson Textbook of Pediatrics*, 20th Edition, Kligman, St. Geme et al. Editors, Elsevier 2016

and shallow respirations (tachypnea) are characteristic of parenchymal pathology. Chest wall, intercostal, and suprasternal retractions are most striking in extra-thoracic airway obstruction as well as diseases of decreased compliance. Inspiratory stridor is a hallmark of extra- thoracic airway obstruction. Expiratory wheezing is characteristic of intrathoracic airway obstruction, either extrapulmonary or intrapulmonary. Grunting is produced by expiration against a partially closed glottis in small airway obstruction (bronchiolitis) to maintain a higher positive pressure in the airway during expiration, decreasing the airway collapse. Grunting is most prominent in alveolar-interstitial disease to help maintain FRC.

4.5 Presentation Profiles of Respiratory Failure in Childhood

When mechanical dysfunction is present (by far, the most common circumstance), arterial hypoxemia and hypercapnia (and hence, pH) are sensed by peripheral (carotid bodies) and central (medullary) chemoreceptors. After being integrated with other sensory information from the lungs and chest wall, chemoreceptor activation triggers an increase in the neural output to the respiratory muscles, which results in the physical signs that characterize respiratory distress. When the problem resides with the respiratory muscles (or their innervation), the same increase in neural output occurs, but the respiratory muscles cannot increase their effort as demanded; therefore, the physical signs of distress are more subtle. Finally, when the control of breathing is itself affected by disease, the neural response to hypoxemia and hypercapnia is absent or blunted and the gas exchange abnormalities are not accompanied by respiratory distress (Fig. 4.1).

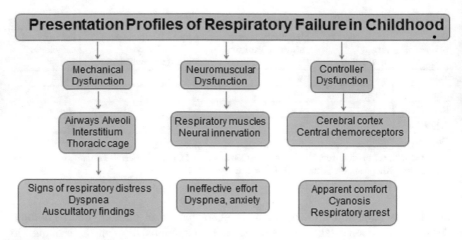

Fig. 4.1 Respiratory failure in children may present in different forms depending on the type of dysfunction

4.6 Respiratory Distress Without Respiratory Disease

Although respiratory distress most frequently results from diseases of lungs, airways, and chest wall, pathology in other organ systems can manifest as respiratory distress and lead to misdiagnosis and inappropriate management (Table 4.3).

Table 4.3 Non-pulmonary causes of respiratory distress

System	Example (s)	Mechanism (s)
Cariovascular	Left-to-right shunt Congestive heart failure Cardiogenic shock	↑Lung blood/water content Metabolic acidosis Baroreceptor stimulation
Central nervous system	Increased intracranial pressure Encephalitis Neurogenic pulmonary edema Toxic encephalopathy	Stimulation of brain stem respiratory centers
Metabolic	Diabetic Ketoacidosis Organic academia Hyperammonemia	Stimulation of central and peripheral chemoreceptors
Renal	Renal tubular acidosis Hypertension	Stimulation of central and peripheral chemoreceptors Left ventricular dysfunction Pulmonary edema
Sepsis	Toxic shock syndrome Meningococcemia	Cytokine stimulation of respiratory centers Baroreceptor stimulation from shock Metabolic acidosis

Respiratory distress resulting from heart failure or diabetic ketoacidosis may be misdiagnosed as asthma and improperly treated with albuterol, resulting in worsened hemodynamic state or ketoacidosis. Careful history and physical examination provide essential clues in avoiding misdiagnosis.

Suggested Reading

1. Malley WJ. Clinical blood gases assessment and intervention, 2nd Edition 2005. Elsevier Saunders, St Louis, Missouri
2. MacIntyre NR, Branson RD. Mechanical ventilation. 2001. W.B. Saunders. Philadelphia, Pennsylvania
3. der Stayy V, Chatburn RL. Advanced modes of mechanical ventilation and optimal targeting schemes. Intensive Care Med Exp. 2018;6(1):30.
4. Chatburn RL, El-Khatib M, Mireles-Cabodevila E. A taxonomy for mechanical ventilation: 10 fundamental maxims. Respir Care. 2014;59(11):1747–63.
5. Dexter AM, Kimberly C. Ventilator graphics: scalar, loops, & secondary measures. Respir Care. 2020;65(6):739–59.

Chapter 5
Monitoring

Shekhar T. Venkataraman

Recent advances have made it possible to monitor a variety of respiratory functions at the bedside in infants and children. These include an assessment of gas exchange, lung mechanics, work of breathing, neuromuscular capacity and the metabolic status of the patient. This chapter will briefly review some of the monitoring that is readily available at the bedside.

5.1 Gas Exchange

5.1.1 Assessment of Arterial Oxygenation

Monitoring of oxygenation includes assessment of (a) gas exchange in the lungs, (b) oxygen transport to the tissues, and (c) oxygen utilization in the tissues (Fig. 5.1). Indexes used to assess the lung as an oxygenator are: (1) arterial O_2 tension (PaO_2), (2) oxyhemoglobin saturation (SaO_2), (3) intrapulmonary shunt fraction (Q_s/Q_t), (4) alveolar-to-arterial O_2 tension difference ($PA\text{-}aO_2$), (5) arterial-to-alveolar oxygen tension ratio (PaO_2/PAO_2), and (6) arterial oxygen tension-to-fraction of inspired O_2 ratio (PaO_2/FiO_2).

Arterial partial pressure of oxygen (PaO_2).

PaO_2, the partial pressure of oxygen in the arterial blood, is measured using a blood gas analyzer, either in a central laboratory or using a hand-held device at the bedside. PaO_2 represents the net effect of O_2 exchange in the lung. At sea level, the normal

S. T. Venkataraman (✉)
Professor, Departments of Critical Care Medicine and Pediatrics, University of Pittsburgh School of Medicine, Pittsburgh, PA, USA
e-mail: venkataramanst@upmc.edu

Medical Director, Respiratory Care Services, Children's Hospital of Pittsburgh, 4401 Penn Avenue, Faculty Pavilion 2117, Pittsburgh, PA 15224, USA

© Springer Nature Switzerland AG 2022
A. P. Sarnaik et al. (eds.), *Mechanical Ventilation in Neonates and Children*,
https://doi.org/10.1007/978-3-030-83738-9_5

55

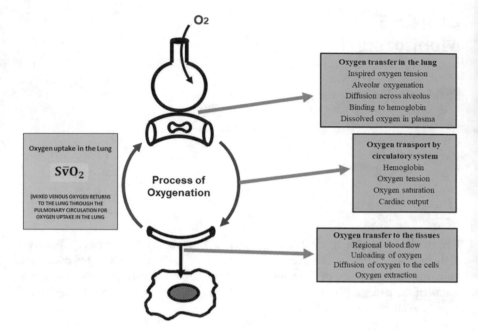

Fig. 5.1 Process of Oxygenation and Assessment of Oxygenation. On the right side is shown oxygen transfer in the lungs, oxygen transport by the circulatory system and oxygen transfer to the tissues with some relevant bedside monitoring variables. On the left side is depicted oxygen saturation in the mixed venous blood returning to the lung to be re-oxygenated

PaO_2 in a newborn infant is between 50 and 70 mmHg, breathing room air. Soon after birth, the range of normal values increases rapidly such that the normal PaO_2 will range between 60 and 80 in room air. With increasing age, the PaO_2 increases until it reaches an adult value of 90–100 mmHg. Hypoxemia is a PaO_2 lower than the acceptable range for age, whereas hypoxia is inadequate tissue oxygenation. For a child, a PaO_2 of < 60 mmHg may be considered hypoxemia, whereas that may be acceptable for a newborn due to the presence of fetal hemoglobin and persistent right to left shunts as a component of transitional circulation. Causes of hypoxemia are: (1) decreased inspired oxygen concentration, (2) hypoventilation, (3) right-to-left intracardiac shunts, (4) diffusion defect, (5) ventilation-perfusion inequality (lung segments with very low ventilation-perfusion ratios), and (6) intrapulmonary shunting. The effect of ventilation-perfusion inequality and intrapulmonary shunting is referred to as venous admixture. It is important to remember that dissolved oxygen contributes only to a small portion of the total oxygen content in normal circumstances. Arterial oxygen tension may be normal in states of inadequate tissue oxygenation due to anemia, cyanide poisoning, methemoglobin toxicity, or carbon monoxide poisoning. Venous admixture as measured by intrapulmonary shunt fraction (Q_s/Q_t) requires a pulmonary artery catheter and measurement of mixed venous oxygen content.

Indices of the lung as an oxygenator

If the lung were a perfect oxygenator, then pulmonary venous PO_2 would be identical to the alveolar PO_2 (PAO_2), and if the right ventricular output traverses the ideal lung, then PaO_2 would be the same as pulmonary venous PO_2. PAO_2 is calculated from the simplified alveolar gas equation, as described in Chap. 1. With venous admixture, PaO_2 is less than PAO_2. Alveolar to arterial oxygen gradient (PA-aO_2), the ratio of arterial PaO_2 to alveolar PO_2 (PaO_2/PAO_2), and the ratio of arterial PaO_2 to the fraction of inspired oxygen (PaO_2/FiO_2) are indices that determine the extent to which the PaO_2 deviates from PAO_2 as a measure of venous admixture. The normal PA-aO_2 is usually less than 20 mmHg in a child, and less than 50 mmHg in a newborn infant. A large PA-aO_2 represents venous admixture. PA-aO_2 is affected not only by venous admixture but also by mixed venous oxygen saturation. A major limitation of this index is that it increases unpredictably with increasing FiO_2. To compare gradients over time, FiO_2 must remain constant. To be reliable, the arterial-to-mixed venous PO_2 difference must also be constant. Unlike PA-aO_2, PaO_2/PAO_2 relationship changes much more predictably with increasing FiO_2. Thus, it is preferred over PA-aO_2 as an index of oxygen transfer in the lung and can be used to predict changes in PaO_2 when FiO_2 is altered. PaO_2/FiO_2 ratio is the easiest index to calculate, and does not require calculation of PAO_2. The disadvantage is that it does not adjust for alveolar CO_2. At high FiO_2, this error becomes quite small. The normal PaO_2/FiO_2 in a child is > 400 mmHg breathing room air at sea level. A PaO_2/FiO_2 ratio of less than 300 is an indication for supplemental oxygen and a ratio of 150 on supplemental O_2 is usually an indication for intubation and mechanical ventilation.

Oxyhemoglobin saturation

SaO_2, the arterial oxygen saturation of hemoglobin, is the percent oxyhemoglobin in the arterial blood. The oxygen dissociation curve describes the avidity with which oxygen binds to hemoglobin. Acidemia, hypercarbia, an elevated temperature and an increased red-cell 2,3- diphosphoglycerate (DPG) level shifts the curve to the right making the oxygen molecules dissociate easily from Hb, thus making it available for the tissues. Alkalemia, hypothermia, fetal hemoglobin and decreased 2,3- DPG shift the curve to the left resulting in greater affinity of Hb to O_2. Cyanosis can be detected in the nailbeds and mucosa when the deoxygenated hemoglobin concentration is at least 5 g/dL. Detection of cyanosis is often imprecise, especially under artificial lighting. As the severity of illness increases, more precise monitoring of SaO_2 becomes essential.

Pulse Oximetry

According to Beer-Lambert law, the optical density of a light-absorbing material is directly proportional to the concentration of the light absorbing material. Hemoglobin acts as a light absorbing material in blood. The pulse oximeter probe has light emitting diodes as well as light absorbing sensors. The probe is usually placed across a vascular bed such as a fingertip or the lobe of the ear. The light

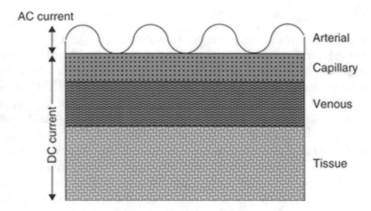

Fig. 5.2 Plethysmographic waveform of light transmission in pulse oximetry. Light transmitted through the vascular bed displays both a pulsatile component (which is assumed to be due to arterial pulsations) and a non-pulsatile component (which is assumed to be through non-pulsatile elements of the vascular bed including the capillaries, veins and tissue)

emitting source in a pulse oximeter has two wavelengths, 660 nm (red region) and 940 nm (infrared region). Deoxyhemoglobin absorbs more light at 660 nm compared to oxyhemoglobin. On the other hand, oxyhemoglobin absorbs more light at 940 nm compared to deoxyhemoglobin.

When light is passed through a vascular bed, a certain amount of light is absorbed and the rest is transmitted. The transmitted light has pulsatile and non-pulsatile components (Fig. 5.2) which are converted to electrical signals. Pulsatile waveform which is represented by the AC current (Alternate Current) is assumed to be due to arterial blood. The non-pulsatile waveform, represented by the DC current (Direct Current), is assumed to be due to light absorption in tissues, veins and capillaries. The amount of light in the pulsatile component is then indexed to the non-pulsatile component of each of the wavelengths. The pulse oximeter then calculates a ratio called R, which is calculated as follows:

$$R = \frac{AC_{660}/DC_{660}}{AC_{940}/DC_{940}}$$

where, R is the ratio of absorbance of the pulsatile and non-pulsatile elements. In the numerator is the ratio of the AC to the DC components for 660 nm and the denominator is the ratio of the AC to the DC components for 940 nm. The more oxygenated the blood, the R decreases in value. A computer algorithm is generated where the R value is correlated to oxygen saturation values obtained from volunteers and programmed into each monitor as a look-up table. When a pulse oximeter is placed on a patient, the monitor assesses the light absorption through the vascular bed and calculates the R value and displays the corresponding oxygen saturation value. The resultant pulse oximetry oxygen saturation (SpO_2) has been found to correlate well with SaO$_2$ in critically ill patients in the range of 70–100%. Below 70%, SpO$_2$ does correlate with SaO$_2$ but there is greater variability. SpO$_2$ can reliably detect hypoxemia, defined as SpO$_2$ < 90%. SpO$_2$ is less sensitive in detecting hyperoxemia. Fetal hemoglobin does not affect SpO$_2$ since the absorption characteristics are similar to that of adult hemoglobin.

Carboxyhemoglobin, absorbs light maximally at 660 nm, but does not absorb light at 960 nm. As carboxyhemoglobin levels increase, SpO$_2$ readings will overestimate SaO$_2$, since it assumes that the increased light absorption at 660 nm is due to oxyhemoglobin. With smoke inhalation, where increased carboxyhemoglobin is possible, co-oximetry should be performed to measure SaO$_2$. Methemoglobin absorbs light almost equally at both 660 nm and 960 nm. This makes the ratio of the light absorbed at the 660 nm/960 nm to be equal to one, which corresponds to SaO$_2$ of 85%. With low methemoglobin levels (<15%), SpO$_2$ underestimates SaO$_2$. With high methemoglobin levels (>30%), the SpO$_2$ overestimates SaO$_2$ reads around 85% despite increasing levels. Bilirubin absorbs light maximally at 460 nm and therefore, it should have no effect on SpO$_2$.

5.1.2 Assessment of Oxygen Transport

Oxygen delivery

Oxygen delivery (DO$_2$) is the amount of oxygen delivered by the cardiovascular system to the tissues every minute. It is calculated by the formula: DO$_2$ = CaO$_2$ x Q, where Q is the cardiac output in L/min. A normal DO$_2$ in a child is ~ 15–17 mL/kg/min. This is increased during exercise, fever, thyrotoxicosis etc. to meet tissue O$_2$ demands. The two major determinants of DO$_2$ are Hb-O$_2$ saturation and cardiac output. Mild hypoxemia can be compensated by increasing either Hb or cardiac output or both. If DO$_2$ is adequate to meet the tissue O$_2$ demands, the absolute PaO$_2$ is not that critical as long as SaO$_2$ remains adequate. Oxygen delivery requires measurement of cardiac output. Invasive techniques of measuring cardiac output include thermodilution and dye-dilution techniques and require invasive vascular catheterization. Noninvasive techniques of measuring cardiac output include using ultrasonography and thoracic electrical impedance.

Assessment of oxygen utilization

Oxygen consumption (VO$_2$) is the amount the oxygen that is utilized by the body in a minute. VO$_2$ can be measured by analyzing the inspired and expired gases using a Douglas bag or by using the Fick equation, where VO$_2$ = Q (CaO$_2$–CvO$_2$). Fever, thyrotoxicosis, and increased catecholamine release or administration increase the metabolic rate and increase VO$_2$. Hypothermia and hypothyroidism tend to decrease VO$_2$. Measurement of VO$_2$ may be important in critically ill patients especially those with moderately severe cardiorespiratory dysfunction. There are currently two methods of measuring oxygen consumption at the bedside. One is using a metabolic cart, which measures the difference between the amount of oxygen inspired and the amount exhaled during minute ventilation. A metabolic cart can be used with both intubated and non-intubated patients. The second method is to measure cardiac output, arterial oxygen and mixed venous oxygen contents and using the formula above calculate the oxygen consumption. This requires placement of a pulmonary artery catheter to obtain mixed venous samples. Superior vena cava sample is sometimes substituted for mixed venous blood which allows methods of cardiac output measurement that do not require a pulmonary artery catheter. Under normal conditions, VO_2 is independent of DO_2. In some patients, VO_2 becomes DO_2-dependent. If clinically possible, DO_2 should be increased until VO_2 is no longer DO_2-dependent.

Mixed venous oxygen saturation (SvO_2) is commonly used as a measure of the balance between O_2 demand and supply (Fig. 5.3). A low SvO_2 usually signifies that DO_2 is decreased and the body is extracting more oxygen from the blood. This is usually true in hypovolemia and cardiogenic shock. In sepsis, where there is maldistribution of peripheral blood flow, SvO_2 may be normal or even high, though there may be oxygen deficits in the tissues. A high SvO_2 is usually seen in hypothermia due to decreased oxygen demand and also from increased hemoglobin

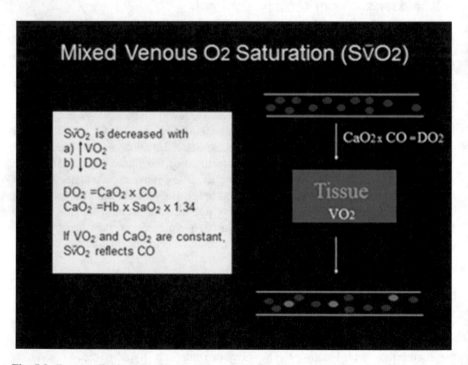

Fig. 5.3 Factors affecting mixed venous saturation. Mixed venous saturation (SvO_2) is decreased with increased tissue oxygen consumption and decreased oxygen delivery. If O_2 consumption and arterial oxygen content remain constant, a decrease in SvO_2 is reflective of decreased cardiac output

affinity for O_2. A high SvO_2 can also be seen in brain death as the brain usually constitutes a major part of the total body oxygen consumption. Other situations where a high SvO_2 is observed are arteriovenous mixing (cerebral arteriovenous fistula, TAPVR and impaired O_2 utilization (cyanide poisoning).

5.1.3 Assessment of Ventilation

Arterial PCO_2

Carbon dioxide (CO_2) produced during metabolism is transported from the tissues to the lungs in the venous blood mainly in three forms: dissolved in plasma, as bicarbonate in the red cells, and bound to hemoglobin (carbamino compound). Dissolved CO_2 is measured as the partial pressure in mmHg or kPa. Serum bicarbonate measures the amount of CO_2 present as bicarbonate in the plasma. The amount of CO_2 bound to hemoglobin is usually small and not measured in usual clinical practice.

In the lungs, CO_2 diffuses from the pulmonary capillaries into the alveolus where minute alveolar ventilation removes the CO_2 from the alveoli. $PaCO_2$ is the PCO_2 in arterial blood and reflects the efficiency of the lung as a ventilator. $PaCO_2$ measurement requires arterial blood sampling either through a puncture or through an indwelling arterial catheter. Capillary sample or arterialized finger-stick sample is sometimes used in small children to approximate $PaCO_2$.

Capnography

Capnography refers to the measurement of carbon dioxide concentration in the exhaled breath and a capnogram is the graphical representation of the carbon dioxide concentration over time, usually expressed as the partial pressure (mmHg or kPa) or fractional concentration over time. There are generally two forms of exhaled CO_2 measurement at the bedside. One is a colorimetric technique where the presence of CO_2 in the exhaled gas changes the color of the filter in the device attached to the endotracheal tube. The other is a continuous recording of CO_2 partial pressure over time during all phases of respiration, the capnogram. The exhaled CO_2 is usually plotted over time and displayed on a monitor. Some devices are capable of plotting exhaled CO_2 against the exhaled volume (volumetric capnography).

Figure 5.4 shows an idealized capnogram. The first phase is the flat part of the capnogram where no CO_2 is detected. This corresponds to the early phase of exhalation consisting of anatomic dead space. The second phase is the upstroke or ascending part. This corresponds to the appearance of CO_2 in the exhaled gas when the alveolar gas mixes with the gas in the airway. The CO_2 concentration rises rapidly during the second phase and reaches a plateau. The third phase is the plateau phase. This corresponds to alveolar gas appearing in the exhaled gas. The termination of the plateau phase is the end of expiration. The CO_2 concentration at this

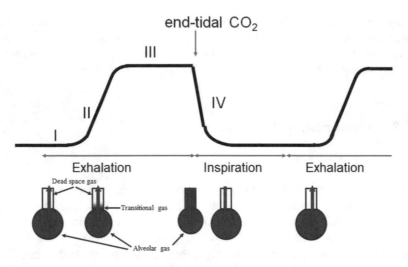

Fig. 5.4 Phases of a capnogram. In Phase I, the CO_2 concentration is very low or zero. In Phase II, the CO_2 concentration increases and in Phase III reaches a maximum. The CO_2 concentration at the end of exhalation is termed end-tidal CO_2 (ETCO$_2$). Phase IV shows a rapid reduction in CO_2 concentration due to inspiration of fresh gas that has little to no CO_2

point is called the "end-tidal CO_2 (ETCO$_2$). If one assumes an ideal lung, the CO_2 tension of the blood leaving the lung should equilibrate with that in the alveoli. Since CO_2 is twenty times as diffusible as oxygen, it is reasonable to assume that the pulmonary venous CO_2 reflects alveolar CO_2. Since the last part of the lung that empties during expiration is the alveolar space, P_{ETCO2} is a reasonable estimate of $PaCO_2$. The fourth phase is the descending part or the down stroke of the capnogram. This is due to fresh gas passing across the sampling site with inspiration.

Technical Details: Capnometers and Capnographs

A Capnometer is a device that provides measures CO_2 concentration of the gas in the airway during breathing. Some capnometers provide only a numerical value of the CO_2 concentration without any graphical display. A portable calorimetric capnometer in use to verify endotracheal or esophageal intubation detects the presence of CO_2 in the exhaled gas by a change in color of a pH sensitive filter paper. The filter paper starts with a purple color and changes to a tan or yellow color in the presence of CO_2. During inspiration, with fresh gas the filter paper will revert back to the purple color. Many intensive care monitors are capable of displaying the capnogram on the screen. There are stand-alone capnometers that have a built-in display of the capnogram. Certain devices can not only display a capnogram but also analyze the respiratory gases to measure CO_2 production as well as physiologic dead space (described later in Volumetric Capnography).

There are two sampling techniques for measurement of CO_2 during breathing – mainstream and side-stream. A mainstream capnometer measures CO_2 directly in the airway or circuit as the exhaled gas passes through.it. A side-stream capnometer

Table 5.1 Differences between Mainstream and Side-stream Capnometers

Features	Mainstream	Sidestream
Location of sensor	At the airway connection	In the machine
Size of connector	Small	Small
Weight	Light + sensor weight	Light + tubing weight
Location of airway connector	Endotracheal tube	Endotracheal tube
Sample Tube	None. Has a cable	Small bore sample tube
Durability	Durable	Varies
Sampling	Airway adapter and sensor	Airway adapter, sample tube, filters, water trap
Airway Connector	Sensor reusable Airway adapter disposable or reusable	Airway adapter disposable or reusable
Use on extubated patients	With a mask or mouthpiece	Nasal prongs

aspirates a small sample of gas from the airway to the measuring device. Another way to think about the difference between these two techniques is that in a mainstream capnometer the sampling site and the measuring sites are the same whereas in a side-stream capnometer the measuring site is distal to the sampling site. The main advantage of the mainstream capnometer is real-time measurement without delay whereas the side-stream capnometer allows for the monitoring of respiratory gases without the additional dead space and weight associated with the more common mainstream adapters. Table 5.1 shows the main advantages and disadvantages of both types of capnometers. The two main techniques of measuring CO_2 concentration are infrared spectroscopy and mass spectroscopy.

In some of the older models, the inspired gas is assumed to contain no CO_2 and therefore the value at baseline is displayed as zero. The CO_2 concentration in the exhaled gas displayed is relative to the baseline and therefore, does not represent the actual ETCO_2. Modern capnographs do not use such assumptions and measures the actual CO_2 concentrations in both inspired and expired gases. The baseline in these capnometers represents the true CO_2 value.

Clinical Applications

ETCO_2 is defined as the peak CO_2 value during expiration and is dependent on adequate pulmonary capillary blood flow. The normal ETCO_2 in healthy subjects is generally < 5 mm Hg lower than the PaCO_2, representing normal total dead space of the respiratory system. An abnormally high baseline during Phase I represents rebreathing of expired carbon dioxide (Fig. 5.5A). This observation will not be seen in capnometers that assume the inspired to contain no CO_2. A slow upstroke during Phase II is due to slow rate of sampling (for example with side-stream analyzers) or uneven emptying of the lung suggesting increased alveolar dead space (Fig. 5.5b).

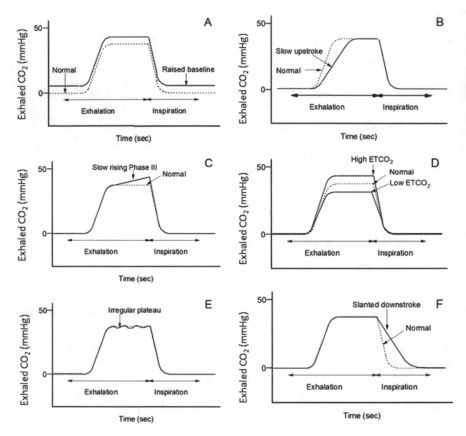

Fig. 5.5 Capnogram waveforms with different conditions. Each phase of the capnogram can be affected by different conditions as shown in the figure and described in the text

A rising Phase III with no plateau is seen with slow emptying of the alveoli, and is usually seen with prolonged exhalation due to lower airway obstruction (Fig. 5.5c). A high $ETCO_2$ indicates an increased metabolic rate or hypoventilation (Fig. 5.5d). An abnormally low plateau indicates hyperventilation, increased alveolar dead space, decreased effective pulmonary blood flow, or contamination with fresh inflow of gas (Fig. 5.5d). An irregular plateau is the result of uneven emptying of the lungs producing fluctuating changes in expired CO_2 concentration (Fig. 5.5e). A slanted down stroke usually indicates rebreathing of exhaled CO_2 (Fig. 5.5f). Normally, arterial-to-end-tidal difference in CO_2 is < 5 mmHg. When alveolar dead space increases, arterial to end tidal difference in CO_2 increases. An increased arterial-to-end tidal CO_2 difference can also be seen with an abnormally low lung perfusion. When end-tidal CO_2 is higher than $PaCO_2$, it usually indicates rebreathing of expired CO_2 or uneven emptying of the lungs.

Practical uses of $ETCO_2$ monitoring in the ICU include:

1. Apnea monitoring
2. ETT ᴨositioning
3. ETT patency
4. Adequacy of alveolar ventilation
5. Diagnosis and management of reversible lower airway obstruction
6. Patient–ventilator system integrity
7. Diagnosis and management of differential lung emptying.

Esophageal intubation is a serious complication of attempted endotracheal intubation and early detection of this inadvertent placement of the ETT using capnography can be life-saving. In addition to its use as a noninvasive measure of $PaCO_2$, $ETCO_2$ is also useful in assessing the efficacy of cardiopulmonary resuscitation. $ETCO_2$ is low with decreased pulmonary blood flow and when cardiac output improves, $ETCO_2$ increases as well. Since lung is the only source of CO_2 elimination, $ETCO_2$ can also be used to detect endotracheal or esophageal intubation. If there is reasonable pulmonary blood flow, a capnometer will detect CO_2 if the tube is endotracheal and will not detect any CO_2 if the tube is esophageal.

Volumetric Capnography

Volumetric capnography provides a measurement of CO_2 production (VCO_2) and enables calculation of alveolar minute ventilation and the ratio of volume of dead space (Vd) to tidal volume (V_T), Vd/V_T ratio. Volumetric capnography is based on the single breath analysis of exhaled CO_2 with superimposition of exhaled volume over the capnogram (Fig. 5.6).

CO_2 concentration is plotted against expired tidal volume. The first part of the capnogram is due to dead space gas and the terminal part is from the alveoli. $ETCO_2$ is the point estimate of CO_2 concentration at the end of exhalation. In volumetric capnography, both the tidal volume and $PaCO_2$ are superimposed. This allows the estimation of the distribution of the tidal volume into airway and alveolar volumes.

Figure 5.7 shows how volumetric capnography can estimate the distribution of the tidal volume into its component values. Panel 1 shows that a vertical line can be drawn on the slope of the capnogram (Phase II) such that two triangles A and B of equal area can be created. The area to the left of the straight line is the anatomic dead space representing the portion of the tidal volume in the airways. The area to the right of the straight line is the portion of the tidal volume filling the alveolar space. Panel 2 shows an area to the right of the straight line that is above the capnogram that has no CO_2 and therefore, represents a portion of the alveolar volume that is not participating in CO_2 elimination. This is referred to as alveolar dead space. Panel 3 shows a shaded area to the left and above the capnogram which is the sum of the anatomic and alveolar dead spaces and is referred to as total dead space. Panel 4 shows a shaded area subtended by the capnogram which is the expired CO_2 volume per breath. Amount of CO_2 exhaled per breath multiplied by

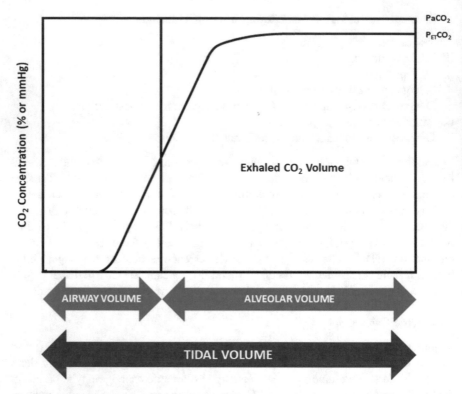

Fig. 5.6 Volumetric capnography. After initial exhalation of airway (dead space) volume, the exhaled CO_2 rises steadily until a plateau is reached when only the alveolar gas is being sampled

the respiratory rate is the amount of CO_2 eliminated in a minute, which in steady state is equal to the CO_2 produced in the tissues per minute.

$ETCO_2$ is assumed to reflect $PaCO_2$ in normal individuals with no lung disease. In clinical circumstances, $ETCO_2$ is often used to titrate mechanical ventilation when arterial blood gases are not available or as a means of reducing the number of blood gas measurements. Normally, $ETCO_2$ is not equal to the $PaCO_2$ but a little lower. The $PaCO_2$-$ETCO_2$ difference with normal lungs and circulation is about 2– 5 mmHg. This is due to the presence of a small amount of alveolar dead space. When alveolar dead space increases, the $PaCO_2$-$ETCO_2$ difference also increases. Alveolar dead space increases in lung segments when its ventilation-perfusion ratio is greater than 1, which means that there is a greater amount of ventilation relative to the perfusion. Conditions where the $PaCO_2$-$ETCO_2$ difference increases are listed in Table 5.2.

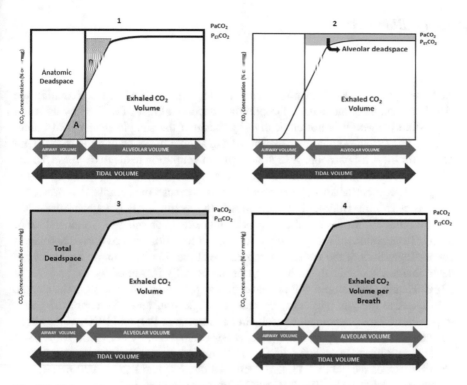

Fig. 5.7 Volumetric capnography depicting the distribution of tidal volume and the measurement of CO_2 per breath. Panel 1 shows the measurement of anatomic dead space; note that areas of A and B are the same. Panel 2 shows alveolar dead space with accounts for the difference between $PaCO_2$ and $P_{ET}CO_2$. Panel 3 shows total dead space which is the sum of the dead spaces measured in Panels 1 and 2. Panel 4 shows the amount of CO_2 exhaled per breath

Table 5.2 Conditions associated with an increased $PaCO_2$-$P_{ET}CO_2$ difference

1. Regional or global hyperinflation
a. Lower airway obstruction
b. High PEEP
c. High mean airway pressures2. Increased V/Q mismatch or increased alveolar dead space
a. ARDS
b. Pulmonary hypertension
c. Pulmonary Embolism3. Decreased pulmonary blood flow
a. Right ventricular failure
b. Cardiac arrest
c. Extreme hypovolemia
d. Decreased effective pulmonary blood flow with single ventricle physiology

5.1.4   *Blood Gases*

An arterial blood sample is useful for determining the effectiveness of the lung as an oxygenator and a ventilator. A venous blood gas is useful in determining the acid–base status of the tissues. A mixed venous blood gas is useful in determining the circulatory status of the patient. Despite the concerns of loss of oxygen by diffusion in plastic syringes, it is not clinically significant if the sample is analyzed immediately. The syringe should be heparinized and should not contain more than 0.1 ml of heparin for 4 ml of blood. A high heparin concentration tends to decrease the pH of the blood sample. Care should be taken not to introduce air bubbles in the sample. The effect of air bubbles would be to decrease the sample PO_2 when the PO_2 is > 150 mmHg, and to increase the sample PO_2 when the PO_2 is < 100 mmHg. Modern analyzers report the results corrected to a temperature of 37 °C. Temperature affects gas solubility, ion dissociation, and oxygen-dissociation curve. Regardless of the patient's temperature at the time the sample for blood gas determination is obtained, the blood gases are actually measured by the analyzer at 37 °C. Heating the sample will increase the gas pressures while cooling the sample will decrease the gas pressures, because of expansion and contraction of gases, respectively. This phenomenon results in an increase in PO_2 and PCO_2 values from what they are in the hypothermic patient. For example, at 37 °C, if the pH is 7.40, the PO_2 is 80 mmHg, and the PCO_2 is 40 mmHg, decreasing the temperature to 35 °C increases the pH to 7.43, and decreases the PO_2 and PCO_2 to 70 mmHg and 37 mmHg, respectively. The lower PCO_2 does not reflect increased alveolar ventilation but effect of temperature on the solubility of CO_2 in blood. For each degree centigrade rise in temperature, there is an increase in PO_2 by 5 torr and PCO_2 by 2 torr, and a decrease in pH by 0.012. A blood gas sample obtained from a hypothermic patient will yield spuriously increased PO_2 and PCO_2 and decreased pH. Similarly, blood gas analysis may yield falsely decreased PO_2 and PCO_2 and increased pH values in a hyperthermic patient. Routinely, blood gas values are not corrected to the patient's temperature but some clinical circumstances such as during cardiac surgery under profound hypothermia, accidental hypothermia, and hyperthermic conditions may warrant such a correction.

5.2   Respiratory Mechanics in Ventilated Patients

Measurements of respiratory mechanics in a relaxed ventilator-dependent patient can be obtained using the technique of rapid airway occlusion during constant flow inflation.

Figure 5.8 shows the pressure–time curve for a constant-flow volume regulated time-cycled breath with an end-inspiratory occlusion maneuver. With an end-inspiratory occlusion maneuver, the inspiratory and expiratory valves in the circuit are closed and the proximal and distal airway pressures equilibrate. The

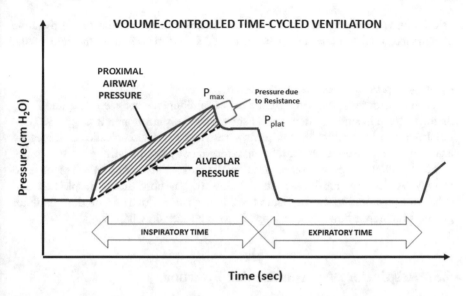

Fig. 5.8 Calculating respiratory mechanics using end-inspiratory occlusion technique. The graph shows the pressure–time tracing with an end-inspiratory occlusion maneuver in volume-controlled time-cycled ventilation. P_{plat} reflects the pressure developed related to compliance and the P_{max}–P_{plat} difference is the pressure related to the total resistance (shaded area)

proximal airway pressure drops from its peak value (P_{max}) to a lower pressure called the plateau or pause pressure (P_{plat}).

As shown in Fig. 5.8, the alveolar pressure rises proportional to the rise in proximal airway pressure. At end-inspiration, the alveolar pressure is lower than P_{max}. With an end-inspiratory occlusion maneuver, the proximal airway pressure equilibrates with the distal alveolar pressure and results in P_{plat}. With normal lungs, where all the alveoli are assumed to have the same mechanics, P_{plat} represents the alveolar pressure throughout the lungs. In the presence of lung or airway disease, P_{plat} represents the weighted average of the alveolar pressures. These pressure values can be used to estimate the dynamic and static compliances, as well as the total resistance of the respiratory system.

Dynamic compliance is measured by dividing the tidal volume by the difference in peak (PIP or Pmax) and baseline pressures (PEEP or total PEEP, which includes auto-PEEP). This includes all the elastic and resistive components of the respiratory system including the ventilator circuit. In order to separate the patient's dynamic compliance from the circuit, the tidal volume and pressures needs to be measured at the hub of the endotracheal tube.

Static compliance is measured by dividing the tidal volume by the pressure difference between the end-inspiratory plateau or pause pressure and baseline pressure (total PEEP, which includes auto-PEEP). Plateau pressure is obtained by airway occlusion which allows for proximal pressure to equilibrate with alveolar pressure in the absence of flow. Thus, the resistive component is removed from the calculation and only the elastic component is determined. Similar to the dynamic compliance, tidal volume and pressures need to be measured at the hub of the endotracheal tube to estimate the patient's total static respiratory system compliance. Chest wall and lung compliances can also be estimated but they require an esophageal pressure measurement.

Total resistance is calculated by the pressure difference between P_{max} and P_{pause} divided by the inspiratory flow and is shown by the shaded area in Fig. 5.8. Total resistance can be partitioned into airflow resistance and viscoelastic resistance by analyzing the pressure decay after inspiratory airway occlusion.

Flow volume-loops are often used to diagnose and monitor the response to therapy. A flow-volume loop plots the flow of gas both during inspiration and exhalation against the corresponding volume change. Analysis of the ventilator graphics including flow-volume loops is covered later in Chap. 9.

5.3   Respiratory Neuromuscular Function

5.3.1   Breathing Pattern

Normal breathing consists of a spontaneous tidal volume of 6–8 mL/kg with a rate that is appropriate for the age with complete thoraco-abdominal synchrony. Abnormal breathing rate consists of apnea, bradypnea (slow for age) and tachypnea (fast for age). Abnormal depth of breathing consists of hypopnea (shallow breathing) and hyperpnea (increased depth of breathing). There are two forms of thoraco-abdominal asynchrony. One is abdominal expansion with a reduction in chest volume during inspiration and the reverse during expiration. This pattern is called see-saw respiration and it is usually due to strong diaphragmatic contraction coupled with a compliant chest wall. The second form of asynchrony is an increase in chest volume with a decrease in abdominal volume during inspiration and the reverse during expiration. This is seen most often with diaphragmatic weakness when inspiration occurs mainly with the action of intercostal muscles. Asynchrony may also be asymmetrical with unilateral diaphragmatic paralysis or paresis. Abnormal breathing pattern may consist of a combination of abnormality in respiratory rate, tidal volume and synchrony.

Rapid shallow breathing is defined as a pattern of breathing where a rapid breathing rate is combined with shallow breaths. This is often seen in patients with pneumonia, pulmonary edema, and ARDS. Rapid breathing may also be associated with normal or increased depth of breathing. Without the presence of lower airway disease, a normal $PaCO_2$ is more indicative of rapid shallow breathing and a low $PaCO_2$ is indicative of hyperventilation. In adults, rapid shallow breathing can be quantified using the following index called the Rapid Shallow Breathing Index (RSBI):

$$RSBI = \frac{RR}{V_T}$$

where, RR is the breathing rate in breaths/min and V_T is tidal volume usually expressed in Liters. A value in the adults greater than approximately 100 is associated with weaning failure. Its utility in infants and children is questionable because the normal absolute values for both breathing rate and tidal volume are different with age and therefore, what is a normal value for an infant may not be a normal value for an older child.

5.3.2 Maximum Inspiratory Airway Pressure

Inspiratory muscle strength can be assessed by measuring maximal inspiratory pressure (MIP) Maximum inspiratory pressure is one of the measurements that is sometimes used to determine suitability to liberate a patient from mechanical ventilation. For example, improvement in a patient who is mechanically ventilated for muscle weakness from Guillain-Barré syndrome may be monitored by daily measurement of MIP. There are several techniques available to measure MIP in intubated patients. The first requirement is that the patient must have spontaneous breathing. In the first method, an expiratory hold is performed. With an expiratory hold, both the inspiratory and expiratory valves are closed and the patient's efforts do not result in any demand flow into the circuit. The inspiratory pressure sensors in the ventilator that are placed distal to the valves measure the pressure generated by the patient. Then, the patient is allowed to be ventilated using the previous settings. In the second method, an occluder is placed between the endotracheal tube and the ventilator circuit with a side port to measure pressure in the endotracheal tube. At end-exhalation, the occluder is closed so that both inspiration and expiration are occluded. In the third technique, an occluder with a one-way valve that allows exhalation but does permit inspiration is placed between the hub of the endotracheal tube and the ventilator circuit. In all methods the occlusions are maintained for 10 breaths or 20 s, whichever comes first. These maneuvers are repeated three times separated by a period that allows stabilization of lung volumes. The most negative value of the three trials is the MIP.

5.3.3 Assessment of Patient Effort

Assessment of effort dependent measures in a non-intubated patient is an important part in determining (a) need for mechanical support and (b) response to therapy. Such an assessment requires patient cooperation and therefore suitable in selected situations. Three simple techniques are readily available at the bedside. These are determination of negative inspiratory pressure (NIP), forced vital capacity (FVC) and peak expiratory flow rate (PEFR).

Maximum negative inspiratory pressure (NIP) that can be generated by a patient is measured by using a digital vacuum manometer attached to a unidirectional expiratory valve and a face mask or a mouth piece. Patients will be able exhale through the valve but inspiration will close the valve and generate a negative pressure. The patient is encouraged to make maximal respiratory efforts. Normal maximum NIP is about -60 to -80 cm H_2O. Indication for intubation is a NIP less negative than -20 cm H_2O. When measuring maximum NIP, care must be taken to eliminate the influence of the action of mouth muscles by using an appropriate mouth-piece so that only the pleural pressure generated by diaphragm and inter-costal muscles is transmitted to the manometer.

Forced vital capacity (FVC) is measured by using a hand-held spirometer that can be attached to a mouth-piece or a face-mask and avoiding any leaks. Patient is encouraged to make a maximal inspiration followed by a maximal exhalation. The exhaled volume from maximal inspiration to exhalation is FVC. Normal FVC is 60–70 mL/kg. FVC less than 15 mL/kg is an indication for mechanical ventilation

Peak expiratory flow rate (PEFR) is very useful to evaluate patients with obstructive lung disease in terms of progression of severity and response to bron-chodilators. The technique is similar to measurement of FVC but instead of a spirometer a hand-held flowmeter is used. The values should be compared to the ones previously observed in the patient or to the age-related normal values.

5.3.4 Esophageal and Gastric Manometry

Esophageal pressure measurements are used in to determine chest wall elastance and calculate lung elastance and transpulmonary pressure (Chap. 1) in mechanically ventilated patients. A dedicated esophageal balloon catheter is then placed in the distal 1/3rd of esophagus to measure tidal variations in esophageal pressure. Instead of a balloon catheter, a fluid-filled catheter may also be used to measure esophageal pressure. Similarly, gastric pressure measurements can be made using a balloon catheter or a fluid-filled catheter. When both esophageal and gastric pressures are measured simultaneously, the difference between the two pressures is called the transdipahragmatic pressure, which is used to measure diaphragmatic strength and endurance in intubated patients, especially during weaning.

Esophageal pressure multiplied by the respiratory rate is called the Pressure Rate Product (PRP). PRP correlates with traditional work of breathing measurements and has been used to evaluate extubation readiness tests such as T-piece breathing, CPAP, and minimal pressure support breathing. Pressure–time index (PTI) or Tension-Time Index of Respiratory Muscles (TT_{mus}) is calculated by using the formula:

$$PTI = \frac{P_{ao}}{P_{max}} \times \frac{T_i}{T_{tot}}$$

where, PTI is the Pressure–Time Index, Pao is the mean pressure of a spontaneous breath, Pmax is the maximal inspiratory pressure, T_i is the inspiratory time of a spontaneous breath and T_{tot} is the total respiratory cycle time of a spontaneous breath. Both the transdiaphragmatic pressure of a spontaneous breath and a maximal inspiratory effort can be substituted in the above equation to yield the Tension-Time Index of the diaphragm (TTI_d). Both the PTI and TTI_d estimate respiratory muscle endurance and low values are often associated with fatigue.

5.3.5 Diaphragmatic Ultrasonography

Point-of-care Ultrasound has become standard of care in intensive care units for a variety of indications such as vascular access, diagnosis of pleural and pericardial effusions, detection of pneumothorax, placement of chest tubes, diagnostic abdominal ultrasound and assessment of trachea and subglottic area. Bedside ultrasound can also be used to assess the diaphragmatic function during spontaneous breathing without any positive pressure for the following:

(1) Whether the diaphragm moves normally and symmetrically
(2) Whether one or both the diaphragms have decreased movement but still move in the normal direction (diaphragmatic paresis or increased intraabdominal pressure)
(3) Whether one or both the diaphragms move paradoxically (diaphragmatic paralysis)
(4) Evaluate the thickness of the diaphragm.

While these are not employed routinely, they are very useful in difficult to ventilate or wean patients to assess the contribution of the diaphragm to the respiratory dysfunction.

Suggested Readings

1. Malley WJ. Clinical blood gases assessment and intervention. 2nd edn. St Louis, Missouri: Elsevier Saunders; 2005.
2. MacIntyre NR, Branson RD. Mechanical ventilation. W.B. Saunders. Philadelphia: Pennsylvania; 2001.
3. der Stayy V, Chatburn RL. Advanced modes of mechanical ventilation and optimal targeting schemes. Intensive Care Med Exp. 2018;6(1):30.

4. Chatburn RL, El-Khatib M, Mireles-Cabodevila E. A taxonomy for mechanical ventilation: 10 fundamental maxims. Respir Care. 2014;59(11):1747–63.
5. Dexter AM, Kimberly C. Ventilator graphics: scalar, loops, and secondary measures. Respir Care. 2020;65(6):739–59.

Chapter 6
Ventilators and Modes

Shekhar T. Venkataraman, Bradley A. Kuch, and Ashok P. Sarnaik

6.1 Basic Concepts and Design

6.1.1 Spontaneous Breathing

Normal breathing is mostly automatic except during activities such as speaking, breath holding, voluntary hyperventilation and voluntary cough. Spontaneous breathing is rhythmic and regulated by neural and chemical mechanisms. The rhythmicity is controlled by neurons in the brainstem which can be modified by higher brain centers, mechanoreceptors in the lungs and upper airways, and chemoreceptors in the brainstem and the carotid body. Arterial oxygen and carbon dioxide tensions and acidity of the blood influence both the rate and depth of the breathing.

A breath is defined as one cycle of flow of gas into the lung (inspiration) and flow of gas out of the lung (exhalation). A breath has 4 phases: (1) breath initiation,

---

S. T. Venkataraman (✉)
Professor, Departments of Critical Care Medicine and Pediatrics, University of Pittsburgh School of Medicine, Pittsburgh, PA, USA
e-mail: venkataramanst@upmc.edu

Medical Director, Respiratory Care Services, Children's Hospital of Pittsburgh, 4401 Penn Avenue, Faculty Pavilion 2117, Pittsburgh, PA 15224, USA

B. A. Kuch
Director, Respiratory Care Services and Transport Team & Clinical Research Associate, Department of Pediatric Critical Care Medicine, UPMC Children's Hospital of Pittsburgh, 4401 Penn Ave, Pittsburgh, PA 15224, USA

A. P. Sarnaik
Professor of Pediatrics, Former Pediatrician in Chief and Interim Chairman Children's Hospital of Michigan, Wayne State University School of Medicine, 3901 Beaubien, Detroit, MI 48201, USA

© Springer Nature Switzerland AG 2022   75
A. P. Sarnaik et al. (eds.), *Mechanical Ventilation in Neonates and Children*,
https://doi.org/10.1007/978-3-030-83738-9_6

(2) inspiratory phase when lungs are inflated, (3) start of exhalation, and (4) expiratory phase when lungs deflate. Trigger is the variable that initiates a breath. Cycling refers to the switch from the end of inspiration to the start of exhalation. For a spontaneous breath, both trigger and cycling are controlled by neural output from the respiratory centers in the brainstem, modified by inputs from mechanoreceptors and chemoreceptors. Neural output stimulates the inspiratory muscles, principally the diaphragm, to contract which causes gas to flow into the lungs. Exhalation is normally passive and starts when the inspiratory neural output is inhibited. The size of the breath is the tidal volume. Inspiratory time is defined as the period from the start of the positive airflow to the start of the negative airflow. Expiratory time is defined as the period from the start of the negative flow to the start of the positive flow. Total cycle time is the sum of inspiratory and expiratory times and is equal to the inverse of breathing frequency. The inspiratory-expiratory (I:E) ratio is defined as the ratio of inspiratory time to expiratory time.

6.1.2   Equation of Motion

In order for gas to flow into and out of the lungs, a pressure gradient has to be generated between the proximal airway and the alveolus, known as the transrespiratory pressure (P_{tr}). During spontaneous breathing, the respiratory muscles create P_{tr} by decreasing the alveolar pressure relative to the proximal airway pressure as a result of negative pressure in the thorax. The pressure generated by the respiratory muscles during spontaneous breathing is expressed as P_{mus} which is a conceptual pressure that cannot be directly measured. Thoracic structures impede lung inflation and therefore, a certain amount of force is required to overcome this impedance. The factors that contribute to this impedance are: (1) Elasticity of the lungs, chest wall, and abdomen, (2) Respiratory system resistance (airflow and tissue resistance) of the lung, chest wall and abdomen), and (3) Inertance of the gas. The equation of motion provides a simple and useful model of the mechanical behavior of the respiratory system which states that P_{tr} required to inflate the lung to a certain volume is equal to the sum of the pressures required to overcome each of the impedance factors. The pressure required to overcome inertance is usually negligible and is ignored. Therefore, P_{tr} required to inflate the lung can then be expressed as a simplified linear equation:

$$P_{tr} = P_{Elasticity} + P_{TotalResistance}$$

or

$$P_{tr} = (Elastance \times Volume) + (Resistance \times Flow)$$

Artificial respiration requires a device to move gas into and out of the lungs. This can be achieved manually or automatically. An example of a manual ventilator is the self-inflating resuscitator bag. Manual compression of the bag causes gas to flow into the lungs by creating a pressure gradient between the bag and patient's lungs. A ventilator, on the other hand, is a device that works automatically to move gas into and out of the lungs. Positive pressure ventilators create P_{tr} by increasing the proximal airway pressure relative to the alveolar pressure. Negative pressure ventilators, conversely, create P_{tr} by decreasing the alveolar pressure relative to the proximal airway pressure. There are three possible ways a P_{tr} may be generated: (1) by the ventilator alone, (2) by a spontaneous breath alone, or (3) a combination of the two. Therefore, the equation of motion can be re-expressed as:

$$P_{tr} = P_{mus} + P_{vent}$$

where P_{vent} is the pressure generated by the ventilator during inspiration and P_{mus} is the theoretical chest wall transmural pressure generated by the inspiratory respiratory muscles that would produce movements identical to those produced by the ventilator. When a ventilator performs all the work of breathing, then $P_{tr} = P_{vent}$. During complete spontaneous breathing $P_{tr} = P_{mus}$. When a spontaneous breath is augmented or supported by a ventilator breath then $P_{tr} = P_{mus} + P_{vent}$. In a sense, a ventilator is a machine that does external work in the form of mechanical breaths and can either replace the patient's work of breathing completely or partially, or augment a patient's breathing efforts.

6.2   Basic Design of a Ventilator

In the pediatric intensive care unit, mechanical ventilation of a patient requires the following components: (1) High pressure gas source, (2) Oxygen blender, (3) Ventilator, and (4) Humidification system. High pressure compressed gas source to power the ventilator can be from tanks, compressors, or wall outlets. Ventilators used in the critical care setting use either compressed gases from the wall outlets or a compressor. Ventilators that use wall outlets have pressure reducing valves internally to modulate the operating pressure of the ventilator. When compressed gas is the input source, the ventilator functions mainly as a controller. The sources for air and oxygen are usually separate so that the inspired concentration of oxygen may be controlled using a blender. The output from the ventilator is a mechanical breath whose size and timing are controlled and determined by pressure and flow waveforms. To achieve this, all ventilators have a control system (pneumatic, electrical or electronic) to regulate the pressure, volume, or flow waveform, a cycling mechanism, and a system to provide end-expiratory pressure.

6.3   Modes of Ventilation

Mode of ventilation is a predetermined pattern of interaction between the patient and the ventilator. It includes the sequence of breaths, breath patterns, control variables within and between breaths, and the schemes used to provide feedback as well as effecting the variables during mechanical ventilation.

6.3.1   Ventilator Breath

Figure 6.1 shows the components of a breath in a pressure-controlled mode. Point 1 is the trigger and initiation of inspiration, 2 is the peak inspiratory flow, 3 is the end of inspiration (cycling), 4 is the peak expiratory flow, 5 is the time taken to fully deflate the lung during expiration, 6 is the end of deflation, and 7 is the expiratory phase before the next inspiration. Inspiratory time = Period between 1 and 3. Expiratory time = Period between 3 and the end of 7. PIP is the peak inspiratory pressure. PEEP is the positive end-expiratory pressure.

A ventilator breath, just like a spontaneous breath, has a trigger to initiate the breath, an inspiratory phase where a tidal volume is delivered, cycling mechanism by which inspiration is terminated, and an expiratory phase initiated. Inspiratory time is defined as the period from the trigger to start inspiration to the point of

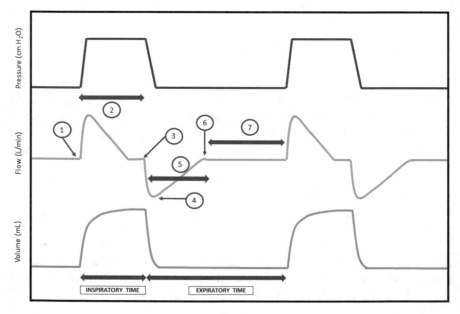

Fig. 6.1 Scalar waveform with pressure, flow and volume over time curves showing different components of a breath for a pressure-controlled time-cycled breath

cycling. Expiratory time is defined as the period from the point of cycling to the trigger for the next mechanical breath. Total cycle time (T_{tot}) is the sum of inspiratory (T_i) and expiratory times (T_e) and is equal to the inverse of breathing frequency. The inspiratory-expiratory (I:E) ratio is defined as the ratio of T_i to T_e. Percent inspiratory time (also called the duty cycle) is defined as the percent of T_{tot} that is spent in inspiration. The tidal volume (V_T) is the integral of flow with respect to time. For constant flow inspiration, this simply reduces to the product of flow and inspiratory time.

6.3.2 Control Variables

During the inspiratory phase of a ventilator breath, pressure, volume, or flow as a function of time may be predetermined. It is important to understand what is meant by the term "control" when it is applied to ventilators and the different modes. Only one variable can be controlled during the inspiratory phase which becomes the independent variable and the other variables vary according to the respiratory system compliance and resistance. Control also refers to the waveform of the variable which is fixed breath to breath. For example, pressure-control refers to the pressure waveform being controlled during inspiration, usually a "square-wave" or rectangular waveform as well as the predetermined pressure limit. With volume control, the shape of the volume waveform as well as the predetermined volume limit is controlled while flow and pressure vary. With flow control, the flow waveform is controlled while volume and pressure vary. The most common flow waveform used in ventilators for pediatric use is rectangular and is referred to as constant-flow inspiration. When constant-flow inspiration is combined with time-cycling, it is identical to volume-control and these terms may be used interchangeably. Time-control is a category of ventilator modes in which the flow, volume and pressure during the set T_i depend on the mechanics of the respiratory system. High frequency oscillatory ventilation (HFOV) and high frequency percussive ventilation are examples of time-controlled ventilation.

6.3.3 Phases of a Breath

All ventilators are equipped with mechanisms to provide four basic functions: (1) initiate lung inflation, (2) inflate the lungs with a tidal volume, (3) terminate lung inflation, and (4) allow the lungs to empty. Trigger is the signal which starts inspiration. Time, pressure, flow, minimum minute ventilation, apnea interval, or electrical signals are used as inspiratory triggers. Cycling refers to the termination of inspiration and the start of exhalation. Time, pressure, volume, flow, and electrical signals are used as cycling signals.

6.3.4 Classification of Breaths

The criteria used to start (trigger) and stop (cycle) inspiration are used to classify breaths. Both triggering and cycling events can be initiated by either the ventilator or the patient. When inspiratory flow starts with a ventilator-generated signal, it is referred to as ventilator-triggering and is independent of a patient-initiated signal. Similarly, when inspiration starts on a patient-generated signal, it is referred to as patient-triggering and is independent of a ventilator-generated signal. The trigger to initiate a breath may be pressure, volume, flow, or time.

Ventilator-cycling refers to ending inspiration based on signals from the ventilator independent of signals based on patient factors. Time-cycling is a common criterion and refers to the time that has elapsed from the start of inspiration and is the same breath-to-breath. Patient cycling occurs when a signal based on the patient's respiratory mechanics, which affects the equation of motion, reaches a threshold value. Similar to the trigger, the variable to cycle a breath from inspiration to exhalation may be pressure, volume, flow, or time.

When the start and end of a breath is determined by the patient, it is referred to as a *spontaneous breath* (Table 6.1). A spontaneous breath is both patient-triggered and patient-cycled. An *unassisted spontaneous breath* refers to a breath where the patient determines both the timing and size of the breath. Normal breathing is an example of unassisted spontaneous breathing. T-piece breathing or breaths during continuous positive airway pressure (CPAP) are also examples of unassisted spontaneous breathing. The size of the breath is determined solely by the effort of the patient with no additional help from the ventilator. An *assisted spontaneous breath* refers to a breath where the ventilator does some of the inspiratory work indicated by an increase in airway pressure above the baseline. For an assisted breath, the patient must initiate a breath, and then the ventilator is triggered to provide a positive pressure breath. With an assisted spontaneous breath, the ventilator contributes to the size of the breath but the patient determines the timing of the breath. Pressure-supported breath is an example of an assisted spontaneous breath. The size of the breath or tidal volume is determined by the effort made by the patient as well as the work done by the ventilator during that breath. A *mandatory breath* is one in which the end of inspiration is determined by the ventilator, independent of the patient. A mandatory breath may be patient-triggered or machine-triggered. The inspiratory time is not under the control of the patient.

Table 6.1 Classification of breaths

Trigger	Inspiratory phase	Cycling	Classification
Patient	Unassisted	Patient	Spontaneous without assist
Patient	Mechanical support	Patient	Spontaneous with assist
Patient	Mechanical support	Ventilator	Mandatory
Ventilator	Mechanical support	Ventilator	Mandatory

The size of the breath is determined either entirely by the ventilator or a combination of the spontaneous effort and the ventilator work.

Trigger

Time-triggered breaths: When a ventilator initiates a breath after a preset time has elapsed from the end of the last exhalation, it is termed as a time-triggered breath. All time-triggered breaths are mandatory breaths. Time to trigger is dependent on the set ventilator rate.

Pressure-triggered breaths: When the ventilator detects a threshold change in pressure from baseline and initiates inspiration, it is termed as pressure triggering. A decrease in circuit pressure is detected by the ventilator pressure sensors and interpreted as a patient effort. While this form of triggering is available in modern ventilators, it has been superseded by flow-triggering.

Flow-triggered breaths: Ventilators that provide flow triggering has a constant bias flow of gas through the circuit during the expiratory phase. When there is no patient effort and with no leaks in the system, there is no difference in the flow across the inspiratory and expiratory flow sensors. Since the difference in flow is zero, no ventilator breath is triggered. Inspiratory effort by the patient or a leak in the system creates a difference in the flow across the inspiratory and expiratory flow sensors. When this difference in flow reaches a preset threshold value, it triggers a breath. This is referred to as flow-triggering.

Trigger Sensitivity

Inspiratory trigger sensitivity refers to the threshold value that needs to be set for patient-initiated breaths and is only applicable to pressure- and flow-triggering since time-triggered breaths are always machine-triggered mandatory breaths. The minimal pressure or flow that needs to be detected in the circuit can be set for any patient-initiated breaths. The actual level of the trigger threshold will depend on the patient's efforts as well as the need to avoid different forms of asynchrony. When the patient is capable of making a strong effort, a higher threshold may be chosen. However, when a patient's inspiratory effort is weak or poor, the threshold should be the lowest that the patient can trigger. A disadvantage of a very low threshold is auto-triggering which is triggering of a breath due to changes in the threshold not created by the patient, such as a leak in the system. A high threshold will increase the trigger work of breathing and may be uncomfortable for the patient. An ideal threshold is one which allows all of the patient's efforts to be triggered without any discomfort or patient-ventilator asynchrony. In most ventilators, the threshold value is the actual value of the trigger such as cm of H_2O for pressure- and L/min for flow-triggering. In some ventilators, the range of threshold values does not represent the actual values, but only degrees of change.

During inspiration, based on the control variable, a preset value is reached before the end of inspiration. Inspiration is pressure-targeted, volume-targeted, or flow-targeted depending on whether a preset value for pressure, volume, or flow is reached before inspiration ends. Cycling may occur due to attainment of preset pressure, volume, flow or time. The criteria for determining the phase variables during a mechanical breath are shown in Fig. 6.2. The above-mentioned description allows one to describe a breath based on the control variable, trigger, targeted variable during inspiration and the cycling mechanism.

6.3.5 Breath Sequences

A breath sequence can be defined as a set of breaths producing minute ventilation. All the breaths delivered by the ventilator may be mandatory or spontaneous or a combination of both. As described above, the spontaneous breaths may or may not be assisted/supported. Therefore, the 3 basic breath sequences that a ventilator delivers are as follows: (1) Continuous Mandatory Ventilation, (CMV), (2) Intermittent Mandatory Ventilation (IMV), and (3) Continuous Spontaneous Ventilation (CSV). CMV refers to a breath sequence when all the breaths are mandatory (Fig. 6.3). During CMV, spontaneous breaths do not occur between mandatory breaths.

Assist-Control refers to a mode of ventilation when a patient can receive either a ventilator-initiated   or   patient-initiated   mandatory   breath   (Fig. 6.4). Machine-triggered   breaths   are   not   preceded   by   a   spontaneous   breath. Patient-triggered breaths are preceded by a spontaneous breath which creates a negative deflection in the pressure–time curve (denoted by the arrows in the Fig. 6.4). While the breaths have different triggers, all the breaths shown are machine-cycled. This breath sequence is also called Assist-Control. In assist-control (AC) mode, every patient breath is triggered by pressure or flow generated by the patient inspiratory effort and "assisted" with either preselected inspiratory pressure or volume. When the patient does not make any effort of breathing such as with neuromuscular blockade, the total number of breaths is equal to the set rate.

Figure 6.4 shows three examples of the total number of breaths in the Assist-Control mode. In this example, the control rate (back-up rate) is set at 24 breaths per minute. When the patient makes no effort, the total number of breaths is 24 breaths/min. When the patient breathes at a frequency of 16 breaths/min, which is less than the set back-up rate, the ventilator will assist all the patient's breaths, and the patient will receive 8 additional machine-triggered breaths/min (Fig. 6.4). When the patient breathes at a frequency of 32 breaths/min, which is higher than the set back-up rate, all the breaths are patient-triggered mandatory breaths. Although useful in some patients, the AC mode cannot be used in the weaning process, which involves gradual decrease in ventilator support.

CSV refers to a breath sequence when all the breaths are spontaneous. During CSV, spontaneous breaths may or may not be supported with positive pressure. Three examples of CSV are shown in Fig. 6.5. Figure 6.5a shows normal continuous spontaneous breathing without any positive pressure support. During inspiration and exhalation, the airway pressures are around atmospheric (0 cm). Figure 6.5b shows CSV with CPAP. During inspiration and exhalation, the airway pressures fluctuate around the CPAP level. No ventilatory assistance is provided.

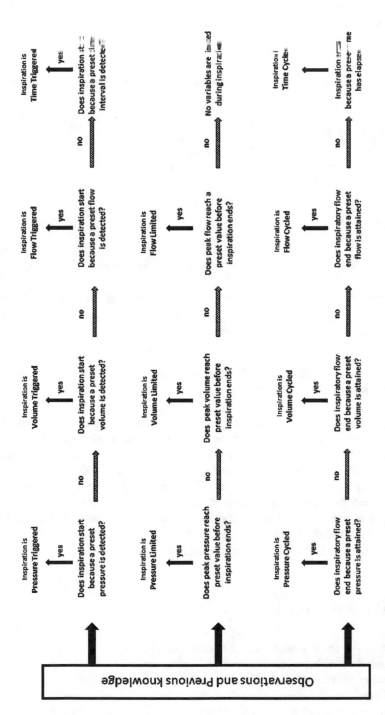

Fig. 6.2 Criteria for determining the phase variables during a ventilator-assisted breath (Reproduced from Chatburn RL: Classification of mechanical ventilators, respiratory care equipment, Philadelphia, 1995, JB Lippincott)

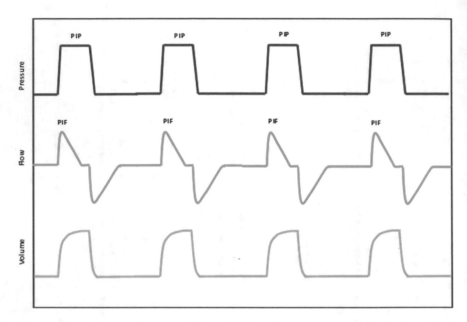

Fig. 6.3 Continuous mandatory ventilation (CMV) with pressure-control ventilation. All the breaths are machine-triggered and machine-cycled

Figure 6.5c shows pressure-support ventilation which is defined as CSV with a positive pressure mechanical assistance with every breath above a baseline level of PEEP.

IMV refers to a breath sequence when spontaneous breaths occur between mandatory breaths. These breaths may or may not be synchronized. When IMV is synchronized to the patient's inspiratory efforts, it is referred to as synchronized IMV (SIMV) (Fig. 6.6). With SIMV, at set intervals, the ventilator's timing circuit becomes activated and a timing "window" appears (shaded area) just before the next mandatory breath is to be delivered. If the patient initiates a breath in the timing window, then the ventilator will deliver a mandatory breath synchronized to the spontaneous breath. If no spontaneous effort occurs, then the ventilator will deliver a mandatory breath at the end of the timing window.

6.3.6 Ventilatory Pattern

A ventilatory pattern is a sequence of breaths (CMV, IMV, or CSV) with a designated control variable (volume control (VC), pressure control (PC) or dual-control (DC). Dual-control modes of ventilation are auto-regulated pressure-controlled modes of mechanical ventilation with a user-selected tidal volume target. Dual control modes use both the pressure and volume signal to control the breath size.

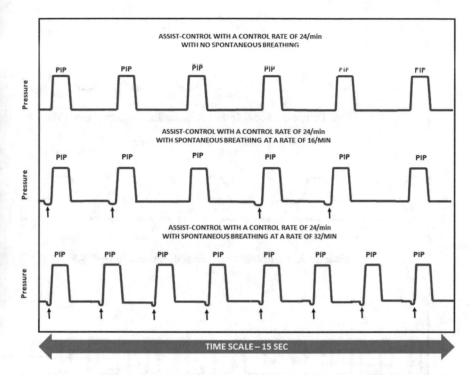

Fig. 6.4 Assist-Control continuous mandatory entilation with pressure-control ventilation. Spontaneous breaths appear as negative deflections in the pressure–time waveform (black arrows)

Out of the 9 theoretical combinations based on 3 breath sequences and 3 control variables, only 8 are operational. These are VC-CMV, PC-CMV, VC-IMV, PC-IMV, PC-CSV, DC-CMV, DC-IMV and DC-CSV. VC-CSV is theoretically not possible because, by definition, all volume-controlled breaths are machine-cycled and therefore, mandatory breaths. These 8 ventilatory patterns are available in most modern ventilators (Table 6.2). Only one ventilatory pattern can be present in a mode of ventilation. Ventilatory patterns can be used as a mode classification system.

6.3.7 Targeting Schemes

The targeting scheme is best defined as the method of feedback control used to deliver a particular pattern of ventilation. There are several types of such feedback control mechanisms. A target can be defined as a predetermined goal of the ventilator output.

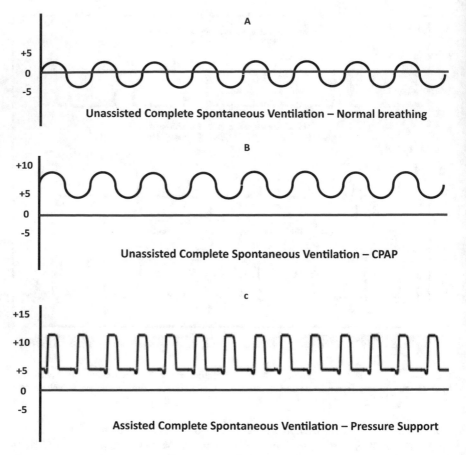

Fig. 6.5 Continuous spontaneous ventilation (CSV). **a** Normal breathing. **b** Spontaneous ventilation with CPAP. **c** Pressure support ventilation with PEEP

Set point: An example of this is Pressure-Control ventilation where a predetermined Pressure Limit is set during inspiration. The ventilator's pressure sensors will provide feedback to a flow regulator which adjusts the flow rate to maintain the set pressure limit. When there is a leak in the system and the pressure limit does not reach its set value, flow will increase to help achieve the set pressure limit.

Dual targeting: An example of this is Volume-Assured Pressure Support. The breath starts with pressure support at a preset pressure limit and when the ventilator senses that the targeted volume will not be delivered within that breath, the ventilator switches to volume control and increases the flow for the remaining portion of the inspiratory time to achieve the volume target.

Servo control: Examples of this are NAVA, Automatic Tube Compensation (ATC) and Proportional Assist Ventilation. In NAVA, for example, the level of

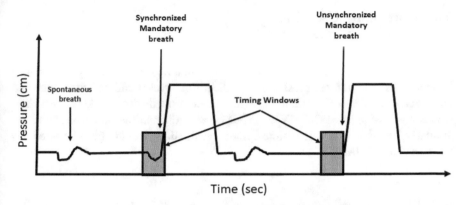

Fig. 6.6 Synchronized intermittent mandatory ventilation (SIMV). Shaded rectangles indicate timing windows with examples of synchronized and unsynchronized mandatory breaths

Table 6.2 Ventilatory patterns by breath control variable and accepted acronym

Breath control variable	Breath sequence	Acronym	Example
Volume	Continuous mandatory ventilation	VC-CMV	Volume-controlled time-cycled ventilation
	Intermittent mandatory ventilation	VC-IMV	SIMV-Volume-control
Pressure	Continuous mandatory ventilation	PC-CMV	Pressure-controlled time-cycled ventilation
	Intermittent mandatory ventilation	PC-IMV	SIMV-pressure-control
	Continuous spontaneous ventilation	PC-CSV	Pressure-support
Dual-Control	Continuous mandatory ventilation	DC-CMV	Pressure-regulated volume control (PRVC)
	Intermittent mandatory ventilation	DC-IMV	SIMV-PRVC
	Continuous spontaneous ventilation	DC-CSV	Volume-support

ventilator support is proportional to the magnitude of the electrical activity of the diaphragm (Edi). A patient's signal is used as servo control to determine the level of support from the ventilator.

Adaptive targeting: This specifically refers to a control system that will adapt the output to changing respiratory conditions using a feedback mechanism. A good example is the pressure regulated volume control (PRVC) mode. The inspiratory pressure is automatically adjusted to achieve an average tidal volume target, and this varies from breath to breath—adapting to the changing compliance.

6.4   Commonly Used Modes

The following is a description of some of the most common modes used in infants and children in more detail. The two most common forms of mandatory modes used in infants and children are pressure-controlled, time-cycled and volume-controlled time-cycled modes of ventilation. Pressure-controlled time-cycled ventilation would be classified as PC-CMV or PC-IMV according to the modern taxonomy. Similarly, volume-controlled time-cycled ventilation would be classified as VC-CMV or VC-IMV.

6.4.1   Volume-Controlled Mandatory Breaths

Volume-controlled ventilation (VCV) can be delivered either by volume-cycled breath, where inspiration is terminated after a preset volume is delivered or by volume-controlled time-cycled breaths, where the cycling mechanism is preset time, and the tidal volume delivered is regulated by adjusting the inspiratory flow rate. The flow waveforms in VCV can be rectangular, decelerating, accelerating and sinusoidal but the tidal volume is delivered throughout inspiration. The peak inspiratory pressure (PIP) is variable and depends on the flow rate, the total resistance, and the total compliance of the ventilator circuit and the patient's lungs. Changes in resistance or compliance will be reflected by a change in PIP, and the ventilator can be set to alarm at a pressure limit that is generally set 5 to 10 cm above the PIP.

The tidal volume delivered by the ventilator is distributed between the ventilator circuit, the airways, and the patient's lungs. The compliances and resistances of the ventilator circuit, the endotracheal or tracheostomy tube, and the patient independently and together affect the distribution of tidal volume delivered by the ventilator. A decrease in the compliance or an increase in the resistance of the ventilator circuit will affect the actual tidal volume delivered to the patient. While most modern ventilators deliver the preset tidal volumes reliably, the tidal volumes delivered to the patient on a breath-to-breath basis may not always be constant. The ventilator circuit includes an internal volume and the external tubing. The actual tidal volume or the effective tidal volume (V_{Teff}) delivered to the patient can be approximated by the following formula:

$$V_{Teff} = V_{Tdel} - V_{Tcircuit}$$

where, V_{Tdel} is tidal volume delivered by the ventilator and $V_{Tcircuit}$ is the volume of gas that is distributed to the ventilator circuit. V_{Tdel} is equal to the inspired tidal volume, when there is no leak in the total respiratory system. When there is a leak in the system, however, such as with the use of uncuffed endotracheal tubes, then

V_{Tdel} is less than the inspired tidal volume. $V_{Tcircuit}$ can be estimated by the following formula:

$$V_{Tcircuit} = C_{vent} \times (PIP - PEEP),$$

where, C_{vent} is the compliance of the ventilator circuit, PIP is the peak inspiratory pressure reached in the circuit during inspiration and PEEP is the level of positive end-expiratory pressure.

During exhalation, expiratory flow curves depend on the type of expiratory resistance or PEEP valve in the system. Changes in pressure, flow, and volume curves in response to changes in compliance and resistance are discussed in the chapter on ventilator graphics (Chap. 9).

6.4.2 Pressure-Controlled Mandatory Breaths

Pressure-controlled, time-cycled ventilation is widely used in infants and children with lung disease. In this mode, inspiratory flow is high at the start of inspiration and the inspiratory pressure rises quickly (Fig. 6.1). In older ventilators, there was a provision to control the inspiratory flow which was usually set at 4–10 L/kg/min. In modern ventilators, the rate of increase in pressure in the early phase of inspiration is controlled by the inspiratory "rise time", which can be adjusted to make the inspiratory pressure rise quickly or slowly. Once the inspiratory pressure reaches the preset limit, the inspiratory valve closes. If the pressure limit were to drift, such as with an endotracheal tube leak, the ventilator will open the inspiratory valve and sufficient flow is allowed to enter the circuit to maintain the pressure limit. During the inspiratory phase with pressure-controlled time-cycled ventilation, the expiratory valve remains closed until the inspiratory time is completed. When the inspiratory time is completed, the expiratory phase begins and the pressure decreases to the baseline positive end-expiratory pressure (PEEP). The tidal volume delivered depends on the compliance and resistance of the respiratory system and the pressure difference between the pressure-limit and PEEP. The inspiratory flow into the lung is a decelerating waveform (high at first and then declining) (Fig. 6.1). When inspiratory time is set to at least 5 times the time-constant of the respiratory system, inflation will be complete and the inspiratory flow will reach zero flow before the end of inspiration. If the inspiratory time is shorter, there will not be full inflation and the inspiratory flow will not reach zero flow when exhalation begins.

6.4.3 Pressure-Regulated Volume Control

Dual-control breath-to-breath mode with mandatory pressure-controlled, time-cycled breath is referred to as pressure-regulated volume control (PRVC) (with Maquet Servo series), adaptive pressure ventilation (APV) (with Hamilton Galileo), autoflow (Evita 4), or variable pressure control (Venturi), depending on the manufacturer. In this form of pressure-regulated, time-cycled ventilation, delivered tidal volume is used as a feedback control for continuously adjusting the pressure limit. All breaths in these modes are time or patient triggered, pressure controlled, and time cycled mandatory breaths.

How it works:

1. First, set the target tidal volume, ventilator rate, inspiratory time, PEEP, FiO_2, trigger sensitivity, and the inspiratory rise time for PRVC
2. Ventilator delivers a volume-controlled time-cycled breath with a 10% inspiratory pause to measure the plateau pressure (P_{plat}).
3. The next breath is a pressure-controlled breath with preset pressure limit or peak inspiratory pressure (PIP) equal to the P_{plat} measured previously.
4. The delivered tidal volume is then measured.
5. If the delivered tidal volume is equal to the set tidal volume, then PRVC is continued with no change in PIP
6. If the delivered tidal volume is less than the set tidal volume, then PIP is increased. The ventilator compares the delivered tidal volume to the set tidal volume and adjusts the PIP until both volumes are equal.
7. If the delivered tidal volume is more than the set tidal volume, then PIP is reduced until the set tidal volume and delivered tidal volume are equal.
8. If there are changes in lung mechanics that affect the delivered tidal volume, adjustments as described above continued automatically to ensure that the set tidal volume is consistently delivered.
9. PIP can only be increased up to 5 cm H_2O below the pressure alarm limit set, at which point it will alarm because the delivered tidal volume will be less than the set tidal volume.
10. There is no lower limit for the reduction in the pressure-limit level. This mode of ventilation appears to be most beneficial when there are rapid changes in lung compliance such as after surfactant administration.

6.4.4 Selection of Parameters for Mandatory Breaths

The following are the parameters of mandatory breaths that are commonly set and titrated: (1) tidal volume or inspiratory pressure limit, (2) ventilator rate, (3) fraction of inspired oxygen (FiO_2), (4) PEEP, (5) inspiratory time and (6) inspiratory rise time. A desirable V_{Teff} for most patients is 6–8 ml/kg. Higher V_T may be required in obstructive lung disease when slower respiratory rates are beneficial. The end-inspiratory alveolar pressure (P_{plat}), measured using an inspiratory hold maneuver should be preferably less than 30 cm H_2O.

Inspiratory rise time refers to the rate at which the ventilator raises the inspiratory pressure (in pressure targeted modes) and flow (in volume targeted flow). It is set as a percent of breath cycle time usually from 0 to 20% or absolute time of 0–0.4 s. The default setting is 5% or 0.15 s. A rapid raise time will achieve the set target (pressure or flow) almost instantaneously while a slower rise time will reach that target more gradually. Very fast rise time may be somewhat uncomfortable for a spontaneously breathing patient and result in turbulence whereas excessively slow rise time may cause "flow starvation" and increased work of breathing.

The initial ventilator rate selected depends on the age of the patient and the ventilatory requirements of the patient. The inspiratory time is selected to provide an inspiratory-to-expiratory time (I:E) ratio of at least 1:2 in most patients. Inspiratory time must be selected to allow sufficient time for all lung segments to be inflated. Adjustments to the inspiratory time may be necessary in certain disease conditions. Similarly, sufficient expiratory time must be provided for all lung segments to empty. If inspiration starts before the lung has completely emptied, this will result in air-trapping and inadvertent positive end-expiratory pressure (Auto-PEEP).

FiO_2 and PEEP are adjusted to maintain an adequate PaO_2. High concentrations of oxygen can produce lung injury and should be avoided. FiO_2 less than 0.5 is generally considered safe. In patients with parenchymal lung disease with significant intrapulmonary shunting, the major determinant of oxygenation is lung volume, which is improved with PEEP.

The optimum level PEEP is the level at which lung compliance is the best with improvement in oxygenation and ventilation without significant hemodynamic side effects.

6.4.5 Pressure-Support Ventilation

A Pressure-Supported breath is one which is patient-triggered, pressure-controlled, and flow-cycled (Fig. 6.7). It is an assisted, spontaneous breath in which the ventilator assists the patient's own spontaneous effort with a mechanical breath with a preset pressure limit. A pressure support breath is triggered either by a negative pressure below PEEP (pressure-triggering) or by a change in flow through the circuit (flow-triggering). The machine delivers high inspiratory flow with a short inspiratory rise time to achieve a peak airway pressure level (pressure support limit) that is selected by the operator and maintains the pressure limit until the inspiratory flow rate decreases to a threshold value (commonly 25 or 30% of the peak inspiratory flow) that can be set in many ventilators. In summary, PSV is patient triggered, pressure controlled, and flow cycled. PSV is entirely dependent on the

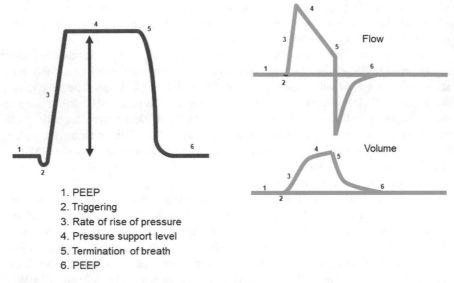

1. PEEP
2. Triggering
3. Rate of rise of pressure
4. Pressure support level
5. Termination of breath
6. PEEP

Fig. 6.7 Components of a pressure-supported breath

patient's effort; if the patient becomes apneic, the ventilator will not provide any mechanical breath. Therefore, PSV is combined with either VC or PC during IMV.

Point 2 is the patient's effort indicated by a negative deflection. Upon sensing this this trigger (change in pressure or flow), the ventilator delivers flow to reach the desired pressure-support level (Point 4) as rapidly as possible. The rate of rise of this pressure can be controlled by adjusting the rise time (Point 3). Ventilator-delivered flow is then servo-adjusted to patient demand to maintain this pressure plateau. During inspiration, the inspiratory flow is maximum at the beginning of the breath and decreases as the lung is inflated and the distal pressures increase. Inspiration is terminated when the flow reaches a pre-set percentage of the peak inspiratory flow (usually 25–30%) (Point 5). Exhalation is passive and returns to the baseline PEEP (Point 6).

6.4.6   Volume Support Ventilation

Volume support is a dual-control continuous spontaneous ventilatory mode (DC-CSV). Spontaneous breaths are supported by pressure support with a targeted volume that is set on the ventilator. The pressure support level required to maintain the set tidal volume is adjusted when the delivered tidal volume differs from the set tidal volume. This is a form of closed loop control using tidal volume as the feedback variable for continuously adjusting the pressure support level. This adjustment of the pressure support level is similar to the adjustment of PIP with

PRVC, which is a mandatory mode of ventilation. With Volume Support, it is also important to set minimum minute ventilation that the patient should receive. The minimum ventilation is set for the ventilator to be a backup PRVC mandatory mode with the set tidal volume and a set ventilator rate with its own inspiratory and expiratory times. As long as the minute ventilation, as determined by the preset target tidal volume and the patient's breathing rate, is higher than the preset minute ventilation, the patient will receive volume-support ventilation. When the minute ventilation is less than the pre-set value, initially the targeted tidal volume will be increased above the preset limit up to a limit. Once that limit is reached, the ventilator will switch to PRVC mode with a mandatory rate (preset) and the preset tidal volume.

6.5 Other Modes

6.5.1 Neurally Adjusted Ventilatory Assist (NAVA)

Neurally Adjusted Ventilatory Assist (NAVA) is a Pressure-Supported Breath where the trigger for initiation of inspiration is the electromyographic activity of the diaphragm (Edi) monitored by a specifically designed catheter. The Edi signal is used to trigger the breath, to determine the level of pressure support, and to cycle from inspiration to exhalation. The pressure support level provided is proportional to the integral of the Edi. For NAVA to work the phrenic nerve needs to be intact and functioning and the primary inspiratory muscle should be the diaphragm. NAVA is designed to improve patient-ventilator synchrony. By allowing better patient-ventilator synchrony, it may be possible to reduce the amount of sedation that needs to be used in these children. The prerequisites and contraindications are presented in Table 6.3 and must be considered prior to initiating NAVA support.

Table 6.3 NAVA prerequisites and contraindications

Prerequisites/Indications	Contraindications
Spontaneously respiration	Insufficient/absent respiratory effort
Intact phrenic nerve	Bilateral diaphragm paralysis secondary to phrenic nerve damage
Anticipation of requiring ventilatory support >48 h	Any contraindications for having an orogastric or a nasogastric tube or need for MRI
Difficult to wean patients	Congenital myopathy
Patients that have ventilator asynchrony problems unless sedated and/or paralyzed	Esophageal atresia or diaphragmatic hernia
Past failed extubations	
Requiring BiPAP support	

The Edi catheter consists of electrical connector, gastric suction port with evacuation holes at the distal end, and an array of 10 electrodes that capture the diaphragmatic signal (Fig. 6.8). The electrodes are arranged in pairs so that they can capture the electrical signals from both hemidiaphragms. The measured Edi signal also provides continuous monitoring of respiratory drive while determining the level of support indicated by the strength of the diaphragm's excitation.

The Edi catheter can be easily placed nasally or orally with the correct size determined by patient size. The ventilator has an Edi catheter position screen to assist with proper placement using QRS waveforms. Proper catheter placement is evaluated and confirmed by the following:

1. As the catheter moves from above the diaphragm to below, QRS waveforms will dampen
2. As the catheter is advanced, the QRS will turn "Blue/Purple", indicating that the electrical sensors are close to the diaphragm.
3. Optimal placement will be shown by the middle 2 waveforms being "Blue/Purple (Fig. 6.9c)".
4. The size of the QRS complexes is largest at the top (proximal) waveform (Fig. 6.9a) since that electrode is closest to the heart. The QRS complexes decrease in size as we go from the top waveform to the bottom (Fig. 6.9b).
5. Correct placement of the Edi catheter is additionally confirmed using a radiograph (Fig. 6.10).

Once in good position, the pressure support level that will result in a desired tidal volume or chest expansion needs to be set. It is set using the equation:

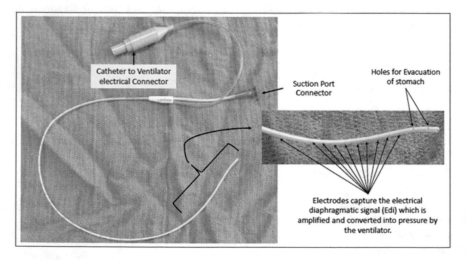

Fig. 6.8 Anatomy of the Edi catheter consisting of a catheter connector, suction port, and electrode array

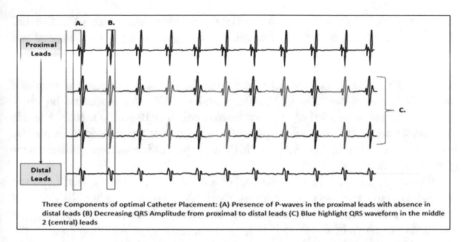

Three Components of optimal Catheter Placement: (A) Presence of P-waves in the proximal leads with absence in distal leads (B) Decreasing QRS Amplitude from proximal to distal leads (C) Blue highlight QRS waveform in the middle 2 (central) leads

Fig. 6.9 QRS waveforms demonstrating correct Edi Catheter placement. Size decrease from the Proximal leads to the distal leads with the smallest QRS in the last lead. Most distal lead has absent P-waves. Middle 2 leads have either Blue or purple waves indicating ideal catheter placement

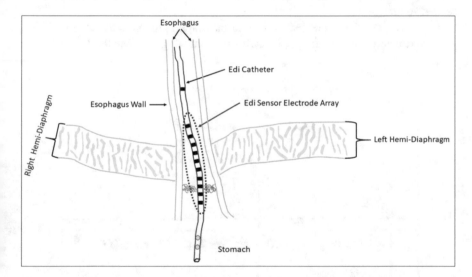

Fig. 6.10 Illustration demonstrating correct Edi catheter placement via the distal esophagus. The Electrode array is positioned between the left and right hemi diaphragm with distal end located in the stomach

$$Pressure\ Support\ Level = NAVA\ level x Edi(Peak - Min)$$

where Edi is the strength of the electrical signal in microvolts (μV) and NAVA is the pressure support per μV of Edi. The Edi_{peak} represents the maximal electrical activity of the diaphragm for a particular breath (in μV). The Edi_{min} represents the electrical activity of the diaphragm between inspiratory efforts (in μV). The Edi signal is monitored > 60 times per second the Edi_{peak} and Edi_{min} are measured at a set interval. The pressure support level provided by the ventilator is set by the NAVA level (set on the ventilator) multiplied by the difference in Edi signals between Edi_{peak} and Edi_{min} (ΔEdi) as shown in the equation above. For example, if the NAVA level is set to 0.5 μV/cmH$_2$O and the ΔEdi for a specific breath is 20 μV, the maximum level of support for that breath is 10 cmH$_2$O. NAVA levels are usually set in the range of 0.5–4 cmH$_2$O/μV. Scalar representation of NAVA support is illustrated in Fig. 6.11. With increase in ΔEdi, additional pressure support is provided.

Normal Edi_{peak} is 10–15 μV. The goal of NAVA is to provide enough support to normalize diaphragm work by adjusting the NAVA level. A higher NAVA level provides more support while decreasing the NAVA level reduces support. An illustrative example of this is a) if Edi_{peak} is consistently above normal range, the patient is working too hard or the ventilator is not providing enough support. In such a case NAVA level should be increased until Edi Peak returns to the normal range. If Edi_{peak} is consistently below the goal, the patient is receiving too much support, and the NAVA level should be decreased until the Edi Peak returns to the desired range.

The Edi_{min} represents the resting tone of the diaphragm. Normal range for Edi_{min} is approximately 2–4 μV. Edi_{min} is useful in evaluating whether the PEEP level is

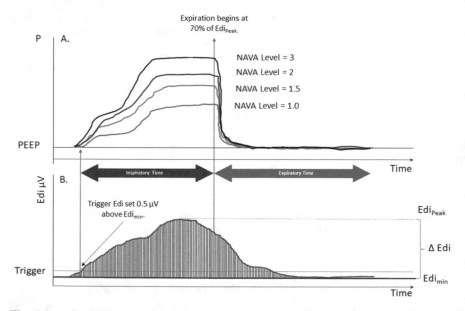

Fig. 6.11 a Pressure over Time illustrating the Pressure wave form increasing with set NAVA Level. **b** Edi Measure over time—Blue line represents individual Edi Measurement associated with pressure support level provided. Green line indicates NAVA trigger level. Red Line is the measured Edi Min

Table 6.4 Effects of PEEP

Beneficial effects
1. Recruitment of collapsed alveoli
a. Improve lung compliance
b. Decrease total dead space
c. Decrease venous admixture
d. Decrease pulmonary vascular resistance (by improving functional residual capacity)
2. Prevention of airway collapse by decreasing the closing capacity
3. Maintaining stability of alveolar segments
a. Shift alveolar fluid into the interstitium (pulmonary edema)
b. Prevent crumpling of alveolar walls
4. Reduce work of breathing
5. Stent the airways open (bronchomalacia)
6. Decrease left ventricular afterload (heart failure)
Adverse effects
1. Over-distention of alveoli
a. Increase total dead space
b. Decrease lung compliance
c. Increase pulmonary vascular resistance
d. Increase venous admixture (with heterogenous lung disease)
2. Air-leaks
a. Alveolar rupture
b. Alveolar rupture
3. Decrease venous return

adequate. For example, if the Edi min is consistently above the desired range, the resting diaphragmatic tone is too high and may signify an attempt by the patient to maintain end-expiratory lung volume. Increasing PEEP, by increasing the end-expiratory lung volume, might decrease the need for the diaphragm to maintain a high tone. Conversely, if the Edi_{min} is consistently below the desired range, the resting tone of the diaphragm is too low and weaning the PEEP should be considered (Table 6.4).

Both Edi_{peak} and Edi_{min} will vary with patient activity. Any clinical situation resulting in an increased work of breathing will increase the Edi_{peak}. The clinician should evaluate whether the episode is a result of discomfort (short-term) or clinical decompensation (long-term, with sustained change in vital signs). If the increase in Edi_{peak} is sustained, the NAVA level should be increased for additional support. Finally, the patient should be challenged daily to facilitate liberation from the ventilator. Challenging the patient will help identify opportunities for ventilator weaning. Once the patient is stable on a NAVA level of 1, extubation may be considered. Non-invasive NAVA (NIV-NAVA) is a mode that can be used for post-extubation support. However, the greatest barrier to NIV-NAVA is finding an interface device that is well tolerated. NIV-NAVA works well with large leaks as the trigging mechanism is the EMG of the diaphragm.

6.5.2 Airway Pressure Release Ventilation

Airway pressure release ventilation (APRV) is a method of mechanical ventilation introduced by Stock and Downs. The original circuit included a CPAP device with unrestricted gas flow allowing spontaneous breathing, and a mechanism to release airway pressure periodically to some desired low pressure. A level of CPAP is provided to keep the lungs open while spontaneous breathing is responsible for maintaining adequate ventilation (Fig. 6.12).

In modern ventilators that provide APRV, there are 4 major variables that determine an APRV breath. These are P_{high}, P_{low}, T_{high}, and T_{low}. P_{high} is defined as the pressure limit of the triggered mandatory breath and T_{high} is the duration that P_{high} is maintained. P_{low} is the release pressure and T_{low} is the time of the pressure release (Fig. 6.8). The top panel of Fig. 6.8 shows the ventilator settings with no spontaneous breathing. With no spontaneous breathing, this mode of ventilation is Pressure-Control CMV with inversed I:E ratio. The bottom panel of Fig. 6.8 shows the same ventilator settings but with spontaneous breathing occurring both during P_{high} and during P_{low}. The mandatory breaths applied by APRV are time-triggered, pressure-targeted, time-cycled breaths. The advantage of APRV in parenchymal lung disease is lung recruitment and improvement in gas exchange with much lower peak alveolar pressures.

APRV is currently seldom used as a primary mode of ventilation when the patient is intubated and initially placed on mechanical ventilation. It is often used after a period of conventional mechanical ventilation. The initial level of P_{high} can be one to provide a mean airway pressure 3–6 cm of H_2O above the conventional ventilation. Subsequent adjustments can be made based on level of chest expansion (visually as well as on a chest radiograph) and by gas exchange parameters. There are two methods to set the P_{low} value. One method is a fixed value similar to PEEP. The second method is to set the P_{low} to be zero; this is usually combined with

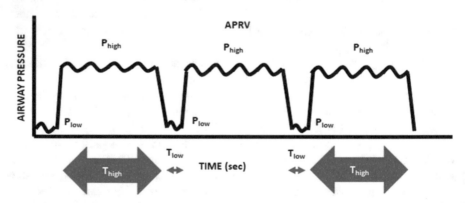

Fig. 6.12 Airway Pressure Release Ventilation. P_{high} is the pressure limit of the ventilator breath, P_{low} is the release pressure, T_{high} is the duration that P_{high} is maintained and T_{low} is the duration of P_{low}. Note that spontaneous breaths (waveform) occur both during P_{high} and P_{low}

setting the T_{low} to terminate when the expiratory flow rate decreases to a predetermined value, usually 30% of the peak expiratory flow. When T_{low} terminates
before the expiratory flow reaches zero flow, pressure in the alveoli is positive and
prevents de-recruitment. This is similar to the auto-PEEP concept with lower airway
obstruction. The degree of ventilatory assistance provided by APRV will be
determined by the difference between P_{high} and the pressure in the lungs at the end
of T_{low}, frequency of pressure release, the duration of pressure release, the patient's
lung-thorax compliance, and flow resistance in the patient's airways. With APRV,
minute ventilation occurs with both spontaneous breaths and the periodic inflation
and deflation that occur with the two levels of airway pressure. Gas exchange can
occur throughout the respiratory cycle. Inspiratory demand flow during spontaneous breathing.

Only 2 parameters are usually used to wean patients from APRV. One is P_{high}
and the other is the ratio between T_{high} and T_{low}. Decreasing P_{high} will decrease the
tidal volume and mean airway pressure and is akin to weaning CPAP. Increasing
the ratio between T_{high} and T_{low} decreases the frequency of pressure release and the
minute ventilation provided by the ventilator. Patients can be either switched to
conventional ventilation or by simply lowering P_{high} to CPAP breathing.

6.6 High Frequency Ventilation

6.6.1 Definitions and Description

High-frequency ventilation (HFV) refers to diverse modes of ventilation characterized in general by supra-physiologic ventilatory frequencies (>60/min) and low
tidal volumes. Commonly used high frequency modes described below are high
frequency oscillatory ventilation (HFOV) and high frequency jet ventilation (HFJV)
(Table 6.5).

The exact mechanism of gas transport in HFV is not fully elucidated. It is
possible that each mode of ventilation may have differing mechanisms of gas flow
from the proximal airway to the alveoli. The mechanisms include increased gas
mixing with agitation of the airway gas, accelerated axial dispersion, increased
collateral flow through pores of Kohn, intersegmental gas mixing or Pendelluft
phenomenon, Taylor dispersion, asymmetrical gas flow profiles, and gas mixing
within the airway due to the nonlinear pressure-diameter relationship of the bronchi.

Table 6.5 Commonly used types of high frequency ventilation		HFJV	HFO
	Usual rate	240–660	300–900
	Vt/kg	2–4	1–3
	Exhalation	Passive	Active
	Entrainment	Yes	Yes

6.6.2 High Frequency Oscillatory Ventilation

HFOV refers to ventilation at frequencies of 170–900 (2.8–15 Hz) cycles per minute, with an alternating positive and negative pressure in the airway. This oscillatory pressure may be produced by a piston pump or a diaphragm with tidal volumes of 1–3 ml/kg. HFOV systems widely used are the Viasys Critical Care 3100A and 3100B ventilators. The main difference between these two ventilators is the age range each of them supports. The 3100A is designed to support HFOV in neonates and small children. The 3100B is designed to support older children and adults weighing more than 35 kg. Input power for both the ventilators requires two pneumatic gas sources and one electrical source. The first pneumatic connection through a blender determines the FiO_2 delivered to the patients. The second pneumatic connection is for cooling the oscillator. The drive mechanism is a square-wave driver which has an electric linear motor and a piston. The stroke of the piston (both positive and negative) determines the amplitude. The position of the piston determines the mean airway pressure of the circuit.

The main controls in HFOV are mean airway pressure, oscillatory pressure amplitude/power, bias flow, frequency, and inspiratory time. With piston-driven oscillators, the piston position should be centered which can be controlled using a knob. Mean airway pressure determines the mean lung volume of the lung. Oscillatory amplitude is the total change in pressure around the mean airway pressure produced by forward and backward displacement of the piston. The pressures developed in the patients' airways are considerably dampened due to the impedance of the endotracheal tube. The pressure profile is further dampened progressively in the distal airways due to the impedance of the proximal airways. If the oscillatory frequency approaches the natural resonant frequency of the lung and airways, there may be amplification of the pressure waves developed in the airways. The oscillatory amplitude determines the volume displacement with each stroke of the piston. For a given amplitude, a lower frequency will result in less attenuation of pressures along the airways and improve gas exchange. Inspiratory time is generally controlled at 33% of the total cycle time. The absolute inspiratory time is thus inversely proportional to the frequency. Bias flow is a continuous flow of fresh humidified gas and allows replenishing oxygen and removing carbon dioxide from the circuit. Determinants of oxygenation during HFOV are mean airway pressure and FiO_2. Minute ventilation during HFOV is directly proportional to the frequency and the square of the tidal volume. Tidal volume is determined by the amplitude and the duration of each stroke. With increased frequency, the time for each stroke is reduced, decreasing the tidal volume. When the ventilatory frequency is decreased, the time for each stroke is increased thus increasing the tidal volume. The primary determinant of ventilation is oscillatory amplitude which is adjusted by the power setting. Decreasing the frequency to reduce pressure attenuation will increase the tidal volume per breath and improve ventilation. But such a maneuver may increase the pressure changes in the alveoli which may not be desirable.

Optimization of HFOV

HFOV may be considered when the mean airway pressure during conventional mechanical ventilation is around 20 cm H_2O. The most common strategy when HFOV is initiated is to set the mean airway pressure to be about 2–5 cm higher than that with conventional ventilation. Amplitude is set by adjusting the power control while observing for adequacy of chest wall vibrations. There are many ways to recruit the lung and optimize HFOV settings. The most common method of alveolar recruitment is incremental increase in mean airway pressure followed by arterial blood gases to determine whether further increase in mean airway pressure is warranted. An optimal recruitment would be manifested by an increase in lung volume on a chest x-ray, and improved oxygenation and ventilation. Adequacy of lung recruitment is usually verified by ensuring that both hemidiaphragms are displaced to the level of the 9th posterior rib on a chest radiograph. Once sufficient recruitment has been achieved, FiO_2 should be decreased. The goal for oxygenation is to employ a mean airway pressure that will allow reduction of FiO_2 to at least 0.6 while maintaining an arterial oxygen saturation of at least 90%. This may require titration of the mean airway pressure from the initial setting. Once an appropriate degree of lung inflation and patency of the endotracheal tube are verified, ventilation needs to be addressed. Arterial $PaCO_2$ can be maintained at the desired level by changing the amplitude or frequency. Ventilation is increased by an increase in amplitude and a decrease in frequency. It is also important to deflate the cuff of the endotracheal tube, if a cuffed tube is used. Increasing the inspiratory time is a less effective strategy to improve carbon dioxide elimination.

Weaning from HFOV to Conventional Ventilation

Once the mean airway pressure is below 20 cm H_2O, the patient may be placed on conventional mechanical ventilation. The rule of thumb is to employ the same mean airway pressure (MAP) as HFOV and make adjustments based on the gas exchange. Most modern ventilators display the approximate MAP values. FiO_2 would be the same as in HFOV and the ventilator rate would be one appropriate for age and adjusted based on gas exchange. An $ETCO_2$ monitor would be very helpful in adjusting the rate when the patient is switched from HFOV to conventional ventilation.

6.6.3 High Frequency Jet Ventilation

High frequency jet ventilation (HFJV) refers to delivery of inspiratory gases through a jet injector at a high velocity into the trachea at a rate of 240–660 cycles per minute. Along with these tiny high velocity jets, additional air from the bias flow is entrained to generate tidal volumes of 2–4 mL/kg. The main indications for HFJV are (1) as a means to support gas exchange in patients with severe parenchymal lung disease, and (2) management of bronchopleural fistula.

Special endotracheal tubes were required for jet ventilation necessitating reintubation which may be hazardous in severe respiratory failure. Adapters with a side port are now available to fit an already present ET tube to deliver jet ventilation without the need for reintubation. These adapters also provide a port to monitor proximal pressures delivered by HFJV. As in HFOV, these pressures are attenuated lower down in the airways and alveoli. The mechanisms involved in gas transport during HFJV are complex and include Taylor dispersion, accelerated axial dispersion, increased collateral flow through pores of Kohn, intersegmental gas mixing or Pendelluft phenomenon, asymmetrical gas flow profiles, and gas mixing within the airway due to the nonlinear pressure-diameter relationship of the bronchi. A conventional ventilator is used in tandem to provide PEEP and sigh breaths. Administration of sigh breaths is important to recruit the lungs and maintain lung volume. Sigh breaths should be at such inflation pressure (lower than the HFJV PIP) so as to not hinder the delivery of the jet pulses. Exhalation on HFJV is passive from elastic recoil.

There are 3 parameters that can be set: PIP, Jet valve time and Rate. The desired level set for PIP is accomplished by automatic adjustment of the internal machine servo pressure. If PIP falls below the desired level (e.g., improved compliance/ resistance), the machine raises the servo pressure to raise the PIP. Conversely, the servo pressure is decreased if the PIP rises (worsening compliance/resistance) to bring the PIP down to the desired level. Changes in servo pressure level for a desired PIP are thus important indicators of the respiratory compliance/resistance. The jet valve time is set at 0.02 s. This refers to the time the jet valve is opened to generate pulses of jet that are delivered to the patient. It is nearly equivalent to T_i. Increasing the jet valve time improves tidal volume but carries the risk of decreasing the exhalation time resulting in air trapping. The rate is generally set at 420/min. Decreasing the rate results in an increase in the exhalation time allowing greater alveolar emptying but decreasing minute ventilation. Increasing the rate will decrease the exhalation time and may result in air trapping.

The parameters that are monitored during HFJV include PIP, ΔP, PEEP, MAP, and servo pressure. PEEP is adjusted through the conventional ventilator. ΔP refers to the difference between PIP and PEEP and it is responsible for generating V_t. MAP can be adjusted by adjusting the PEEP. The servo pressure, measured in PSI, is an indicator of the internal system pressure that is necessary to generate the desired PIP. Larger patients and those with compliant (and low resistant) lungs will need a higher servo pressure.

6.6.4   Clinical Applications

Both modes of high frequency ventilation have been used to treat severe respiratory failure due to parenchymal lung disease where the major pathophysiology includes atelectasis, intrapulmonary shunting, ventilation-perfusion mismatching and decreased compliance.

All three modes of high frequency ventilation have been reported to improve oxygenation with adequate recruitment of the lung. HFJV is particularly useful with air leaks, especially bronchopleural fistula that precludes use of high airway pressures. HFJV has been successful in supporting gas exchange in patients with bronchopleural fistula while keeping the fistula flow to be low.

HFJV is especially suited for patients who have a significant component of intrathoracic airway obstruction in addition to their alveolar-interstitial pathology. Figure 6.13 shows comparison of HFOV and HFJV in a patient with airway obstruction. The top panel shows the lung and airway pressures during HFOV. A large proportion of the negative pressure generated during active exhalation is transmitted to the site of obstruction while the pleural and alveolar pressure remains positive. This creates an excessively high transmural pressure favoring dynamic airway collapse and airway obstruction exacerbating the already existing hyperinflation and air trapping. The bottom panel shows the same patient with HFJV. Since exhalation is passive, intraluminal pressure does not fall below PEEP. The

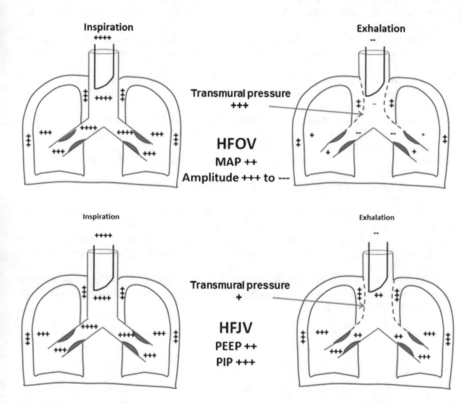

Fig. 6.13 Transmural pressures in the airways in a patient with lower airway obstruction with HFOV (top panel) and HFJV (bottom panel). During exhalation, the proximal airway pressure during HFOV is negative compared to intrathoracic pressures beyond the obstruction causing dynamic airway collapse. In HFJV, the intraluminal pressure doesn't fall below the PEEP. The transmural pressure during exhalation resulting in airway collapse is not as high in HFJV as in HFOV

transmural pressure favoring airway collapse is not as strikingly elevated as in HFOV. HFJV may therefore be a preferred option compared to HFOV in management of patients with obstructive airway disease such as bronchiolitis.

Suggested Readings

1. Sarnaik AP, Bauerfeld CP, Sarnaik AA. Mechanical ventilation. In: Kliegman RM, Stanton BF, St Geme JW, Schor NF, editors. Nelson textbook of pediatrics, 21st ed. Philadelphia: Elsevier.
2. Sarnaik AP, Daphtary K, Meert KL, Lieh-Lai MW, Heidemann SM. Pressure controlled ventilation in children with status asthmaticus. Pediatr Crit Care Med. 2004;5:133–8.
3. Gama de Abreu M, Belda FJ. Neurally adjusted ventilatory assist: letting the respiratory center take over control of ventilation. Intensive Care Med. 2013;39:1481–3.
4. Ducharme-Crevier L, Du Pont-Thibodeau G, Emeriaud G. Interest of monitoring diaphragmatic electrical activity in the pediatric intensive care unit. Crit Care Res Pract. 2013;Article ID 384210:7 pages.
5. Valentine KM, Sarnaik AA, Sandhu HS, Sarnaik AP. High frequency jet ventilation in respiratory failure secondary to respiratory syncytial virus infection: a case series. Front Pediatr. 2016;30(4):92.
6. Pappas MD, Sarnaik AP, Meert KL, Hasan RA, Lieh-Lai MW. Idopathic pulmonary hemorrhage in infancy: clinical features and management with high frequency ventilation. Chest. 1996;110:553–5.
7. Sarnaik AP, Meert KM, Pappas MD, Simpson PM, Lieh-Lai MW, Heidemann SM. Predicting outcome in children with severe acute respiratory failure treated with high-frequency ventilation. Crit Care Med. 1996;24:1396–402.
8. Corrado A, Gorini M. Negative-pressure ventilation: is there still a role? Eur Respir J. 2002;20:187–97.
9. Hess DR. Noninvasive ventilation in neuromuscular disease: equipment and application. Respir Care. 2006;51(8):896–912.
10. Hassinger AB, Breuer RK, Nutty K, et al. Negative-pressure ventilation in pediatric acute respiratory failure. Respir Care. 2017;62(12):1540–9.
11. Sarnaik AA, Sarnaik AP. Noninvasive ventilation in pediatric status asthmaticus: sound physiologic rationale but is it really safe, effective, and cost-efficient? Pediatr Crit Care Med. 2012;13(4):484–5.
12. Miller AG, Bartle RM, Feldman A, Mallory P, Reyes E, Scott B, Rotta AT. A narrative review of advanced ventilator modes in the pediatric intensive care unit. Transl Pediatr. 2020. https://doi.org/10.21037/tp-20-332.

Chapter 7
Mechanical Ventilation Strategies

Ashok P. Sarnaik and Shekhar T. Venkataraman

When a decision is made to initiate invasive mechanical ventilation, the clinician is required to determine the components of the patient's respiratory system that are failing and require to be supported. It is important to recognize that mechanical ventilation does not offer cure to the underlying disease process. The goal is to buy enough time until the dysfunctional tissues recover either on their own or through pharmacologic means. The objective of mechanical ventilation is to maintain sufficient oxygenation and ventilation to ensure tissue viability and to minimize the inevitable complications of the treatment itself.

7.1 Pathophysiologic Considerations

When instituting mechanical ventilation, it is important to recognize that "one size does not fit all". The underlying pathophysiologic derangements are remarkably different in an individual patient and indeed they may change from time to time in

---

The original version of this chapter was revised with correct missing text at Figure 7.7. The correction to this chapter can be found at https://doi.org/10.1007/978-3-030-83738-9_14

A. P. Sarnaik (✉)
Professor of Pediatrics, Former Pediatrician in Chief and Interim Chairman Children's Hospital of Michigan, Wayne State University School of Medicine, 3901 Beaubien, Detroit, MI 48201, USA
e-mail: asarnaik@med.wayne.edu

S. T. Venkataraman
Professor, Departments of Critical Care Medicine and Pediatrics, University of Pittsburgh School of Medicine, Pittsburgh, PA, USA
e-mail: venkataramanst@upmc.edu

Medical Director, Respiratory Care Services, Children's Hospital of Pittsburgh, 4401 Penn Avenue, Faculty Pavilion 2117, Pittsburgh, PA 15224, USA

© Springer Nature Switzerland AG 2022, corrected publication 2022   105
A. P. Sarnaik et al. (eds.), *Mechanical Ventilation in Neonates and Children*,
https://doi.org/10.1007/978-3-030-83738-9_7

the same patient. The challenge to the clinician is to tailor the mechanical ventilation strategy to suit the patient's changing respiratory function in the least injurious fashion. To accomplish this, one should consider the respiratory support as a type of a pharmacologic agent. The "dose" of the support should be titrated to the patient's need for ventilation and oxygenation and utilize the appropriate strategy not to normalize the gas exchange, but to maintain it in a safe and adequate range suitable for recovery to occur. Two major targeted components are: a) alveolar ventilation to eliminate CO_2 and 2) arterial oxygenation to maintain sufficient O_2 delivery to the tissues.

7.1.1 Alveolar Ventilation (V_A)

Overall minute ventilation is represented as a product of tidal volume and the rate (V_T X Rate). Part of the tidal volume consists of dead space which is made up of conducting airways which do not contribute to the gas exchange. The amount of air contributing to gas exchange is alveolar ventilation, calculated as $V_A = (V_T - V_D)$ X Rate. This equation assumes, as a matter of convenience, gas movement is in the form of bulk flow which suggests that the first part of the tidal volume comprises the previously exhaled gas occupying the conducting airway (V_D) and therefore useless as far as bringing the atmospheric gas into the alveoli (see Chap. 3, Fig. 3.2). The determinants of V_A, therefore, are tidal volume (V_T), dead space (V_D) and respiratory rate.

The alveolar ventilation equation can be rewritten as: $V_A = (V_T$ X Rate$) - (V_D$ X Rate$)$. One can surmise that the most efficient means of increasing V_A is to increase the V_T as opposed to the rate. Table 7.1 illustrates the effect of various combinations of V_T and respiratory rate on total minute ventilation and V_A. With a constant anatomic dead space, at multiple combinations of V_D and V_T that provide the same amount of overall minute ventilation, there will be greater V_A at a higher V_T and a lower rate. Both V_T and the rate have important limitations. At higher V_T, the risk of volutrauma is a concern, while at higher respiratory rate adequacy of inspiratory and expiratory times to deliver the prescribed V_T to alveoli may be compromised. Depending on the altered pathophysiology, the clinician must decide which combination is least injurious and most efficient in delivering the dose of V_A to attain a desired $PaCO_2$.

The concept of bulk flow model for V_A is not entirely accurate. This is because of frictional resistance and asymmetric velocities especially at higher respiratory rates and lower tidal volumes as in high frequency ventilation (see Chap.3, Fig. 3.2).

Table 7.1 Relationship of V_T, V_D and the Respiratory Rate on V_A

V_T (mL)	V_D (mL)	$V_T - V_D$ (mL)	Respiratory Rate/Min	Minute Ventilation (L/min)	V_A (L/ Min)
200	100	100	30	6	3
250	100	150	24	6	3.6
300	100	200	20	6	4
350	100	250	17	≈ 6	4.25
400	100	300	15	6	4.5

Because of frictional resistance, gas molecules move with asymmetric velocities rather than in blocks. The molecules in the center move faster than those in the periphery. Thus, volume of gas moving in and out of alveoli is in fact higher than what can be predicted by pure bulk flow movement.

7.1.2 Time Constant

Delivery of gas occurs from a higher pressure to lower pressure. Gas flow continues as long as pressure gradient exists and it ceases after proximal pressure equilibrates with the distal end. Once proximal and distal pressures equilibrate, the flow ceases and no additional volume is delivered. The pressure equilibration does not occur instantly. It takes time. The amount of time taken for pressure to equilibrate from proximal end to distal end is directly proportional to compliance (opposite of elastance) and resistance (opposite of conductance). Pressure equilibration is faster when compliance is decreased as the alveoli oppose expansion to a greater extent and fill up quickly. On the other hand, the pressure equilibration time is longer when resistance is increased. The product of compliance and resistance (C X R) is referred to as time constant (TC) which is a reflection of the amount of time it takes for a certain percentage of the volume change. With a constant inflation pressure, 63%, 95% and 99% of the maximal tidal volume will be delivered in 1, 3 and 5 time constants, respectively. Similarly, during exhalation, 63%, 95% and 99% of the initial volume will be exhaled with 1, 3, and 5 time constants, respectively (see Chap. 2, Fig. 2.2). Normally, the expiratory time constant (TC_E) is greater than the inspiratory time constant (TC_I) since airways get narrower during exhalation resulting in increased airway resistance. With decreased compliance, TC is decreased and the TC_E is closer to TC_I. With increased resistance, both TC_I and TC_E are prolonged but TC_E is prolonged much more than TC_I. (see Chap. 2, Fig. 2.3).

Most pulmonary disorders requiring mechanical ventilatory support are of two types; a) decreased lung compliance (decreased time constant) and b) increased resistance (increased time constant). Disease states with decreased lung compliance (ARDS, pneumonia, pulmonary edema etc.) have quicker approximation of pressure for alveolar filling and emptying. However, lung disease is rarely homogenous. While the composite TC may be either decreased or increased, areas with increased and decreased TC may co-exist in the same patient and may indeed change in their respective contributions at different times. The clinician must determine which component is the dominant one. The effect of time on delivered (or emptied) volume in lungs with differing time constants is shown in Chapter 2, Fig. 2.4. Increasing the time during inspiration or exhalation will result in greater volume change in areas with increased TC (increased resistance) but will have little to no effect in changing lung volume in areas with short time constant (decreased compliance).

7.1.3 Functional Residual Capacity

While the atmospheric air is brought into the alveoli only during inspiration, gas exchange between the alveolar gas and pulmonary capillary blood is continuous. During inspiration alveolar PO_2 (PAO_2) rises as fresh atmospheric gas with higher PO_2 is brought in. During exhalation O_2 continues to be removed by deoxygenated pulmonary arterial blood. PAO_2 rises during inspiration and declines during exhalation. Alveolar PCO_2 ($PACO_2$) on the other hand, falls during inspiration as it is diluted by the atmospheric gas containing negligible amount of CO_2, and rises during exhalation as CO_2 is being added from the pulmonary circulation. The fluctuations in alveolar gas composition during inspiration and exhalation are buffered by functional residual capacity (FRC) which is the gas left in the lung at end-exhalation. The changes in PAO_2 and $PACO_2$ during the respiratory cycle are only a few torr (Fig. 7.1).

Pulmonary capillary circulation is in a state of equilibration with the FRC by the process of diffusion. Mean PAO_2 and $PACO_2$ are approximately 100 and 40 torr respectively. During inspiration PAO_2 rises to 102 torr and during exhalation it falls to 98 torr. $PACO_2$ likewise rises to 41 torr during exhalation and falls to 38 torr during inspiration. Under normal circumstances, the systemic venous blood brought to the alveoli by pulmonary capillaries will have a PO_2 of 40 torr and PCO_2 of

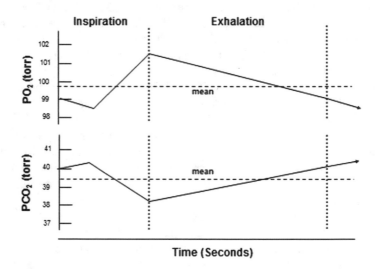

Fig. 7.1 Alveolar PO_2 and PCO_2 fluctuate throughout the respiratory cycle. During inspiration PAO_2 rises and $PACO_2$ declines as fresh atmospheric gas enters the alveoli. During exhalation the PAO_2 decreases and $PACO_2$ rises as O_2 continues to get removed and CO_2 is added by the pulmonary arterial circulation. Note that during the early part of the inspiration PAO_2 continues to decline as $PACO_2$ rises because of the entry of the dead space (previously exhaled gas). The degree of fluctuations in alveolar gas tensions is buffered by the FRC. *(Modified from Comroe JH: Physiology of respiration, ed 2, Chicago, 1974, Year Book Medical Publishers, p 12.)*

46 torr. FRC represents the environment available for pulmonary capillary blood for gas exchange at all times. As the pulmonary capillary blood flows across the alveoli it gets arterialized to a PO_2 of 100 torr and PCO_2 of 40 torr. The major pathophysiologic effect of decreased FRC is hypoxemia. Reduction in FRC results in a sharp decline in PAO_2 during exhalation because limited volume is available for gas exchange. PO_2 of pulmonary capillary blood therefore falls excessively, approaching venous PO_2 during exhalation leading to decline in arterial PO_2. When FRC is reduced and the patient is breathing room air, any increase in PAO_2 during inspiration cannot compensate for decreased PAO_2 during exhalation due to the sigmoid shape of the O_2 dissociation curve. Since most of the O_2 in blood is combined with Hb, it is the percentage of oxyhemoglobin (SaO_2) that gets averaged rather than the PaO_2. The steep O_2 desaturation of Hb during exhalation results in overall arterial desaturation and hypoxemia. In situations where FRC is severely depleted, hypoxemia becomes resistant to administration of supplemental O_2 administration. Since CO_2 dissociation curve is relatively linear, decreased FRC does not significantly affect $PaCO_2$ as long as V_A is maintained. Two strategies can be employed during mechanical ventilation to ameliorate the hypoxemia secondary to decreased FRC. The first one is an "open lung" strategy in an attempt to increase FRC by application of positive end expiratory pressure (PEEP). The second strategy is to increase the inspiratory time (T_I) fraction of the respiratory cycle allowing for longer exposure of pulmonary capillary blood to higher O_2 and shorter exposure to lower O_2 during expiratory time (T_E). In order for the increased T_I to produce a favorable result, one must ensure that the decreased T_E is still sufficient to allow for adequate alveolar emptying. Such a strategy requires the expiratory time constant to be reduced such as in disease states with decreased compliance. Inverse ratio ventilation (IRV) and airway pressure release ventilation (APRV) are extreme examples of such a strategy.

7.1.4 Pressure–Volume (P–V) Relationship

Real time changes in volume as inflation pressure is applied is an important consideration during mechanical support of ventilation (Fig. 7.2). Collapsed or atelectatic alveoli require considerable amount of pressure to open. Once open, the alveoli require relatively less pressure for continued expansion. The process of opening collapsed alveoli is called lung recruitment and it is intended to increase the FRC. Opening the atelectatic alveoli and keeping them in an expanded state during tidal respiration is termed "open lung" strategy. Repetitive opening and closing the alveoli during tidal respiration, referred to as "tidal recruitment", is injurious to the lung and it is an important component of ventilator induced lung injury. The brunt of pressure applied to atelectatic alveoli is experienced at the delicate terminal airway-alveolar junctions causing atelectotrauma. Also, pressure delivery to maximally open alveoli cause them to over-distend and resulting in volutrauma. Most atelectatic lung diseases (e.g. ARDS) are heterogeneous in

Fig. 7.2 Pressure–volume relationship in ARDS versus normal lung. Pulmonary compliance is reduced in ARDS with a narrow zone of "safe" ventilation (green rectangle) where the dynamic compliance is at its maximum. Ventilation at lung volume below the lower P_{Flex} (critical opening pressure) results in tidal recruitment and atelectrauma. Ventilation at lung volume above upper P_{Flex} results in volutrauma

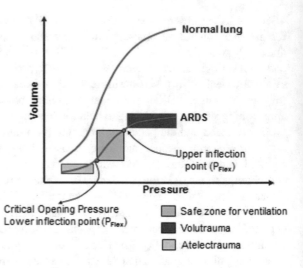

nature. Each of the millions of alveoli has its own mechanical characteristics; however, a composite pressure–volume relationship for the entire lung is useful to conceptualize.

Compared to the normal lung, the ARDS lung is less compliant resulting in a PV curve with a decreased slope (Fig. 7.2). At the beginning of inspiration, the atelectatic alveoli are being forced open requiring a large change in pressure for a relatively small change in volume (lower horizontal part of PV curve). Once these alveoli are opened, further increase in volume requires a relatively smaller change in pressure (middle vertical part of PV curve). After the alveoli are maximally distended, their PV curve again resumes horizontal nature indicating opposition to further volume change with added pressure. The point at which the alveoli open up to accept greater volume change for increase in pressure is termed lower inflection point (lower P_{Flex}) and the point at which added pressure yields less volume change is called the (upper P_{Flex}). The goal of mechanical support of ventilation should be to keep PEEP above the lower inflection point and to keep the peak alveolar pressure (PIP with PCV and plateau pressure with VCV) below the upper inflection point, the so called "safe zone" of ventilation. If PEEP is below the lower inflection point, the alveoli whose critical closing pressure is above the level of PEEP are likely to collapse and reinflate during subsequent inspiration, a process termed "tidal recruitment" that is injurious to lung due to the stress experienced by terminal airway-alveolar junctions. If the peak alveolar pressure is higher than the upper inflection point, overdistension of alveoli is likely to occur resulting in volutrauma and barotrauma. The strategy to avoid inflation pressure that includes lower P_{Flex} is to leave the lungs at a constant state of recruitment with appropriate amount of PEEP. Inclusion of upper P_{Flex} during inflation is avoided by delivering relatively small amount of V_T.

7.2   Planning of Mechanical Ventilation in Individual Situations

The technologic details of ventilator functioning are described in Chap. 6. Following is a suggested approach for the clinician to consider at the bedside.

Pathophysiologic considerations When strategizing mechanical ventilation for an individual patient, certain physiologic parameters need to be assessed (Fig. 7.3). These are FRC, time constant and critical opening pressure. Since reliable measurements are not readily available for any of these variables, the clinician must make reasonable assumptions based on the type of the disease process, clinical findings, blood gas analyses, and imaging studies.

7.2.1   Phases of Respiratory Cycle

Four phases of the respiratory cycle should be taken into consideration when tailoring the strategy for a given situation (Fig. 7.4). These are (1) Initiation of inspiration and a variable that is controlled, often referred to as the mode; (2) Inspiratory phase characteristics, which determine the duration of inspiration and how the pressure or volume is delivered; (3) Termination of inspiration, often referred to as the cycle; and (4) Expiratory phase characteristics which mainly consists of application of PEEP. Decision should also be made regarding the extent and the nature of patient-machine interaction that should be allowed in an individual situation.

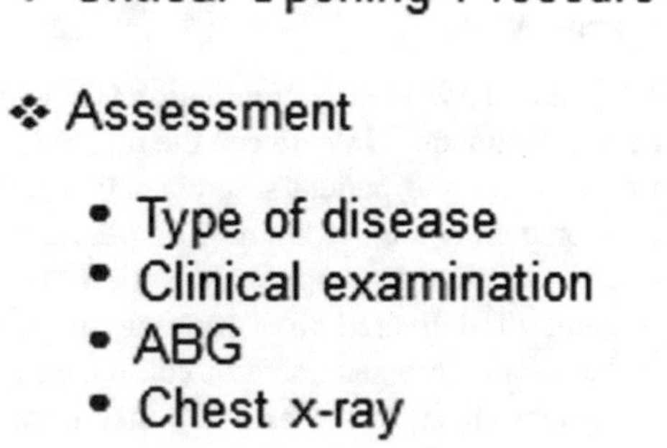

Fig. 7.3 Pathophysiologic considerations in mechanical ventilation

❖ FRC

❖ Time Constant

❖ Critical Opening Pressure

❖ Assessment

  • Type of disease
  • Clinical examination
  • ABG
  • Chest x-ray

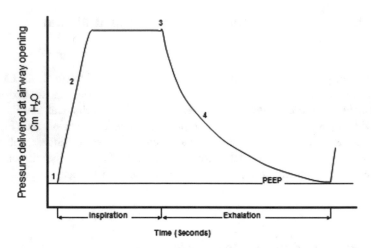

Fig. 7.4 Four phases of a pressure-controlled time-cycled mechanically delivered breath. (1) Initiation of inspiration, (2) Inspiratory phase characteristics, (3) Termination of inspiration, and (4) Expiratory phase characteristics

7.2.2 Initiation of Inspiration and the Control Variable (Mode)

The initiation of inspiration can be set to occur at a predetermined rate and time interval regardless of patient effort, or it could be timed in response to patient effort. Once the inspiration is initiated, the ventilator breath is either delivered by precisely set volume or pressure parameters (volume control or pressure control mode) or supports the patient's effort to a predetermined inspiratory volume or pressure target (volume support or pressure support mode). Advances in technology have allowed greater patient-ventilator synchrony to occur. The ventilator may be set to be "triggered" by the signal it receives as a result of the patient effort. This signal may be in form lowering of either pressure (pressure trigger) or the base flow (flow trigger) in the ventilator circuit generated by the patient's inspiratory effort. If no such signal is received, the ventilator delivers a breath at an interval selected by the operator.

Control Modes

Intermittent Mandatory Ventilation (IMV) mode In IMV, the inspiration is initiated at a set frequency. In between the machine delivered breaths a fresh source of gas is provided for the patient's spontaneous breaths. Once initiated the inspired gas is delivered at a pre-set amount of pressure (Pressure control) or volume (Volume control). Patient's respiratory system compliance and resistance determine the amount of delivered tidal volume in pressure control mode or the amount of inflation pressure generated in volume control mode. The delivered IMV breath can be synchronized to the patient's inspiratory effort (SIMV).

Assist-Control (AC) Mode In AC mode, every spontaneous breathing effort by the patient triggers a machine delivered breath, either as pressure or as volume controlled. Once initiated, the inspiratory characteristics are according to the pre determined parameters. A back-up control rate is set to ensure the minimum number of breaths delivered if there is insufficient number of patient trigger events. Since every spontaneous breath triggers a machine delivered breath, this mode is not suitable for patients as a weaning strategy.

Control Variable Once initiated, either the V_T or the inflation pressure is controlled. The mechanical breath is described as either volume controlled when a predetermined machine-delivered tidal volume is delivered or pressure controlled when a predetermined inflation pressure is generated at the airway opening. Adjusting the flow rate determines the inspiratory time (T_I) over which V_T is delivered in volume-controlled ventilation (VCV) whereas in pressure-controlled ventilation (PCV) T_I is directly pre-set as the time over which the inflation pressure will be administered. The inflation pressure generated during VCV and V_T delivered during PCV are secondary variables dictated by the respiratory system compliance and resistance.

VCV and PCV have their own advantages and disadvantages (Table 7.2). In patients with un-uniform time constants where some lung units fill up quickly (diseases with reduced compliance) and some take much longer for pressure equilibration to occur (diseases of increased resistance), PCV offers an advantage of raising the inflation pressure quickly, allow the areas of short time constants to fill up in early part of inspiration and let the areas of prolonged time constant fill in the later part of inspiration (Fig. 7.5).

Table 7.2 Characteristics of PCV and VCV

	Pressure-Controlled Ventilation	Volume-Controlled Ventilation
Control variables	- Inflation Pressure - Inspiratory time - Rise time	- Tidal volume - Flow rate - Inspiratory flow pattern (constant vs decelerating)
Machine-delivered volume	Depends on respiratory system compliance and resistance	Constant
Inflation pressure	Constant	Depends upon respiratory system compliance and resistance
Inspiratory time	Precisely set	Depends on flow rate adjustment
Endotracheal tube leak	Somewhat compensated	Part of delivered volume leaked during inflation
Distribution of ventilation	More uniform in lungs with varying time constant units	Less uniform in lungs with varying time constant units
Weaning process	Inflation pressure adjustment required to deliver desired tidal volume	Tidal volume remains constant, inflation pressure automatically weaned
Patient comfort	Possibly compromised	Possibly enhanced

Table 7.3 General recommendations for mechanical ventilation for patients with severely decreased respiratory system compliance (e.g., ARDS, pneumonia)

Age (Years)	Rate ("Rapid")	Tidal volume ("Shallow")	I:E ratio
0.1–2	30–40/min	6 mL/Kg	(1.5–1):2
2–4	25–30/min	6 mL/Kg	(1.5–1):2
5–12	20–25/min	6–7 mL/Kg	(1.5–1):2
13–18	20/min	6–7 mL/Kg	(1.5–1):2

Titrate PEEP ($\geq$ 6 cm H_2O) for improving PaO_2/FiO_2. Monitor C_{dyn}

Table 7.4 General recommendations for mechanical ventilation for patients with severe obstructive lung disease (e.g., status asthmaticus).

Age (Years)	Rate ("Slow")	Tidal volume ("Deep")	I:E ratio
1–4	18–20/min	10 mL/Kg	1:3
5–8	14–18	10–12 mL/Kg	1:3
9–12	12–14	12 mL/Kg	1:3.5
13–18	8–12	12 mL/Kg	1:4

Add sufficient PEEP to counteract Auto-PEEP. Monitor C_{dyn}

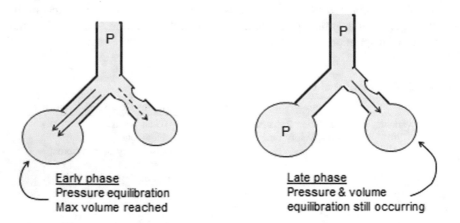

Early inspiration - Areas with short time constants fill up quickly and equilibrate with proximal airway pressure.

Late inspiration - Areas with prolonged time constants receive more volume with slower equilibrium of pressure.

Result More even gas distribution compared to volume-controlled ventilation especially in obstructive lesions

Fig. 7.5 Pressure-control Ventilation

Areas with low resistance and high compliance
are preferentially filled throughout inspiration
(both early and late) resulting in uneven
ventilation especially in obstructive lesions

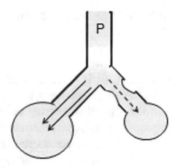

Fig. 7.6 Volume-control Ventilation

This limits excessive rise in inflation pressure and forces more uniform distribution of tidal volume. In VCV, the areas of shorter time constant will be preferentially filled with the delivered volume throughout the inspiration resulting in uneven distribution of ventilation and a rise in inflation pressure and a decrease in C_{DYN} (Fig. 7.6). VCV is more advantageous in patients with relatively normal or recovering lungs as a reliable V_T can be delivered. In such situations, the inflation pressures fall automatically with improving compliance and resistance. With PCV, the delivered V_T can change significantly with rapid changes in compliance and resistance requiring frequent manipulations of inflation pressure.

Pressure Regulated Volume Control (PRVC)

The advantage of PRVC over PCV is a more consistent tidal volume delivery over time since it targets a set tidal volume per breath. When the delivered tidal volume is lower than the set tidal volume, the ventilator automatically increases the peak inspiratory pressure required to meet the target tidal volume up to a certain limit. When the delivered tidal volume is larger than the set tidal volume, when there is an improvement in compliance, the peak inspiratory pressure is automatically decreased to maintain the set tidal volume. The disadvantage is that in PRVC, with severe lung disease, the peak inspiratory pressure may be increased above the upper inflection point to maintain the tidal volume. Therefore, in PRVC, peak inspiratory pressure changes need to be monitored more closely.

Support Modes

Pressure-support ventilation (PSV) and Volume support ventilation (VSV) Support modes are designed to support patient's spontaneous respiratory efforts. With PSV, the patient's spontaneous respiratory effort is supported by a rapid rise in in ventilatory pressure to a pre-selected level. The inspiration is continued until the inspiratory flow falls to a pre-set level (generally 25%) of peak flow rate as the lungs fill up. Thus the T_I is controlled by the patient's own efforts and the pulmonary mechanics. With VSV, all spontaneous breaths are supported by generation of inflation pressure to deliver a pre-set tidal volume. They are frequently combined with SIMV so that any breath above the SIMV rate is supported by either PSV or VSV.

Inspiratory phase characteristics Once initiated, the T_I, the inspiratory flow waveform, and the pressure rise time can be adjusted to suit the pulmonary mechanics. In PCV, T_I is directly set in seconds. In VCV, the T_I is adjusted by adjusting the inspiratory flow (volume over time). Increasing the flow rate will decrease T_I and decreasing the flow rate will increase it. I:E ratio depends on the respiratory rate which determines the duration of the total respiratory cycle. Both T_I and T_E should be considered individually. Increase in T_I will increase MAP and also the duration of time the pulmonary capillary blood is exposed to higher PO_2 resulting in improved oxygenation. This strategy is helpful in situations where FRC is decreased such as in ARDS or pulmonary edema. Increasing T_I will also increase V_T in PCV without increasing the inflation pressure if inspiratory flow has not ceased at the end inspiration. T_E must be sufficient to allow for expiratory flow to return to baseline or close to it. Decrease in respiratory rate may be required if T_E is insufficient for adequate exhalation.

Inspiratory flow waveform can be adjusted in VCV mode as either a constant flow (square waveform) or a decelerating flow (descending ramp waveform). With a square waveform the flow is kept constant throughout inspiration. In a descending waveform, flow is maximal at the start of inspiration and steadily declines to zero at end inspiration.

In PCV and PSV, the predetermined inflation pressure is achieved through delivery of airflow. Pressure rise time reflects the rapidity with which the ventilator achieves the target pressure. Rise time is adjusted to a value that is most comfortable for a patient who is awake and also to prevent a rapid rise and pressure overshoot that could be injurious to the lung.

Termination of inspiration (Cycle) Cessation of inspiration is effected by 3 mechanisms depending on the mode used; time-cycling, volume-cycling, or flow-cycling. PCV is "cycled off" when a predetermined T_I elapses (time-cycled), VCV inspiration is terminated after the prescribed volume is delivered, and PSV is cycled off after inspiratory flow declines to a pre-selected percentage of peak flow. Volume cycled breath can be pressure-limited to prevent a rise in pressure beyond a certain limit. In such a situation, an inspiratory hold is created as the excess volume is popped off in the expiratory circuit. While this strategy prevents undesirable elevation in the inflation pressures, less than predetermined volume is delivered to the patient.

Expiratory phase maneuvers The most useful expiratory phase maneuver is the application of PEEP. The most important clinical benefits of PEEP are to recruit atelectatic alveoli and to increase FRC in patients with alveolar-interstitial lung disease thereby improving oxygenation. Even briefly disconnecting the ventilator and allowing the alveolar pressure to reach zero results in substantial de-recruitment and loss of FRC that takes a period of time to recover from after reapplication of PEEP. In patients with obstructive disease where insufficient exhalation time results in auto-PEEP, application of extrinsic PEEP, can delay airway closure and improve ventilation. Other salutary effects of PEEP include displacement of alveolar fluid to

Fig. 7.7 Effect of FRC on PVR. Pulmonary vascular resistance (PVR) is the lowest at normal FRC. At too low (atelectasis) and too high (overdistension) FRC, the PVR is proportionately elevated

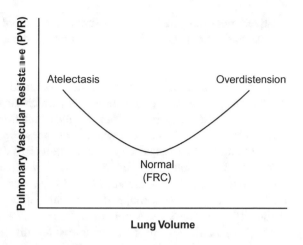

extra-alveolar spaces, decrease in left to right shunt and stabilization of chest wall. Effect of PEEP on lung compliance is variable and it depends on the patient's pulmonary mechanics. By shifting the ventilation to a more favorable part of the pressure–volume curve, PEEP may recruit more alveoli and improve lung compliance. Excessive PEEP on the other hand will result in alveolar overdistension and reduction in compliance. (Fig. 7.2). The effect of FRC on pulmonary vascular resistance (PVR) is parabolic. PVR is at the lowest at a normal FRC. PVR is increased at excessively low (atelectasis) and excessively high (overdistention) FRC. (Fig. 7.7). Elevated PVR increases right ventricular afterload and impairment of cardiac output. At low FRC, there is increased intrapulmonary right to left shunting past the hypoventilated, atelectatic alveoli whereas at high FRC, there is increase in dead space ventilation because of decreased pulmonary perfusion. Efforts directed at achieving normal FRC is the goal of the mechanical ventilation strategies.

Airway Pressure Release Ventilation (APRV) APRV is utilized to improve oxygenation in patients with diffuse atelectatic process such as ARDS. This modality delivers high level continuous positive pressure (P_{high}) to the respiratory system through most of the breath cycle (3–5 s) with intermittent release of the pressure without allowing it to return it zero (P_{low}) for brief periods (0.3–0.5 s) of time. P_{high} is aimed at recruiting alveoli and maintaining satisfactory lung volume while P_{low} is to allow alveolar gas to escape for CO_2 elimination while still maintaining positive alveolar pressure at end expiration to maintain satisfactory FRC. P_{high} is akin to PIP and P_{low} is similar to setting PEEP. The patient is allowed to breathe during both the P_{high} and P_{low} phases. The long P_{high} phase is tolerated because of the active expiratory valve in the ventilatory circuit making spontaneous respiration possible.

High Frequency Ventilation (HFV) HFV is another approach used especially in children with hypoxemic respiratory failure. The strategy is to recruit lung volume using supraphysiologic respiratory rates at high mean airway pressure (MAP) and relatively minor fluctuations in pressure around it to deliver small V_T. The aim is to protect the lung from excessive tidal stretch which is responsible for ventilator induced lung injury. Two forms of HFV are most commonly in vogue. Both are commonly used as rescue therapies when conventional ventilation is likely to be ineffective or injurious. High frequency oscillation (HFO) employs to and fro oscillations with a parallel bias flow from which air is entrained. Air is pushed in during inspiration and sucked out during exhalation. The main determinants of oxygenation are MAP and FiO_2 whereas changes in pressure (amplitude) determine the ventilation. High frequency jet ventilation (HFJV) tiny amounts of gas (jets) at high velocity are introduced into the bias flow causing entrainment of additional gas. Unlike HFO, the exhalation in HFJV is passive due to the elastic recoil of the lungs and the chest wall. Major determinants of oxygenation are FiO_2 and PEEP while PIP determines the ventilation. In our experience, HFOV is an effective strategy for predominantly alveolar interstitial disease such as ARDS and pneumonia. However, in patients with significant airway obstruction (e.g. bronchiolitis, pertussis), the use of HFOV may exacerbate airway collapse during exhalation (Fig. 6.13) because of the generation of negative pressure in the airway. In such situations, HFJV may be the preferred option.

Conventional Ventilator Settings

Fraction of inspired oxygen (FiO2) The shape of the hemoglobin-O_2 dissociation dictates that most of the oxygen attaches to the hemoglobin at PaO_2 of around 70 torr at which hemoglobin-O_2 saturation (SO_2) is 94% under normal circumstances. Higher PaO_2 levels contribute little to increase O_2 content while exposing the patient to the risk of O_2 toxicity. Unless higher PaO_2 is required temporarily for select situations such as CO poisoning, pulmonary hypertensive crisis and severe anemia, a PaO_2 that yields SaO_2 in the mid 90's should be adequate. In most situations, a PaO_2 value around 70 torr is a reasonable goal. Whenever possible, FiO_2 should be decreased to < 0.50 as long as SaO_2 remains in the mid 90's. FiO_2 concentrations less than 0.5 are generally considered safe.

Mode The choice of mode of ventilation depends upon the disease entity that is treated and how much ventilator-patient interaction is desired. Patients with normal lungs with ability to trigger the machine are best managed with SIMV in a volume control mode or either PSV or VSV as a support mode. The emphasis should be placed on the mode that provides maximum comfort. Patients with abnormal lungs, either obstructive or restrictive nature, will require more precise ventilatory strategies. Generally, VCV is preferable since it is the V_T that determines the alveolar ventilation rather than inflation pressure which effects a change in volume as a secondary variable. In more severe alterations with respiratory units of different time constants, PCV is the preferred choice for effecting a more uniform distribution of V_T. Regardless of the choice of the mode, the exhaled VT (VT_E) and PIP should be monitored on an ongoing basis.

Tidal Volume and Rate The dose of alveolar ventilation (V_A) is calculated as ($V_T - V_D$) X Rate. The anatomic V_D is generally estimated to be 2.2 mL/kg. The manner in which V_A is administered should be based according to the patient's pathophysiologic alterations. The most important consideration is that of time constant, a product of compliance and resistance.

In patients with normal lungs, time constant can be assumed to be normal. V_T can be chosen as 8–10 mL/kg with age appropriate respiratory rate. In such patients (such as those being ventilated for status epilepticus, traumatic/metabolic encephalopathies, neuromuscular dysfunction etc.), alveolar ventilation should be adjusted to maintain a desired $PaCO_2$ as monitored by $ETCO_2$ or blood gas analysis.

In patients with reduced lung compliance (e.g. ARDS, pulmonary edema, interstitial pneumonia), the time constant is shorter than normal. Pressure equilibration occurs more rapidly. Also, larger tidal volumes and higher inflation pressures are injurious to the lungs. Such patients are best ventilated at relatively lower V_T (6–7 mL/kg) and higher respiratory rates to maintain adequate V_A. When using PCV, an appropriate inflation pressure (PIP-PEEP) should be selected to deliver the desired volume. If VCV or PRVC is used, the end inspiratory pressure should be kept under less than 30 cm H_2O if possible.

In patients with increased airway resistance (e.g. asthma), the time constant is prolonged, necessitating longer time for pressure to be equilibrated and volume to be delivered to the distal end. Such patients should be ventilated at slower rates providing sufficient time for inflation and deflation to occur. To compensate for slower rates, V_T needs to be increased up to 12 mL/kg as necessary (Tables 7.3 and 7.4).

Inspiratory Time (TI) and Expiratory Time (TE) Both T_E and T_I need to be set to allow for satisfactory inflation and deflation to occur. In addition to considering the I:E ratios, T_I and T_E should also be considered independently of each other in terms of adequacy for pressure equilibration to occur. This most certainly depends on the time constant. The total time available for each respiratory cycle is determined by the respiratory rate (RR). Thus $T_E + T_I$ is 5 s at RR of 12/min and 3 s for RR of 20/min. In a normal respiratory pattern the exhalation is twice as long as inspiration with pressure equilibration occurring at the end of either of these phases. With diseases of compliance, as the time constant is short, pressure equilibration is rarely a problem allowing for faster rates and smaller V_T. Prolongation of T_I is often practiced to improve oxygenation by (a) increasing MAP and (b) allowing greater duration for pulmonary capillary blood to be exposed to higher PAO_2. In diseases of increased airway resistance the time constant is prolonged. However, the TC_E is prolonged much more than TC_I necessitating not only a slower rate but prolongation of exhalation with I:E ratios of 1:3 or more. The best way of determining the effective T_I, T_E and I:E ratios is to observe flow time relationship on ventilator wave form and the VT_E. The flow should be nearly complete especially at end exhalation and VT_E should be sufficient for adequate V_A. T_I is set directly on the ventilator setting in PCV and PRVC while in VCV, it is a function of inspiratory flow rate which is set to distribute the V_T over the duration of T_I.

Positive End-Expiratory Pressure (PEEP) The most important application of PEEP is in alveolar-interstitial disease to increase FRC above the critical opening pressure or lower P_{Flex} and allowing ventilation to occur in the relatively safe zone, improving C_{dyn} and avoiding tidal recruitment (Fig. 7.2). Increase in FRC results in improved oxygenation and decrease O_2 requirements. Choosing the ideal PEEP is often based on PaO_2/FiO_2 values. The adverse effects of PEEP on venous return compromising cardiac output should also be taken into account. In diseases of increased resistance, application of PEEP delays airway closure and reduce air-trapping. This effect can be monitored by measuring the auto-PEEP before and after application of PEEP. A decrease in auto-PEEP is desired after application of PEEP through the ventilator. Presence of an ET tube prevents the patient's ability to grunt by exhaling with a partially closed glottis. Grunting results in maintaining positive pressure at end expiration to maintain alveolar volume. All intubated patients, even those with normal lungs, should therefore have, at a minimum, a small amount of PEEP (2–4 cm H_2O) to maintain FRC.

The optimum PEEP is the level at which there is an acceptable balance between the desired goals and undesired adverse effects. The desired goals are (1) reduction in inspired oxygen concentration to "nontoxic" levels (usually < 50%); (2) maintenance of PaO_2 or SaO_2 (arterial oxygen saturation) of more than 60 mmHg or more than 90%, respectively; (3) improvement of lung compliance; and (4) maximal oxygen delivery.

7.3 Weaning and Extubation

Mechanical ventilation, while life-saving, can be associated with undesirable side effects and complications. Therefore, it is important that, as soon as the patient is capable of comfortably sustaining adequate gas exchange with spontaneous breathing, mechanical ventilation is discontinued. When weaning the patient off mechanical ventilation, it is important to consider decreasing the most injurious part of the support. Often it is the FiO_2, inflation pressure (or V_T), and respiratory rate in that order. Also, greater reliance on support modes over mandatory modes is preferred for patient comfort and safety.

7.3.1 The Weaning Process

Weaning from mechanical ventilation is the transition from ventilatory support to complete spontaneous breathing. During this transition, the patient assumes increasing responsibility for effective gas exchange while positive pressure support is reduced. Weaning is complete and is defined as a success when a patient maintains adequate gas exchange with complete spontaneous breathing, while remaining comfortable without any mechanical assistance. Weaning is defined as a failure when spontaneous efforts are incapable of sustaining effective gas exchange without mechanical support. The timing of extubation generally coincides with an assessment that the patient is capable of maintaining acceptable gas exchange without ventilator support. Extubation failure is defined as the need for reintubation within 48 h of extubation.

7.3.2 Initiation of Weaning

Weaning should start when: (1) the underlying disease process is improving; (2) the gas exchange is adequate; (3) no conditions exist that impose an undue burden on the respiratory muscles, such as cardiac insufficiency, severe malnutrition, and muscle weakness; and (4) the patient is capable of sustaining spontaneous ventilation as ventilator support is decreased without expending an excessive amount of energy. Improvement of the underlying disease process can be assessed by measurement of gas exchange, respiratory system mechanics, and x-ray findings. Patients cannot be arbitrarily forced to wean because it is the patient who dictates the pace of the weaning process. Patient's ability to breathe effectively depends on several factors: (1) respiratory muscle strength, (2) stability of the cardiovascular system, (3) work of breathing, (4) general nutritional status of the patient, and (5) the absence of an underlying hypercatabolic state (e.g., sepsis).

7.3.3 Weaning Techniques

Weaning practice ranges from abrupt withdrawal to gradual withdrawal from ventilatory support. Most common practice is gradual reduction in ventilator settings which involves reducing the mechanical minute ventilation, FiO_2, and PEEP in steps while assessing the patient's ability to tolerate the change. Currently, most children are weaned with SIMV with or without added pressure support, or with pressure support alone. At the end of weaning, patients may or may not be tested with an extubation readiness test (ERT) before liberation from mechanical ventilation. An ERT is defined as a trial that tests the ability of complete spontaneous breathing to maintain gas exchange with or without minimal assistance. The criteria for passing and terminating an ERT are shown in Table 7.5.

Studies have shown that in children, when the criteria to initiate weaning are met, 50–75% of the patients can be liberated from mechanical ventilation after passing an ERT without undergoing a gradual reduction in ventilator settings. The premise underlying the more rapid withdrawal is that many patients are ready to be liberated as soon as they meet the criteria to initiate weaning and therefore, do not require a prolonged weaning process. If patients meet the criteria as outlined in Table 7.6, they can be subjected to an ERT. If the ERT is successful, then the patient can be liberated from mechanical ventilation. If a patient fails an ERT, mechanical ventilation can be continued at a level that keeps the patient comfortable with no increased work of breathing. If invasive mechanical ventilation in continued, the ERT can be repeated in 24 h. Alternatively, the patient can be extubated

Table 7.5 Criteria for initiating an Extubation Readiness Test (ERT)

Eligibility for an ERT
1. Improvement or resolution of the underlying cause of acute respiratory failure
2. Adequate oxygenation
• $PaO_2 > 65$ mmHg
• $SpO_2 > 95\%$
• $F_IO_2 < 0.4$
• PEEP < 7 cmH$_2$O
3. Adequate ventilation
• $PaCO_2 < 45$ mmHg with no chronic respiratory failure
• $PaCO_2 > 45$ mmHg with acceptable arterial pH with chronic respiratory failure
4. A core temperature below 38.5 °C
5. Alert mental status after removal of sedative agents
6. Minimal to no vasoactive agent requirement
• There should be no planned procedures for next several hours
• Enteral feeds should be stopped for 4 h before ERT
• Maintenance fluid are being given IV in infants and small children

Table 7.6 Criteria for passing an extubation readiness test

• Can maintain $SpO_2 > 95\%$ during the test
• Is breathing comfortably without significant retractions or paradoxical breathing
• Respiratory rate within the range: (a) age < 6 months - 20–60/min
(b) 6 months-2 years - 15–45/min
(c) 2–5 years - 15–40/min
(d) > 5 years - 10–35/min
• Spontaneous tidal volume > 5 mL/kg
• No hemodynamic instability during the trial

to noninvasive mechanical ventilation, if appropriate and eligible. If the decision is to extubate to noninvasive positive pressure support, then it would be prudent to test the patient on a level of pressure support that is necessary to maintain gas exchange and decrease the work of breathing (Table 7.6).

7.3.4 ERT Trials

There are three commonly employed ERT methods: CPAP provided through the ventilator, T-piece breathing, and minimal PSV with PEEP. During a CPAP trial, the patient is placed on a low level of CPAP (usually 5 cm H$_2$O) with or without supplemental oxygen and without any pressure support. With a T-piece trial, the patient is removed from the ventilator and humidified supplemental oxygen is provided to the airway. In this system, a corrugated tubing from the nebulizer/humidifier attaches to one end of the T-piece, and an extension of corrugated tubing attaches to the other end of the T-piece. The flow rate is adjusted to produce a constant mist coming from the extension piece on the T-tube both during inspiration and expiration so that the patient's minute ventilation is matched by the device. This corresponds to approximately at least three times the patient's minute ventilation There is some concern that the endotracheal tube increases the work of breathing. Therefore, a low-level PSV (5–10 cm H_2O) has been advocated as an ERT based on the hypothesis that this overcomes the resistance to breathing through the artificial airway. Several studies have shown that an appropriately sized endotracheal tube with an adequate inspiratory flow through a T-piece circuit does not increase the inspiratory work of breathing. The duration of an ERT can range from 30 min to 2 h. An ERT is terminated if any of the criteria listed in the Table 7.6 is not present. Instead of a specific level of pressure support, some ventilators such as the Servo-I have a volume-targeted pressure-support mode called volume support that can guarantee a minimal tidal volume and minute ventilation. When the pressure support level decreases to a predetermined low level usually < 8 cm H_2O while maintaining a tidal volume of at least 5 mL/kg, then the patient can be liberated from mechanical ventilation. Most clinicians prefer either a CPAP or a pressure support with PEEP trial.

7.3.5 Extubation

The patient must be awake, alert, and have airway protective reflexes. Breathing must be effective and without undue exertion. Adequate gas exchange with a relatively low FiO_2 must be established. Cardiovascular function with satisfactory perfusion is a prerequisite. When the ERT is deemed successful, the patient can be extubated and be liberated from mechanical ventilation to entirely spontaneous breathing without any positive pressure support. When the patient fails an ERT, he/she can still be extubated to noninvasive ventilation if they are suitable candidates. For patients to be candidates for non-invasive mechanical ventilation, they must have adequate airway protective reflexes and tolerate the necessary nasal mask or facemask. In infants, extubation to nasal CPAP may be an option. It is important to remember that while they have been liberated from endotracheal intubation, they have not been liberated from positive pressure support. Noninvasive ventilation, therefore, can be viewed as a transitional step toward complete liberation from positive pressure support.

Extubation failure is defined as the requirement for reintubation within 48 h after extubation.

Factors that prolong the weaning process are (1) slow resolution of the underlying disease process, (2) ventilatory pump failure, and (3) psychological factors. Ventilatory pump failure can be due to increased respiratory work load, decreased respiratory muscle capacity, or a combination of both. Decreased ventilatory drive may result from respiratory center dysfunction caused by sedative agents; neurological dysfunction, and metabolic alkalosis. Phrenic nerve injury, chest wall splinting and instability are contributing factors after cardiovascular surgery. They increase the work of breathing.

7.4 Ventilator Induced Lung Injury

Ventilator-induced lung injury (VILI) is a term that encompasses many aspects of injury caused by mechanical ventilation. Alveolar rupture can occur from over-distended alveoli. Pneumothorax, pneumomediastinum, pneumoperitoneum, pneumopericardium, interstitial emphysema and subcutaneous emphysema are all examples of overt ventilator-induced lung injury. These examples of extra-alveolar air can be life-threatening due to cardiovascular compromise. A bronchopleural fistula is a track that develops between the bronchus and the pleural space resulting in an almost continuous flow of air from the airway into the pleural space. Ventilator-induced lung injury can be minimized by protective lung ventilation.

7.4.1 Airway Injury

An endotracheal tube traversing the upper airway can be associated with significant airway injury. Tight taping can cause pressure injury leading to ulceration of the angle of the mouth (orotracheal tube) or ala nasi (nasotracheal tube). Palatal injury can range from simple ulceration to deep grooves including traumatic cleft palate in severe cases. Newborns and young infants are especially vulnerable because of their softer tissues. Laryngeal injury may extend from minor swelling to ulceration of the mucosa involving supraglottic structures and the vocal cords. A common injury seen in infants and children is in the subglottic region and may range from minor swelling to major ulceration. Scarring and granuloma formation can result in significant airway obstruction. The factors that increase the risk of tracheal injury are the size of the endotracheal tube, high cuff pressure, decreased tissue perfusion, upper respiratory tract infection, duration of intubation, and head/neck movement. Suctioning to keep the airways patent and clear secretions can also cause injuries if done vigorously. Tracheal injuries can lead to tracheal stenosis and/or tracheomalacia.

7.4.2 Biotrauma, Atelectrauma, Oxytrauma

Large V_T delivered at pressures with increased frequency cause cyclic strain, which may lead to disruption of the tight junctions between the alveolar epithelial and capillary endothelial cells and intracapillary blebs. The resultant biotrauma may cause the release of proinflammatory cytokines that further injure the lung and enter the systemic circulation, leading to multiorgan failure. Evidence shows that in patients with ARDS, avoidance of $V_T \geq$ 10 mL/kg and $P_{plat} \geq$ 30 cm H_2O limits alveolar damage. An barotrauma is a direct stress on the alveolar walls caused by cyclic opening and closing of the alveoli. Keeping PEEP above the lower P_{Flex} prevents repetitive alveolar collapse. It is important that alveolar units are neither overdistended nor collapsed. Careful adjustments of PEEP are also useful in lowering the FiO_2 another source of lung injury (oxytrauma). Although the FiO_2 value below which there is no risk of O_2 toxicity is unknown, a value < 0.6 is prudent.

7.4.3 Ventilator-Associated Pneumonia

The pathophysiology of ventilator-associated pneumonia (VAP) is multifactorial. Aspiration of oral and/or gastric secretions, colonization of ET tube, suppression of cough and impediment to mucociliary clearance play a collective role. New-onset fever and leukocytosis accompanied by demonstration of a newly observed infiltrate on chest radiograph are consistent with a diagnosis of VAP. Occurrence of VAP results in worsened gas exchange, increased duration of ventilation, and even death. Elevation of the head of the bed to 30 degrees after initiation of mechanical ventilation and oral decontamination measures during mechanical ventilation are effective means of reducing the risk for VAP. The most effective strategy to minimize any of the aforementioned complications is regular assessment of extubation readiness and liberation from mechanical ventilation as soon as clinically possible.

7.5 Heart–Lung Interactions

While anatomically the heart lies between two lungs, functionally the lungs are in between two types of heart circulations; systemic and pulmonary. It is hardly a surprise that alteration in one organ influences the function of the other. Heart-lung interactions can be classified as neural, humoral, functional, and mechanical. Neural interactions refer to the changes in the respiratory or cardiovascular system when the other system is perturbed due to neural connections between the two systems. For example, hypoxemia stimulates peripheral chemoreceptors and cause hyperpnea and hyperventilation. Lung inflation can induce reflex changes in heart rate. Humoral interactions are mediated through substances that are released by the lung during lung inflation which affects the cardiovascular system. Functional interactions refer to the effect of dysfunction of one system on the other. Heart failure can affect gas exchange and breathing. Chronic lung disease can result in pulmonary hypertension which can affect right ventricular function. These are referred to as functional heart–lung interactions. Mechanical interactions are due to the changes in lung volume and intrathoracic pressure affecting cardiovascular function.

7.5.1 Mechanical Heart–Lung Interactions

During inspiration, there is change in lung volume as well as a change in intrathoracic pressure. Intrathoracic pressure is negative during spontaneous breathing and negative pressure ventilation, while positive pressure ventilation increases the intrathoracic pressure during inspiration. Heart–lung interactions involve changes in lung volume or intrathoracic pressure affecting heart rate, preload, contractility and afterload of one or both ventricles. Lung inflation at normal tidal volumes increases heart rate by inhibiting the vagus nerve.

Spontaneous breathing increases venous return and right ventricular preload by increasing the gradient for venous return. Positive pressure ventilation on the other hand, decreases right ventricular preload by decreasing the gradient for venous return. The effect of positive pressure on venous return is exacerbated in shock, especially due to hypovolemia. This effect can be mitigated by bolus fluid administration. Pulmonary vascular resistance (PVR) is lowest at normal functional residual capacity. PVR increases when lung volume is below or above the functional residual capacity (Fig. 7.7). With atelectasis, there is local hypoxic pulmonary vascular resistance and kinking of vessels which leads to an increase in PVR. Hyperinflation of the lungs results in alveolar vessel compression and a rise in PVR. During spontaneous inspiration, right ventricular preload increases. The increase in right ventricular end-diastolic volume leads to a decrease in left ventricular end-diastolic volume and compliance and reduced left ventricular filling. The effects on afterload are different in right and left ventricle. Changes in intrathoracic pressure are shared equally by the right ventricle and pulmonary circulation, but while these changes are experienced by the left ventricle, a large part of systemic circulation is outside the thorax and not subjected to them. The left ventricular afterload is thus increased during inspiration while breathing spontaneously as it must generate greater cavity tension to overcome systemic vascular resistance. The decreased preload and increased afterload during inspiration is thought to be the mechanism for pulsus paradoxus during obstructed breathing such as with croup and asthma.

Practical Applications of Heart–Lung Interactions

The clinician has to consider several practical applications of heart–lung interactions when managing patients with mechanical ventilation. Many factors may influence decision making during invasive ventilation, the weaning process and thereafter.

Oxygen Cost of Breathing

Under resting conditions, oxygen cost of breathing is minimal, about 5% or less of the total oxygen consumption. A patient with normal cardiovascular function has a large reserve capacity to increase the cost of breathing such as with exercise. But with heart failure, the oxygen cost of breathing increases, and around 15% or greater, patient becomes dyspneic. When the demand of the respiratory muscles outstrips the cardiovascular system's ability to supply O_2, the respiratory muscles are prone to fatigue resulting in respiratory pump failure. Mechanical ventilation reduces the work of breathing and the oxygen cost of breathing, thereby reducing the fraction of blood flow needed for the respiratory muscles. During weaning, spontaneous breathing increases and may unmask cardiac dysfunction by a reduction in central/mixed venous oxygen saturation and an increase in lactate production.

Preload Responsiveness of the Heart

With a normal heart, which is preload-dependent, there is a cyclic variation in systolic blood pressure during mechanical ventilation. The normal difference between the peak increase and peak decrease is about 5–10 mmHg. This magnitude is increased with hypovolemia or a compromise in venous return such as with application of PEEP. The greater the magnitude, greater is the response to a fluid bolus. Thus, in a patient with circulatory shock, systolic pressure variation during mechanical ventilation can be used to determine whether a patient will respond to a fluid bolus. On the other hand, in heart failure where the heart is preload-independent, systolic blood pressure variation may be minimal or absent.

Improvement in Cardiovascular Performance in Heart Failure

In patients with heart failure, mechanical ventilation may improve cardiovascular performance by several mechanism: (1) increasing stroke volume by reducing the left ventricular afterload, (2) decreasing PVR by normalizing FRC, (3) reducing the demand on the heart by reducing the work of breathing, and (4) decreasing lactate production by respiratory muscles, and (5) improvement in gas exchange by decreasing alveolar edema and recruitment of alveoli.

Hemodynamic stability in Functionally Univentricular Lesions

Following a Fontan procedure for tricuspid atresia where pulmonary blood flow is passive, increase in intrathoracic pressure will not only decrease venous return but also increase the PVR. The end result is a decrease in the driving pressure for pulmonary blood flow and a decrease in cardiac output. Early extubation and spontaneous breathing are to be encouraged. Some patients may develop atelectasis and may need lung inflation or a distending pressure to maintain adequate lung volumes. Negative pressure ventilation offers an attractive alternative to these patients by creating a negative intrathoracic pressure which will recruit the lungs and increase the gradient to pulmonary blood flow.

In patients with univentricular physiology where the pulmonary and systemic blood flows are dependent on a single pumping chamber such as after Norwood procedure, a switch from positive pressure ventilation to spontaneous respiration may pose a formidable challenge after transitioning from positive pressure ventilation to spontaneous respirations after surgical repair. Increased afterload for the systemic circulation compared to that for the pulmonary circulation, may direct the cardiac output from the single pumping chamber preferentially to the pulmonary circulation resulting in potentially life-threatening systemic hypoperfusion syndrome and lactic acidosis. Such patients may benefit from reinstitution of either invasive or noninvasive positive pressure ventilation.

Suggested Readings

1. Sarnaik AP, Bauerfeld CP, Sarnaik AA: Mechanical ventilation. In: Kliegman RM, Stanton BF, St Geme JW, Schor NF, editors. Nelson textbook of pediatrics. 21st edn. Philadelphia: Elsevier.
2. Sarnaik AP, Daphtary K, Meert KL, Lieh-Lai MW, Heidemann SM: Pressure controlled
3. Ventilation in children with status asthmaticus. Pediatr Crit Care Med. 2004;5:133–8.
4. Gama de Abreu M, Belda FJ. Neurally adjusted ventilatory assist: letting the respiratory center take over control of ventilation. Intensive Care Med. 2013; 39:1481–1483
5. Ducharme-Crevier L, Du Pont-Thibodeau G, Emeriaud G. Interest of monitoring diaphragmatic electrical activity in the pediatric intensive care unit. Crit Care Res Pract. 2013; Article ID 384210:7.
6. Valentine KM, Sarnaik AA, Sandhu HS, Sarnaik AP. High frequency jet ventilation in respiratory failure secondary to respiratory syncytial virus infection: a case series. Front Pediatr. 2016 ;30(4):92.
7. Pappas MD, Sarnaik AP, Meert KL, Hasan RA, Lieh-Lai MW. Idopathic pulmonary hemorrhage in infancy: clinical features and management with high frequency ventilation. Chest. 1996;110:553–5.
8. Sarnaik AP, Meert KM, Pappas MD, Simpson PM, Lieh-Lai MW, Heidemann SM. Predicting outcome in children with severe acute respiratory failure treated with high-frequency ventilation. Crit Care Med. 1996;24:1396–402.
9. Corrado A, Gorini M. Negative-pressure ventilation: is there still a role? Eur Respir J. 2002;20:187–97.
10. Hess DR. Noninvasive ventilation in neuromuscular disease: equipment and application. Respir Care. 2006;51(8):896–912.
11. Hassinger AB, Breuer RK, Nutty K, et al. Negative-pressure ventilation in pediatric acute respiratory failure. Respir Care. 2017;62(12):1540–9.
12. Sarnaik AA, Sarnaik AP. Noninvasive ventilation in pediatric status asthmaticus: sound physiologic rationale but is it really safe, effective, and cost-efficient? Pediatr Crit Care Med. 2012;13(4):484–5.
13. Miller AG, Bartle RM, Feldman A, Mallory P, Reyes E, Scott B, Rotta AT. A narrative review of advanced ventilator modes in the pediatric intensive care unit. Transl Pediatr 2020 https://doi.org/10.21037/tp-20-332

Chapter 8
Mechanical Ventilation for Neonates

Nithi Fernandes and Sanjay Chawla

Common indications for the need for respiratory support in neonates include respiratory distress syndrome (RDS) due to surfactant deficiency, apnea of prematurity, bronchopulmonary dysplasia (BPD), meconium aspiration syndrome, transient tachypnea of the newborn, pulmonary hypoplasia due to congenital diaphragmatic hernia, congenital heart disease, and encephalopathy affecting respiratory drive and airway control.

There is a significant variation in the size (350 G to 10 kg), maturity (22 to 42 weeks gestation), and age (0–1 year) of patients admitted to Neonatal Intensive Care Units (NICU). Development of alveoli and pulmonary vasculature continues many years after birth. Pulmonary mechanics continue to evolve with age both in healthy infants and in those with underlying morbidity. It is important to consider the changing pulmonary mechanics and to understand the goals for optimal oxygenation and ventilation when deciding the appropriate respiratory support for an individual patient in NICU. The underlying differences in anatomy and physiology of the respiratory system of neonates, as compared to older children, need to be taken into account while providing respiratory support: (a) small mouth, relatively large tongue and a more superior laryngeal position make the laryngoscopy and endotracheal intubation more challenging, (b) the short tracheal size increases the risk of accidental extubation, as well as right main bronchus intubation, (c) a more compliant chest reduces functional residual capacity (FRC) and ventilatory efficiency in neonates with parenchymal lung disease, (d) a more horizontal insertion of diaphragm in the ribcage makes it work less efficiently, (e) the smaller airways increase airflow resistance, (f) the small endotracheal tube increases risk of tube obstruction and the risk of dampening of pressure with any small bend in the endotracheal tube, (g) the addition of flow sensors to the circuit carries a clinically

N. Fernandes · S. Chawla (✉)
Central Michigan University, Division of Neonatology, Children's Hospital of Michigan and
Hutzel Women's Hospital, 3901 Beaubien Boulevard, Detroit, MI 48201, USA
e-mail: schawla@dmc.org

© Springer Nature Switzerland AG 2022
A. P. Sarnaik et al. (eds.), *Mechanical Ventilation in Neonates and Children*,
https://doi.org/10.1007/978-3-030-83738-9_8

significant risk of increasing the total dead space, and (h) the high respiratory rate can make the end-tidal CO_2 (ETCO$_2$) readings to be inaccurate due to insufficient time for equilibration.

8.1 Respiratory Distress Syndrome (RDS)

Respiratory Distress Syndrome (RDS) is common among preterm infants. The diagnosis of RDS is based on the clinical features (tachypnea, nasal flaring, intercostal and subcostal retractions, head bobbing, grunting and apnea). Classic radiographic findings include low lung volume, generalized opacification of lungs, diffuse reticulogranular pattern and ground-glass appearance, and air bronchograms (Fig. 8.1).

8.1.1 Pathophysiologic Considerations

RDS occurs due to deficiency of surfactant which is associated with an increase in the surface tension at the air-fluid interface, increasing the risk of asymmetric lung

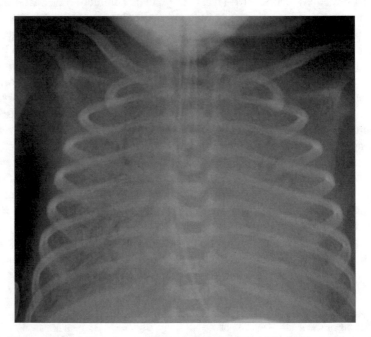

Fig. 8.1 Chest radiograph depicting classical findings of RDS with low lung volume, and diffuse reticulogranular pattern and ground-glass appearance with air bronchograms (Image courtesy of Dr. Sheena Saleem, Staff Radiologist, Children's Hospital of Michigan, Detroit)(Image courtesy of Dr. Sheena Saleem, Staff Radiologist, Children's Hospital of Michigan, Detroit)

expansion with multiple areas of atelectasis with some over-distended alveoli. The main pathophysiologic consequences include decreased FRC, decreased compli-ance, short time constant, and increased critical opening pressure. Ventilation perfusion mismatch along with poor lung compliance associated with atelectasis, causes hypoxemia and hypercarbia. Injury to the lungs and the airways is exacer-bated by mechanical ventilation, oxygen toxicity, patent ductus arteriosus (PDA) and infection.

8.1.2 Prevention of RDS

In pregnant women at risk of spontaneous preterm birth, use of progesterone is associated with decreased rates of preterm delivery. Antenatal steroids reduce the risk of RDS, mortality and intracranial hemorrhage in preterm infants. All pregnant women who are at risk of delivery within a week and fetal gestation between 23 and 34 weeks should receive antenatal steroids. Antenatal steroids help reduce the severity and incidence of RDS by increasing synthesis and release of surfactant, improving clearance of fluid from the lungs, and facilitating the maturation of fetal lung architecture (Fig. 8.2).

8.1.3 Delivery Room Stabilization

Neonatal Resuscitation Program (NRP) guidelines include achieving normothermia starting from the delivery room, maintaining environmental temperature of 25 °C, use of a plastic bag to cover the neonate and use of a chemical warming mattress. Following admission to NICU, preterm infants should be managed in the incubators with a high relative humidity to reduce insensible water losses. Every attempt should be made to provide a neutral thermal environment (NTE) defined as envi-ronmental conditions that allow for maintenance of body temperature with the least amount of O_2 consumption and energy expenditure.

8.1.4 Respiratory Support in the Delivery Room

There are insufficient data to guide optimal initial FiO_2 for preterm neonate based on gestational age. European Consensus Guidelines on the management of respi-ratory distress syndrome published in 2019 recommend using initial FiO_2 of 0.30 for neonates < 28 weeks' gestation, 0.21–0.30 for neonates between 28 and 31 weeks, and 0.21 for > 31 weeks of gestation. For spontaneously breathing preterm infants, initial respiratory support can be provided by continuous positive airway pressure (CPAP) delivered via nasal prongs or face mask. A large

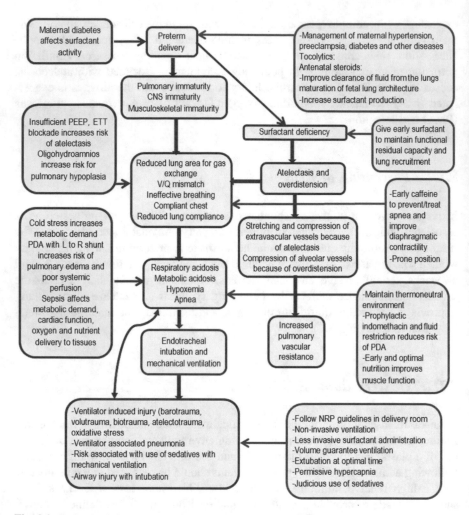

Fig. 8.2 Pathophysiology, prevention and management of RDS

randomized controlled trial (RCT) (GA 24–27 6/7 weeks, n = 1316) noted no significant difference in the primary outcome of death or BPD with prophylactic CPAP, as compared to intubation and early surfactant use for extremely preterm infants. Secondary analyses noted that use of CPAP was associated with a reduced rate of intubation, use of postnatal corticosteroids and a shorter duration of mechanical ventilation (MV), as compared with intubation and surfactant administration.

8.1.5 Respiratory Support During Hospital Stay

The goals of mechanical ventilation (MV) for preterm infants with RDS include provision of a stable airway, adequate lung recruitment, avoidance of hypoxemia and hypercarbia with the use of the lowest necessary tidal volume and peak inspiratory pressures. Approximately 80 to 90% of extremely preterm (gestational age < 28 weeks) infants receive MV to maintain oxygenation and ventilation. The indications for endotracheal intubation and MV among preterm infants include (a) lung immaturity, (b) surfactant deficiency, and (c) inability of the respiratory muscles to sustain large elastic workload. A longer duration of MV has been associated with an incremental increase in the risk of BPD. Volume-targeted mode is beneficial in patients with RDS due to auto-weaning of peak inspiratory pressure with a change in the respiratory compliance over time as the disease evolves and after surfactant administration. For preterm infants with RDS, volume targeted ventilation has been noted to be associated with lower rates of BPD or death and intracranial hemorrhage and a lower duration of mechanical ventilation, when compared to pressure-controlled ventilation. Significant hypocarbia, hypercarbia, as well as rapid fluctuations in $PaCO_2$ should be avoided to reduce the risk of intraventricular hemorrhage. In the initial days after birth, continuous monitoring of $PaCO_2$ may be helpful. Elective high frequency ventilation for preterm infants, as compared to conventional ventilator has been associated with an increased risk of pulmonary air leaks (gross air leaks or pulmonary interstitial emphysema), small but inconsistent reduction in risk of BPD, with no difference in mortality. High frequency ventilation may be better suited for patients with severe RDS needing high peak inspiratory pressure to maintain optimal ventilation and oxygenation to reduce the risk of air leaks.

Extubation of preterm infants to non-invasive respiratory support

A long cumulative duration of MV in preterm infants has been associated with higher rates of death and various neonatal morbidities, including upper airway injury, airway edema, subglottic stenosis, granulation tissue, neurodevelopmental impairment, and nosocomial infections. Appropriately timed extubation may reduce the risk of some of these complications. However, about 25 to 35% of elective extubations in preterm infants are not successful. Preterm neonates may fail extubation for various reasons such as increased work of breathing, apnea and bradycardia, low SPO_2, respiratory acidosis, and upper airway narrowing. A significant proportion (15%-20%) of extremely-low-birth-weight infants may be exposed to multiple courses of MV before discharge. Failed extubation has been independently associated with an increased risk of mortality, incidence of BPD, severe intracranial hemorrhage, longer hospitalization, and longer duration of supplemental oxygen and ventilator support.

Factors associated with extubation failure

Lower gestation, lower weight, male sex, prolonged ventilation (>2 weeks), low pre-extubation blood pH, and extubation from higher ventilatory settings have been noted to be associated with extubation failure. In addition, the presence of other morbidities, such as hemodynamically significant patent ductus arteriosus (PDA) and pulmonary hemorrhage, may reduce the likelihood of successful extubation. Because of the lack of a good prediction tool for extubation success, clinicians use different criteria for extubation and the timing of extubation is often based on the clinician's preference. Recently, Gupta et al. developed an extubation readiness estimator based on a study at our institution that included infants with birth weights $\leq$ 1,250g. Of 621 infants, 312 underwent elective extubation within the first 60 days of age. Extubation succeeded in 73%. Adjusted factors associated with successful extubation included greater gestational and chronological age, higher pre-extubation pH, and lower pre-extubation Fio_2, along with lower peak respiratory severity score (RSS) in the first 6 h of age. These data were used to develop an extubation readiness estimator that provides the probability of extubation success for an individual preterm infant (http://extubation.net).

Non-invasive respiratory support

Noninvasive respiratory support includes CPAP, humidified high-flow nasal cannula (HFNC), and non-invasive/nasal intermittent positive pressure ventilation (NIPPV). If feasible, noninvasive respiratory support is considered the preferred method to manage preterm neonates with RDS.

Continuous Positive Airway Pressure (CPAP)

CPAP involves delivering heated, humidified gas, with a constant, controlled pressure throughout the respiratory cycle. Potential benefits of CPAP for preterm neonates with RDS include splinting of the upper airway and maintenance of lung volume by prevention of atelectasis. The increase in FRC helps improve oxygenation. CPAP should be started after birth in all preterm neonates at risk of RDS (< 30 weeks' GA) who do not get intubated.

Non-invasive positive pressure ventilation (NIPPV)

NIPPV is frequently used for preterm infants with RDS. A recent meta-analysis (10 trials, n = 1,061) noted lower rates of respiratory failure, need for endotracheal intubation, with no difference in BPD and mortality associated with early NIPPV vs early CPAP. Use of NIPPV has also been shown to reduce the risk of extubation failure, as compared to CPAP in preterm infants.

Heated humidified high flow nasal cannula (HHFNC)

With HFNC, heated, humidified gas is delivered with nasal catheters at a flow rate that is at least 0.5 L/kg/min. The nasal catheters are small enough not to occlude the nostrils and therefore, generate inconsistent levels of CPAP which varies based on the flow rate as well as the size of the cannula and the leak around it. A potential benefit of HFNC is washout of carbon dioxide from the nasopharyngeal space. In a large multicenter trial, use of HFNC as the primary support for RDS resulted in significantly higher rate of treatment failure, compared to CPAP (25.5 vs. 13.3%). HFNC may not be as effective as CPAP as the initial support for extremely preterm infants but may be used as an alternative to CPAP for some infants during the weaning phase with the advantage of less nasal trauma. HFNC has similar rates of efficacy compared to nasal CPAP or respiratory support after intubation for preventing treatment failure [and reintubation. However, majority of studies excluded extremely preterm infants with GA < 28 weeks. There is insufficient evidence to support the use of HFNC as the primary mode of respiratory support after extubation of extremely preterm infants.

Neurally Adjusted Ventilatory Assist (NAVA)

In NAVA, a special orogastric tube with sensors is used to detect the electrical activity of the diaphragm (Edi or electrical activity of the diaphragm). The ventilator provides assists to spontaneous breaths by delivering a proportional pressure as determined by the NAVA level. The PIP delivered is proportional to the amount of Edi. Among intubated preterm infants, use of NAVA has been associated with reduced patient-ventilator asynchrony, lower PIP and FiO_2 requirement, and reduced need for sedation. No significant differences have been noted in the total duration of MV, rate of BPD, pneumothorax or intraventricular hemorrhage with the use of NAVA, compared with conventional ventilation. Suggested respiratory settings for neonates with RDS are shown in Table 8.1.

8.1.6 Role of Surfactant in Patients with RDS

Patients with RDS benefit from administration of exogenous surfactant. There are various types of synthetic and animal-derived surfactants. Figure 8.3 shows two adjacent alveolar units of different sizes. With surfactant deficiency, surface tension is elevated to the same degree in both units. According to Laplace's law ($P = 2 T/R$; where P is pressure, T is surface tension and R is the radius), the pressure in the smaller alveolus will be greater than that in the larger alveolus (Fig A). The smaller alveolus will tend to empty into the larger one leading to atelectasis and uneven ventilation. After surfactant administration (Fig B), the surface tension in the smaller unit will be lower than that in the larger unit due to higher concentration of surfactant (surfactant per unit surface area). Lower surface tension will counterbalance the effect of smaller radius resulting in reduction and equilibration of pressures (P1 and P2), and stability of alveoli.

Timing of surfactant

Neonates who are intubated for RDS should receive surfactant as soon as possible. Rescue surfactant should be considered early in the course for preterm neonates with RDS who have worsening clinical course when FiO_2 is more than 30% on CPAP pressure of at least 6 cm H_2O. With greater experience and availability of non-invasive ventilation for preterm infants starting in the delivery room along with greater use of antenatal steroids, the need for endotracheal intubation for prophylactic surfactant has decreased.

Table 8.1 Respiratory support for patients with RDS

Type of respiratory support	Range of respiratory support*
Non-invasive Support	
HFNC	2–4 L/minute
CPAP	4–8 cm H_2O
NIPPV	PEEP: 4–6 cm H_2O PIP: 15–30 cm H_2O Rate: 20–40/min I time: 0.4–0.5 s
Conventional Ventilation via ETT	
Pressure control	PEEP: 4–6 cm H_2O PIP: 14–25 cm H_2O Rate: 30–60/min I time: 0.30–0.40 s
Volume control	PEEP: 4–6 cm H_2O Tidal volume: 4–6 ml/Kg Rate: 14–60/min I time: 0.3–0.40 s
High Frequency Ventilation via ETT	
HFOV	MAP: 9–15 cm H_2O Amplitude: 18–40 cm H_2O Frequency: 12–15 Hz
Jet ventilator	PEEP: 7–12 cm H_2O HFJV PIP: 15–45 cm H_2O HFJV Rate: 420/min HFJV I time: 0.02 s IMV rate: 0–2/min IMV PIP: 16–35 cm H_2O

HFNC: High flow nasal cannula, CPAP: Continuous positive airway pressure, NIPPV: Nasal Intermittent positive pressure ventilation, HFOV: High frequency oscillatory ventilator, PEEP: Positive end expiratory pressure, MAP: Mean airway pressure; HFJV: high frequency jet ventilator, IMV: Intermittent mandatory ventilation, PIP: Peak inspiratory pressure
* In some patients, higher respiratory support may be needed. Consider switching to a different mode of ventilation if goals for oxygenation and ventilation not met

Techniques of surfactant administration

There are currently two methods to administer surfactant, the Intubation-Surfactant Administration-Extubation (IN-SUR-E) and Less Invasive Surfactant Administration (LISA) techniques. IN-SUR-E procedure involves intubation, surfactant administration and extubation. Earlier studies noted some benefit of INSURE, compared to rescue surfactant administration in reducing the duration of mechanical ventilation. However, patients often are pre-medicated with opioids which affect respiratory drive. Endotracheal intubation may be associated with patient discomfort, traumatic airway injury, lung atelectasis, infection, hemodynamic instability, and altered brain function as monitored with

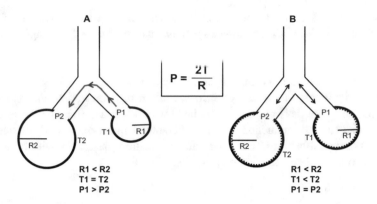

$$P = \frac{2I}{R}$$

Fig. 8.3 With deficiency of surfactant, according to Laplace's law, at a similar surface tension, the smaller alveolar units will generate higher pressure (P1 > P2) and tend to empty into the larger ones (Fig. A). The end result is atelectasis and uneven distribution of alveolar gas. With surfactant administration (Fig. B), not only is the surface tension decreased, but it is decreased to a greater extent in the smaller alveoli as the surfactant is more concentrated in a smaller surface area. The end result is that the surface tension in smaller alveoli (T1) is reduced to a greater extent than in the larger ones (T2), resulting in pressure equalization (P1 = P2) and alveolar stability

electroencephalography. Endotracheal intubation may be technically challenging, and only half of the first intubation attempts by trainees are successful, resulting in adverse events including severe oxygen desaturations. A recent meta-analysis (9 clinical trials, n = 1,551 neonates) compared outcome of infants treated with IN-SUR-E or CPAP alone. There were no differences between early IN-SUR-E and CPAP group for all neonatal morbidities including BPD, death, air leaks, severe intracranial hemorrhage and neurodevelopmental delay. Current evidence does not support that early IN-SUR-E is superior to CPAP alone. There is concern that even a brief period of invasive mechanical ventilation may be associated with lung injury.

A modified IN-SUR-E technique, also known as LISA (less invasive surfactant administration) involves surfactant administration using a small feeding tube (3.5 to 5 French) placed 1 cm below the glottis in a spontaneously breathing neonate without any premedication.

A recent systematic review and meta-analysis (6 RCTs, n = 895) noted that preterm neonates randomized to less invasive surfactant administration (LISA) had lower rate of composite outcome of death or BPD, less invasive mechanical ventilation within 72 h of birth, and need for mechanical ventilation anytime during NICU stay, as compared to those randomized to standard method of delivering surfactant via an endotracheal tube.

Role of caffeine

Caffeine for Apnea of Prematurity (CAP) trial showed that caffeine was associated with earlier extubation, reduction in BPD and reduction in neurologic impairment at 18 months of age. A few observational studies have noted that the early use of caffeine is associated with a reduction in BPD. The standard dose of caffeine citrate is a loading dose of 20 mg/kg, followed by maintenance dose of 5–10 mg/kg per day.

Fluid management and Nutrition

It is important to assess the fluid balance frequently as extremely preterm infants may have significant insensible water loss. Fluid restriction in premature infants in the initial postnatal days has been associated with a reduced risk of PDA and NEC with a trend towards reduction of BPD. Parenteral nutrition should be started as soon as possible after birth. Minimal enteral nutrition preferably with breast milk should also be initiated as soon as possible.

8.2 Bronchopulmonary Dysplasia

Bronchopulmonary dysplasia (BPD) is an acquired chronic lung disease that occurs because of premature birth. BPD is diagnosed in nearly 50% of children born before 28 weeks' GA and nearly 90% of infants born before 24 weeks of GA.

There are multiple published criteria for the diagnosis and classification of severity of BPD. Most widely used definition was proposed by the National Institute of Health in 2000. A more recent definition proposed by Jensen et al. (2019) classifies BPD into 3 grades based on the level of respiratory support administered at 36 weeks' postmenstrual age, regardless of fraction of supplemental oxygen. Based on the receipt of respiratory support at 36 weeks' postmenstrual age, infants are classified into:

1. No BPD—No respiratory support
2. Grade 1 ($\leq$ 2L/min flow)
3. Grade 2 (>2L/min flow or CPAP or NIV)
4. Grade 3 or Severe BPD (invasive mechanical ventilation).

8.2.1 Pathophysiology of BPD and Approach to Respiratory Support

BPD is a chronic disease that evolves with time and is affected by the interplay of ongoing lung injury, body's response to injury, repair mechanism and continued lung maturation and growth over a period of months to years after birth. In contrast to a relatively homogenous lung disease noted in RDS involving the alveoli, lung disease in patients with BPD is more heterogenous, with involvement of both large and small airways in addition. Chest radiograph in a patient with BPD may show coarse, linear densities due to fibrosis or atelectasis, lucent cystic foci, or overall hyper-expansion of lungs due to air trapping (Fig. 8.4).

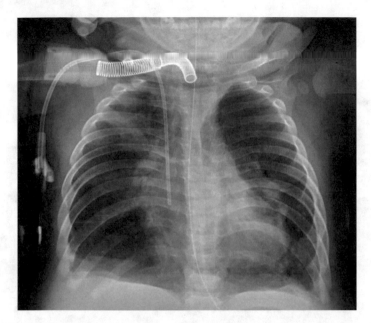

Fig. 8.4 Chest radiograph depicting classical findings of BPD with coarse, linear densities, lucent cystic foci, and overall hyper-expansion of lungs (Image courtesy of Dr. Sheena Saleem, Staff Radiologist, Children's Hospital of Michigan, Detroit, MI)

Patients may have varying degrees of subglottic stenosis and/or tracheobron-chomalacia, especially noted among patients with grade 3 BPD. Two segments within the same lung may have significant variability in airway resistance and lung compliance. In addition, most infants have varying severity of pulmonary hypertension. The management must consider the differences in pathophysiology such as changes in FRC, and time constants that are unique to each patient. Considerable individual variations in pathophysiology means that the management needs to be tailored to the needs of each patient.

While the management in each patient may be different due to the underlying pathophysiology, the general principles of respiratory management are to optimize gas exchange, minimize dead space, avoid intermittent hypoxemia, reduce oxidative and ventilator induced injury and minimize patient discomfort. A patient with BPD with significant tracheobronchomalacia may benefit from higher positive end expiratory pressure (PEEP) to match the collapsing pressure of the airway to reduce the risk of hyperinflation and inadvertent PEEP. A patient with BPD with primarily lung parenchymal disease may need just enough PEEP to prevent atelectasis.

There are limited data to suggest target oxygen saturations in patients with established BPD. The BPD collaborative group suggests targeting oxygen saturations between 92 and 95%. Patients with pulmonary hypertension may benefit with higher saturation target which may prevent an increase in the pulmonary vascular resistance. Up to 25% of patients with BPD have pulmonary hypertension. Patients

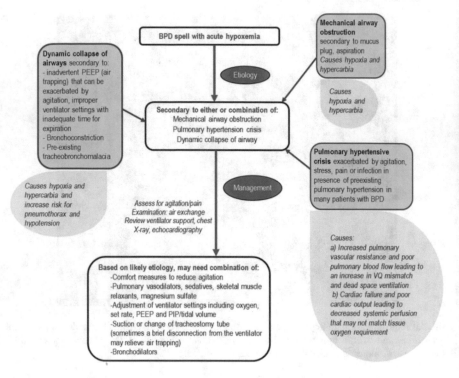

Fig. 8.5 Pathophysiology and management of a BPD spell (Hypoxic Spell)

with BPD sometimes have sudden episodes of desaturations described as BPD/ hypoxic spells. These episodes could occur secondary to airway collapse, bronchospasm, pulmonary hypertension or a combination of all three. It is important to understand the pathophysiology of BPD spell for each patient for optimal management (Fig. 8.5).

8.2.2 Respiratory Support for Patients with BPD

Based on the severity of lung, airway and vascular disease, patients may require oxygen and respiratory support for a prolonged duration. Many patients can be successfully supported via CPAP, HHFNC, or low-flow nasal cannula if they are able to show adequate growth and development with no/minimal increase in the work of breathing. Invasive mechanical ventilation may be required if non-invasive ventilatory support is inadequate. For all patients, general principles to guide respiratory support for patients with established BPD include (a) targeting oxygen saturations between 92 and 95%, (b) use of large tidal volume to account for dead space, (c) adequate PEEP to avoid atelectasis and prevent airway collapse, (d) low

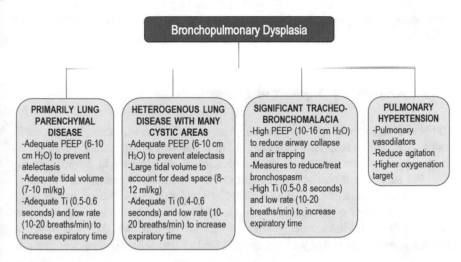

Fig. 8.6 Respiratory support of a patient with BPD based on primary pathophysiology. *For all patients, general principles to guide respiratory support for patients with established BPD include: (a) targeting oxygen saturations between 92 and 96%, (b) use of adequate tidal volume to account for dead space, (c) adequate PEEP to avoid atelectasis and prevent airway collapse, (d) low set rate and high inspiratory time due to long time constant, (e) tolerance of higher $PaCO_2$, and (f) monitoring for pulmonary hypertension

set rate and high Inspiratory time due to high time constant, and (e) tolerance of higher $PaCO_2$ (Fig. 8.6).

Due to heterogeneity of the disease and an increased dead space in patients with BPD, a larger tidal volume (8 to 12 ml/kg) may be necessary, as compared to infants with RDS, where a tidal volume of 4 to 6 ml/kg is used. In some patients, PIP needed to achieve this tidal volume may reach 30–45 cm H_2O. Generally, patients with BPD have a long time constant and they can benefit from lower set rates (< 20 breaths/minute) and longer inspiratory times (0.6–0.8 s) with adequate pressure support for spontaneous breaths. In contrast to patients with RDS who generally need a PEEP of 4–6 cm H_2O, patients with BPD often need a higher level of PEEP due to the tendency for collapse of large and small airways during exhalation secondary to tracheobronchomalacia. Higher ventilatory rates may predispose to auto-PEEP and hyperinflation due to incomplete emptying of the alveoli. Patients with BPD often have high airway resistance secondary to bronchospasm and a tendency for collapse of large and small airways during exhalation due to tracheobronchomalacia. The prolonged time constant necessitates greater exhalation time for adequate alveolar emptying. Higher ventilatory rates may result in air trapping manifested as hyperinflated lungs on chest radiographs (Fig. 8.4). Selection of optimal PEEP is based on clinical examination for air exchange, chest radiograph to assess degree of lung inflation, monitoring the change in compliance and resistance at different PEEP settings, the use of expiratory pause maneuver on the ventilator (to evaluate the auto-PEEP level), and occasionally with the help of bronchoscopy to assess the distending pressure needed to avoid large airway collapse.

8.2.3   Respiratory Support at Home

The goal is to wean patients to room air prior to discharge. However, some patients continue to require respiratory support at home that can range from supplementary oxygen by low-flow nasal cannula to mechanical ventilation via a tracheostomy tube. For safe patient care at home, appropriate instruction of caregivers for care of the infant about medications, feeding, cardiopulmonary resuscitation, use of home ventilator and other monitoring devices needs to be done. As the lung development continues into childhood, many patients can be weaned off the ventilator and decannulated over first few years of age. (Refer to Chap. 12 on chronic ventilation).

8.3   Meconium Aspiration Syndrome (MAS)

8.3.1   Pathophysiology

Meconium, an infant's first stool, contains bile acids, bile pigments, mucopolysaccharides, fatty acids, pancreatic enzymes, vernix, lanugo and swallowed fetal cells. The incidence of meconium-stained amniotic fluid (MSAF) increases with gestational age causing respiratory distress in a subset of infants, defined as meconium aspiration syndrome (MAS). Children who survive MAS may have a higher incidence of exercise-induced airway hyper-reactivity later in life.

The aspiration of meconium either before or during birth can lead to several physical, chemical and biological effects. These include surfactant deactivation, inflammation, and a variable obstructive component often referred to as the ball-valve effect of air-trapping (Fig. 8.7). This leads to over-inflation in some areas and atelectasis in others and is reflected in the patchy chest roentgenogram in cases of MAS (Fig. 8.8). In MAS, end-expiratory lung volume is decreased due to atelectasis in some areas and increased due to hyperinflation in other areas. Compliance is decreased at extremes of FRC (Fig. 8.9). Time constants are variable in different areas, decreased due to atelectasis and prolonged due to increased resistance.

Pulmonary vascular resistance (PVR) is high in the fetal circulation and decreases over the first few days after birth. PVR often remains elevated in MAS for two reasons; (a) coexistence of hypertrophy of medial musculature of smaller acinar pulmonary arterioles and (b) pulmonary vasoconstriction due to hypoxia and acidosis. Additionally, PVR increases with atelectasis, and with hyperinflation. To manage both of these extremes, ventilation goals include adequate PEEP and

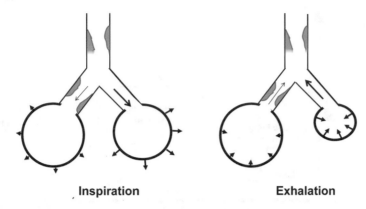

Inspiration   **Exhalation**

Fig. 8.7 Ball-valve phenomenon: Meconium in the airway leads to air trapping on expiration. During inspiration, air entry in meconium-obstructed lung units is decreased but it is unimpeded in those that are unobstructed. During exhalation, the air is trapped by the ball-valve effect of the meconium in the obstructed segment while unobstructed segment empties normally. The obstructed segment is hyperinflated but hypoventilated while the unobstructed segment is normally aerated and ventilated

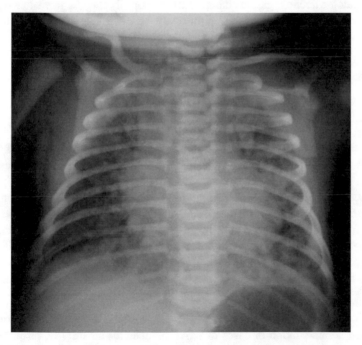

Fig. 8.8 Chest X-ray depicting classical findings of meconium aspiration syndrome with hyperinflated lungs and patchy infiltrates overlying lung parenchyma (Image courtesy of Dr. Sheena Saleem, Staff Radiologist, Children's Hospital of Michigan, Detroit)

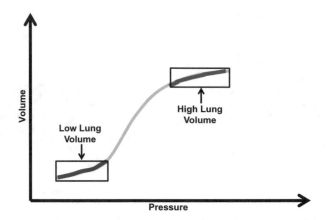

Fig. 8.9 Lung compliance is decreased at extremes of lung volume. MAS results in variable lung volume changes depending on the extent of airway obstruction. Incomplete obstruction results in air-trapping and complete obstruction causes atelectasis

PIP. Meconium obstruction in the distal airways leads to ventilation-perfusion (V/Q) mismatch affecting gas exchange further contributing to persistence of pulmonary hypertension. An altered pulmonary vascular reactivity exacerbates the presentation, leading to severe hypoxemia. Ventilation strategies in MAS need to optimize oxygenation while avoiding worsening over-distension.

8.3.2 Management at Delivery

The presence of MSAF classifies a delivery as high-risk and a team capable of neonatal resuscitation should be present. The most recent Neonatal Resuscitation Program (NRP) guidelines do not advocate tracheal suctioning of meconium prior to resuscitative efforts. Routine stimulation, bulb suctioning and attention to respiratory effort are warranted. If needed, a larger suction catheter should be used to remove any obstructive meconium in the pharynx. Deep, gastric suctioning is not recommended. If positive pressure ventilation is required based on the NRP algorithm, total pressures should be monitored closely as excessive pressures can increase the risk of pulmonary air leak syndromes, particularly pneumothorax.

Surfactant Therapy

The presence of meconium in MAS can deactivate endogenous surfactant. Surfactant administration in cases of MAS reduces the severity of respiratory distress and is widely used to improve oxygenation. A meta-analysis has shown a reduction in the progression to Extracorporeal Membrane Oxygenation (ECMO), without a statistically significant effect on air leak complications or mortality.

8.3.3 Approach to Ventilation

The goals of ongoing respiratory support in these infants are to increase oxygenation and reduce V/Q mismatch by optimizing lung recruitment while minimizing over-inflation.

Oxygen is a potent pulmonary vasodilator which should be used judiciously to maintain a pre-ductal PaO_2 of 50–70 mm Hg. Oxygen hood or tents are not recommended because of the risk of alveolar collapse from the absence of PEEP, which can worsen the intrapulmonary shunt or V/Q mismatch. Excess oxygen can also lead to toxicity, potentially worsening pulmonary vascular resistance and oxidative stress. Table 8.2 summarizes parameters to monitor infants with MAS and target ventilation.

Non-invasive Respiratory Support

Non-invasive respiratory support including NIPPV is the preferred initial modality in an infant with MAS with respiratory distress. Of note, NIPPV in the setting of MAS does not eliminate the risk of air leak syndromes particularly that of pneumothorax. Peak inspiratory pressures, chest X-rays and the infant's clinical status must be closely monitored.

High Flow Nasal Cannula

There are limited outcome data assessing the role of this therapy in the setting of MAS. Initial flow rates may be higher (4–6 L/min) than with other infants who have mild distress to achieve adequate oxygenation. When FiO_2 exceeds 0.30 and flow requirement exceeds 6L/min, CPAP/NIV should be considered.

CPAP CPAP decreases upper airway resistance, augments spontaneous respiration, increases transpulmonary pressure and maintains FRC, thereby improving lung compliance and decreasing the need for intubation. While distending large airways, it supports the expiratory phase of breathing by avoiding air trapping or the ball-valve phenomenon. With airway obstruction, there is a risk of "intrinsic" or "inadvertent" PEEP. Adequate level of extrinsic PEEP will help stabilize the airways without impeding expiratory flow and worsening hyperinflation. Extrinsic PEEP overcomes the intrinsic or inadvertent PEEP of air-trapping on expiration, ameliorating airway obstruction while improving work of breathing. Some infants respond to CPAP, if applied early in the course resulting in decreasing the need for mechanical ventilation. These infants may require CPAP for a week or more.

Table 8.2 Target respiratory parameters when managing infants with MAS.

Respiratory parameter	Target
PaO_2 (pre-ductal)	50-70 mmHg
Saturations (pre-ductal)	90–95%
P_aCO_2	45-55 mmHg

NIPPV NIPPV reduces work of breathing by generating a distending airway pressure, washing out nasopharyngeal dead space and recruiting collapsed alveoli to establish FRC. By adding a rate and inspiratory pressure, NIPPV has been shown to be superior to CPAP in avoiding intubation in late preterm and term infants. It augments spontaneous respiratory effort by providing a positive pressure breath. Synchronized NIPPV (synchronized with the infant's inspiratory efforts) is more effective at avoiding unintended PEEP or overexpansion. It can be synchronized using a flow sensor to detect spontaneous inspiratory flow or NAVA electrical activity of the diaphragm. Unsynchronized NIPPV may also achieve effective tidal volumes for gas exchange but needs to be more closely monitored for over or under-expansion. Monitoring the infant's improvement in oxygenation and blood gases suffices while on NIPPV. Chest radiographs are not routinely obtained. Initial rates of 30–40/min are recommended as these higher rates lead to better respiratory muscles unloading. PEEP should start at 5 cm H_2O, with PIP targeted to 20–25 cm H_2O. Persistent respiratory acidosis ($PaCO_2 > 60$ torr) and/or FiO_2 requirement > 0.40 suggests the need for intubation and invasive MV.

MECHANICAL VENTILATION The reasons for intubation include clinical deterioration demonstrated by (1) worsening clinical distress (2) increased oxygen requirements (3) worsening hypoxemia/acidosis (4) clinical instability and (5) intolerance of CPAP. Either pressure or volume-targeted ventilation can be utilized. Positive pressure ventilation can compromise hemodynamics if intrathoracic pressure is too high from air-trapping and this should be kept in mind when increasing pressures to target ventilation and oxygenation.

SIMV CMV can be started with either pressure-controlled or volume-targeted ventilation. To address the pathophysiology of MAS resulting in obstructive airway disease, ventilation goals include low ventilator rate (30/min), adequate expiratory time to minimize air-trapping and as minimal PEEP as needed to achieve sufficient oxygenation. "Gentle ventilation" strategies are employed with the premise of minimizing lung injury by avoiding high pressures (barotrauma), allowing the lung to heal from the inflammatory effects of meconium, while delivering adequate oxygen. Higher tidal volume and minute ventilation is required in MAS due to increased dead space. Volume-targeted ventilation of 4–6 mL/kg, targeting initial PIP limited to 25 cm H_2O, with PEEP of to 5 cm H_2O. To avoid air trapping, there should be adequate expiratory time, by setting the inspiratory time (T_i) to 0.3–0.4 s. The initial rate is generally 30/min and increased as needed. Reducing the respiratory rate will allow for greater expiratory time to address air-trapping. Mean airway pressures should be observed on the conventional ventilator to infer compliance. If oxygenation is limited despite increasing PEEP to 7 cm H_2O and/or PIP to more than 25 cm H_2O to achieve a higher MAP, the infant likely needs more respiratory support and high frequency ventilation should be considered. The choice of HFOV or HFJV depends on the clinician's expertise and comfort as there is no clear consensus on which is superior in MAS.

HFOV High frequency oscillatory ventilation uses a set MAP to control oxygenation, generally selected to be 2–3 cm H_2O higher than that generated by the prior CMV settings. Chest X-rays should be obtained when switching ventilator

Table 8.3 MAS initial ventilation strategies

Ventilation	CPAP	NIPPV	PC	VT	HFOV	HFJV
PIP (cm H₂O)		20	23	20 (limit)		20
T$_i$ (s)		0.5	0.3	0.3	1:2	0.02
Rate (breaths/min)		40	30	30		420
V$_T$ exhaled (ml/kg)				4–5		
PEEP (cm H₂O)	5–6	5–6		5–6		
Mean P$_{AW+}$ (cm H₂O)					10–12*	8–10
Amplitude					25	
Frequency (Hz)					10–12	

* Mean P$_{AW}$ is generally 2 cm H₂O more than the MAP on CMV

modalities to help avoid hyper-expansion with a target rib expansion of 8–9. Frequency often varies with the size of the infant with lower frequencies often set for larger infants. A lower frequency increases expiratory time which will help in MAS. Amplitude is adjusted based on the chest movement and PCO_2.

HFJV Since targeting MAP and ultimately the oxygenation is the goal in managing MAS, PEEP is the essential variable in jet ventilation. It usually starts higher than CMV, 8–12 cm H₂O. The back-up rate or "sigh breaths" should remain between 0 and 2. HFJV frequency is set at 420/min. Adequate PIP varies according to PCO_2. It can start at 20 cm H₂O with Ti 0.02, adjusted for PCO_2 45–55 torr and adequate chest movement. If PIP more than 45 is necessary, the inspiratory time should be increased.

Table 8.3 summarizes initial ventilation strategies for infants with meconium aspiration syndrome. The oxygenation index (OI) is often used to gauge the extent of hypoxemia in the infant.

Using arterial blood gases (ideally pre-ductal) the following calculation can be used whereby FiO₂ is expressed as a fraction or decimal (if you use the fraction, you have to multiply by 100, otherwise use FiO₂ in percent), MAP is the mean airway pressure on either on CMV, HFOV or HFJV:

$$OxygenationIndex = \frac{FiO_2 \times MAP}{PaO_2}$$

For example, a patient receiving 0.8 FiO₂ with MAP of 20 cm H₂O, and a PaO₂ of 64 torr, has OI of $(0.8 \times 20 \div 64) \times 100 = 25$. An OI > 15–20 suggests the need for inhaled nitric oxide and > 40 is when ECMO should be considered.

8.3.4 Ventilator Weaning Strategies in MAS

It may take several days and sometimes weeks for the PVR to gradually decrease enough for ventilation parameters to be weaned. Weaning should be gradual so as not to compromise lung excursion. If on HFOV, reduce MAP by 1 cm H_2O or amplitude by 2 cm H_2O every 6 h as tolerated. There is no absolute requirement to wean from the oscillator to conventional ventilation prior to extubation. It is possible to wean ventilation support on the oscillator to very low settings (MAP 8 cm H_2O, 15 Hz, Amplitude < 25 cm H_2O) and extubate directly from the oscillator. Synchronized NIPPV or CPAP can bridge the support after extubation. FiO_2 < 0.40 and consistently lower PCO_2 < 45 mm Hg are reasonable extubation parameters. CPAP can be weaned off to HFNC or room air when FiO_2 is consistently < 0.3 with SpO_2 > 90%.

8.4 Congenital Diaphragmatic Hernia

Congenital diaphragmatic hernia (CDH) is a malformation resulting in the migration of intra-abdominal organs into the thoracic cavity during fetal development (Fig. 8.10). This compromises fetal lung development, leading to pulmonary

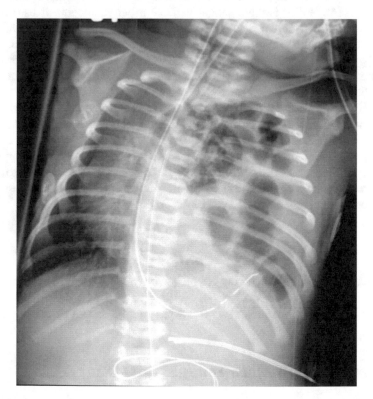

Fig. 8.10 Chest X-ray depicting left-sided congenital diaphragmatic hernia with gas-filled intestinal loops in the left hemithorax with mediastinal shift to the right (Image courtesy of Dr. Sheena Saleem, Staff Radiologist, Children's Hospital of Michigan, Detroit)(Image courtesy of Dr. Sheena Saleem, Staff Radiologist, Children's Hospital of Michigan, Detroit)

hypoplasia with involvement of both ipsilateral and contralateral lungs. Pulmonary hypoplasia is worse on the ipsilateral side. Altered vascular reactivity and reduction in the pulmonary vasculature commonly leads to pulmonary hypertension. The most common defect is posterolateral (Bochdalek hernia), followed by anteromedial (Morgagni hernia).

8.4.1 Prenatal Diagnosis and Fetal Surgery

Prenatal ultrasound is the gold-standard diagnostic test for CDH, but it identifies less than two-thirds of CDH pregnancies. Characteristic findings include displaced intestinal contents, or indirect signs such as mediastinal shifts, polyhydramnios or a change in the cardiac axis.

With earlier diagnosis, in-utero therapeutic intervention aims to counter the potential effects of lung hypoplasia by occluding the trachea. Tracheal occlusion allows for retention of fetal lung fluid to improve alveolar growth. Prolonged tracheal occlusion however can decrease type II pneumocyte maturation and lead to surfactant deficiency. A percutaneous sono-endoscopic approach to the plug-unplug sequence has replaced traditional fetal surgical methods to occlude the trachea, optimally performed between 27 and 29 weeks.

Despite an increased rate of prenatal diagnosis, overall survival in CDH remains low, approximately 65–72%. The observed-to-expected lung area to head circumference ratio (O/E LHR), best obtained between 18 and 38 weeks of gestation, can predict survival and neonatal outcomes in isolated CDH. Additionally, the presence of the stomach and/or liver within the thoracic herniated contents carries a poor prognosis.

8.4.2 Pathophysiology

Pulmonary hypoplasia is pathognomonic of CDH. The severity of pulmonary insufficiency in CDH depends on the degree of pulmonary hypoplasia, which in turn depends on the size of the defect, and how early in gestation the abdominal contents were displaced. Impaired branching morphogenesis, acinar hypoplasia, decreased terminal bronchioles and failed alveolarization all contribute to decreased compliance and FRC. Gas exchange is impaired leading to severe hypoxemia. Time constant is reduced due to reduced compliance. Effective ventilation targets adequate end-expiratory pressures so as to maintain FRC, with adequate mean airway pressure to achieve oxygenation.

Due to vascular remodeling, the physiological decline in pulmonary vascular resistance (PVR) does not occur in CDH. As a large cross-sectional area is required to achieve a low resistance, a reduced cross-sectional area limits the ability of the lungs to lower vascular resistance after birth. High PVR causes dilation and hypertrophy of the right ventricle (RV), often leading to RV diastolic dysfunction. Reduced pulmonary venous return reduces preload for the left ventricle, with high afterload for the right ventricle. LV hypoplasia and dysfunction often seen in left-sided CDH is exacerbated by right-sided dysfunction. Pulmonary hypertension remains persistent and severe, often complicated by systemic hypotension due to cardiac dysfunction and decreased cardiac output. Thus, both left and right ventricular outputs often remain dependent on persistent fetal shunts (foramen ovale and ductus arteriosus) demonstrated in Fig. 8.11. Pulmonary vascular remodeling and hypertrophy are often irreversible and pulmonary hypertension is refractory to therapy. Due to classically seen LV dysfunction, nitric oxide is not routinely used in the management of hypoxemia as it can worsen post-capillary or pulmonary venous hypertension. However, brief trials with NO therapy can offer some short-term benefits..

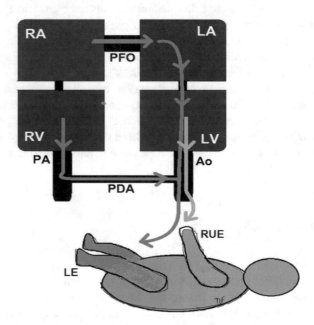

Fig. 8.11 With postnatal pulmonary hypertension, systemic circulation depends on shunting through persistent foramen ovale (PFO) and patent ductus arteriosus (PDA). Part of the right atrium (RA) blood is diverted through the PFO and mixes with the oxygenated blood in the left atrium (LA) to be pumped through the left ventricle (LV) and aorta (Ao) to the head and upper extremities. The remaining part of the RA blood is pumped through the right ventricle (RV), and a significant portion is shunted across the PDA into the descending Ao to the lower part of the body. This results in differential oxygenation with SpO_2 being higher in upper extremities compared to lower extremities

8.4.3 Management at Delivery

Perinatal management is an essential determinant to survival. Without an antenatal diagnosis, a scaphoid abdomen with bowel sounds auscultated in the chest and heart sounds on the right should raise a high suspicion of CDH. A gastric tube to continuous suction should be immediately placed for decompression to avoid intestinal insufflation resulting in compromised bowel perfusion and increased intrathoracic extra-pulmonary pressure. Non-invasive ventilation is not recommended with known CDH. Bag-mask ventilation should be avoided to minimize peak pressures delivered to the lungs; instead the Neopuff™ T-piece resuscitator with nasal prongs can be used to control inspiratory pressures during initial stabilization. If the infant is spontaneously breathing, they may be observed closely. Saturations in the newborn period are often referred to as "pre-" or "post"-ductal in reference to the arterial branching relative to the location of the ductus arteriosus. Pre-ductal perfusion tends to be higher in oxygen content due to the preferential flow of oxygenated blood to the upper body (Fig. 8.11). Post-ductal saturations represent mixed venous and arterial blood with lower SpO_2 in the lower extremities. Immediately after birth, pre- and post-ductal saturations should be closely monitored, with pre-ductal > 70% tolerated if infant is relatively stable and improving. Figure 8.11 displays the differential saturations, a result of increased right sided cardiac pressures (due to high PVR).

Surfactant deficiency specifically in CDH relates to lung size as opposed to the deficiency in preterm infants. In term infants with CDH, there is no clear benefit of routine surfactant administration for CDH and many current guidelines do not recommend it.

8.4.4 Approach to Ventilation

Invasive ventilation strategies have been attempted to be standardized to decrease morbidity amongst survivors of CDH. A clear superiority of either HFOV or CMV has not been established although outcome measures such as the need for ECMO and ventilator days might favor CMV. The "gentle ventilation" strategy with intermittent mandatory ventilation (IMV) is recommended in neonates with CDH requiring ventilatory support.

Permissive hypercapnia ($PaCO_2$ 46–60 torr) is frequently practiced along with lower target preductal SaO_2 (85–95%) and pH 7.25–7.40. Lower peak inspiratory pressures (< 25 cm H_2O) are best to avoid pneumothorax. Mean airway pressures (MAP) can range from 12 to 18 cm H_2O and tend to depend on the gestation, weight and extent of hypoxemia in the infant. It's reasonable to use $PaCO_2$ and OI as primary indices to drive ventilator management.

A few centers have used HFOV for hypercapnia or hypoxia/hypoxemia either as an initial or rescue therapy after CMV did not improve clinical status. Post-ductal

SaO_2 can be tolerated as low as 60% as long as pre-ductal SaO_2 is > 85% and there is evidence of adequate post-ductal perfusion. Hypoxemia can improve over time with decline of PVR. Close monitoring of hemodynamic status and adequate sedation are important.

High-frequency jet ventilation (HFJV) is often reserved for the most critical infants who fail CMV, require iNO and ECMO. In other pathologies, HFJV has been shown to use lower pressures to achieve similar blood gases, possibly contributing to improved systemic and pulmonary venous return. Animal studies have shown that cardiovascular parameters, including pulmonary hypertension can improve on HFJV, but there is a lack of human randomized clinical trials.

Obtaining a chest X-ray after switching between ventilator modalities is a useful way to monitor lung over-expansion to avoid a pneumothorax. Since lung hypoplasia is very common, rib expansion may not be a useful guide and instead attention should be on the unaffected diaphragm to observe for flattening. Table 8.4 summarizes ventilation strategies with different modalities.

Table 8.4 CDH ventilation strategies: summary table

Monitoring parameters	pH	7.25–7.4
	$PaCO_2$	46–60 torr
	Pre-ductal SaO_2	$\geq 85\%$
	Post-ductal SaO_2	No clear recommendations *Due to ductal shunting, can tolerate low (≤ 70 torr) if pre-ductal SaO_2 and post-ductal perfusion remain adequate*
CPAP/NIPPV	PEEP	≤ 6 cm H_2O
CMV	MAP	Variable based on lung excursion and FiO_2 requirements *Gradually increase PEEP to target optimal MAP for oxygenation. Consider HFOV or HFJV if > 10 cm H_2O required in first day of life (term)*
	PIP	≤ 25 cm H_2O
	Volume Targeted	4–6 mL/kg
HFOV	I:E ratio	1:2
	Frequency (Hz)	10–15 *Higher Hz for smaller infants*
HFJV	PIP	Variable based on $PaCO_2$
	"sigh" breaths	≤ 2/min

8.4.5 Pulmonary Hypertension in MAS and CDH

Although the fetus is expected to remain in a state of pulmonary hypertension, the neonate's respiratory status depends on a gradual reduction of PVR in the first 24 to 48 h after birth. The fall in PVR is greatest soon after birth due to pulmonary vasodilation so that the mean pulmonary arterial pressure is 50% of mean systemic artery pressure at 3 days of age in a full-term newborn. PVR continues to decline subsequently because of involution of the pulmonary arterial musculature until 2–3 months of age when it is about 15–20% of SVR. Persistent pulmonary hypertension (PPHN) ensues when pulmonary vasculature fails to adequately dilate after birth such as in CDH and MAS. PPHN is defined as the peak pulmonary artery (PA) pressure to systemic blood pressure ratio ≥ 0.75. To overcome PPHN, mean arterial blood pressure (BP) > 40 mmHg is recommended, with the use of dopamine, dobutamine or epinephrine as needed. Figure 8.11 depicts the mechanisms by which these increased right-sided cardiac pressures cause a right upper to lower extremity oxygen saturation difference. At the extreme, SpO_2 can differ up to 20–30% at these two sites.

While it is important to achieve appropriate oxygenation, hyperoxia (persistent PaO_2 > 80 torr) in cases of PPHN can generate reactive oxygen species (ROS). ROS is known to cause vascular remodeling, decreased eNOS expression and increase phosphodiesterase-5 activity, thus blunting cGMP and nitric oxide mediated vasodilatation. Hyperoxia also reduces response to inhaled nitric oxide (iNO) in the presence pulmonary vasoconstriction. Oxygen weaning protocols can be useful to ensure careful monitoring of FiO_2 as the infant shows signs of improvement as indicated by less differential saturations and improving systemic blood pressures and PaO_2.

INHALED NITRIC OXIDE (iNO) Soluble guanylate cyclase (sGC) is responsible for the enzymatic conversion of guanosine-5-triphosphate (GTP) to cyclic guanosine – 3'5'monophosphate (cGMP) (Fig. 8.12). Nitric oxide (NO) and cGMP together comprise a range of signal transduction mechanisms including smooth muscle relaxation. Inhaled NO by upregulating cGMP via guanylyl cyclase reduces vascular tone and inhibits proliferation, offering a potent and selective pulmonary vasodilatory effect. There has been a steady increase in the use of iNO over the last two decades. Two major trials led to FDA approval of iNO for term and late preterm infants with hypoxemic respiratory failure, significantly reducing the need for ECMO therapy.

Inhaled nitric oxide is used to manage pulmonary hypertension. It is beneficial in cases of MAS or idiopathic PPHN, however routine use in CDH is not recommended. With an OI of > 20–25, a trial of iNO may be attempted, but in classic CDH, the response is less predictable than other causes of PPHN such as in MAS. A meta-analysis of randomized clinical trials evaluated rescue use of iNO in CDH and observed a higher rate of ECMO or death.

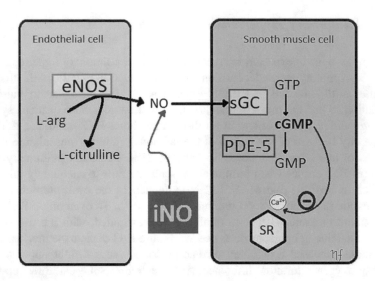

Fig. 8.12 Mechanism of action of inhaled nitric oxide: upregulation of guanylyl-cyclase (sGC) causing increased production of cGMP, which inhibits Ca^{2+} release from the sarcoplasmic reticulum, resulting in smooth muscle vasodilation. Sildenafil inhibits phosphodiesterase-5 (PDE-5), also increasing cGMP

PaO$_2$ and OI as primary indicators for weaning and discontinuation of iNO may not be reliable in PPHN to determine clinical stability. Weaning iNO and/or FiO$_2$ should be done cautiously and gradually. There are other pharmacological agents to lower PVR such as sildenafil which inhibits phosphodiesterase-5 (PDE-5).

8.5 Consideration of Extracorporeal Membrane Oxygenation (ECMO)

Despite meticulous consideration to ventilation and hemodynamics, some infants may require ECMO. MAS is the most common reason an infant is placed on ECMO with good outcomes. Several neonates with CDH may also require ECMO to improve oxygenation. ECMO or extracorporeal life support (ECLS) is a therapy that uses modified partial cardiopulmonary bypass, allowing time for pulmonary and/or cardiac recovery. Term or near-term newborns with potentially reversible respiratory failure tend to have improved survival when ECMO is employed. ECMO criteria can differ between institutions. It is often reserved for severe hypoxemia refractory to ventilation and hemodynamic instability. Usual indication is OI > 40. It should also be considered with an OI between 20 and 40 if the infant has additional signs of clinical deterioration (poor perfusion, air leak syndromes, and decreased cardiac output) on optimal ventilator management. Veno-arterial (VA) ECMO drains blood from the right atrium (RA) and returns blood to the thoracic aorta. It provides both cardiac and pulmonary support. Veno-venous (VV) ECMO drains blood from the RA using a double lumen catheter, returning it back to the right atrium, directed to the tricuspid valve. This mode requires adequate cardiac function but decreases complications from accessing the carotid or femoral arteries as is the case in VA ECMO. VA ECMO tends to be more commonly used in the neonatal period due to the coexisting cardiac and pulmonary dysfunction. This is often the indication for ECMO in this group where the cardiac output needs to be supported by the bypass. During ECMO, low ventilator and FiO_2 parameters are used to allow the lungs to recover, with adequate PEEP delivery to avoid atelectasis. Oxygenation through the extracorporeal circuit as well as through the patient's native pulmonary circulation contributes to improvement in gas exchange.

Suggested Readings

1. Textbook of Neonatal Resuscitation (NRP), 7th ed. American Academy of Pediatrics, 2016.
2. Chandrasekharan PK, Rawat M, Madappa R, Rothstein DH, Lakshminrusimha S. Congenital diaphragmatic hernia—a review. Matern Health Neonatol Perinatol. 2017;3:6. https://doi.org/10.1186/s40748-017-0045-1.
3. El Shahed, AI, Dargaville PA, Ohlsson A, Soll R. Surfactant for meconium aspiration in term and late preterm infants. Cochran Database Syst Rev. 2014; CD002054. https://doi.org/10.1002/14651858.CD002054.Pub3.
4. Lakshminrusimha S, Konduri GG, Steinhorn RH. Considerations in the management of hypoxemic respiratory failure and persistent pulmonary hypertension in term and late preterm neonates. J Perinatol. 2016;36(Suppl 2):S12–9. https://doi.org/10.1038/JP.2016.44 PMID: 27225960.
5. Sweet DG, Carnielli V, Greisen G, et al. European consensus guidelines on the management of respiratory distress syndrome - 2019 Update. Neonatology. 2019;115(4):432–50.
6. Finer NN, Carlo WA, Walsh MC, et al. Early CPAP versus surfactant in extremely preterm infants. N Engl J Med. 2010;362(21):1970–9.
7. Jensen EA, Dysart K, Gantz MG, et al. The diagnosis of bronchopulmonary dysplasia in very preterm infants: An evidence-based approach. Am J Respir Crit Care Med. 2019 sep 15; 200 (6) 751–759.
8. Laughon MM, Langer JC, Bose CL, et al. Prediction of bronchopulmonary dysplasia by postnatal age in extremely premature infants. Am J Respir Crit Care Med. 2011;183 (12):1715–22.
9. Klingenberg C, Wheeler KI, McCallion N, Morley CJ, Davis PG. Volume-targeted versus pressure-limited ventilation in neonates. Cochrane Database Syst Rev. 2017;10:CD003666.
10. Gupta D, Greenberg RG, Sharma A, et al. A predictive model for extubation readiness in extremely preterm infants. J Perinatol. 2019;39(12):1663–9.
11. Idana-Aguirre JC, Pinto M, Featherstone RM, Kumar M. Less invasive surfactant administration versus intubation for surfactant delivery in preterm infants with respiratory distress syndrome: a systematic review and meta-analysis. Arch Dis Child Fetal Neonatal Ed. 2017;102(1):F17–F23.
12. Kinsella JP, Steinhorn RH, Mullen MP, et al. The left ventricle in congenital diaphragmatic hernia: Implications for the management of pulmonary hypertension. J Pediatr. 2018;197:17–22.

Chapter 9
Ventilator Graphics

Shekhar T. Venkataraman and Bradley A. Kuch

Modern ventilators are capable of graphically displaying pressure, flow and volume. In most ventilators, pressure, flow and volumes are measured by inspiratory and expiratory sensors located inside the ventilator. Some ventilators measure these variables at the hub of the endotracheal tube. It is important to understand that these variables are not measured at the alveolar level. There are two types of waveforms - Scalar Waveforms and Loops. Scalar waveforms refer to the real-time display of pressure, flow or volume plotted over time. Loops are the real-time display of pressure with volume or flow with volume. Scalar waveforms are analyzed by examining the phases of a mechanical breath, while loops are analyzed by examining the shape and characteristics of the curves during inspiration and exhalation (Figs. 9.1, 9.2, and 9.3). Waveforms allow the bedside clinician to: (1) identify the mode of ventilation, (2) recognize and measure respiratory system mechanics, (3) examine and evaluate patient-ventilator interactions, and (4) trouble-shoot suboptimal ventilator performance. Waveforms and loops can also be used to optimize ventilator support based on the patient's pathophysiology.

S. T. Venkataraman (✉)
Professor, Departments of Critical Care Medicine and Pediatrics, University of Pittsburgh School of Medicine, Pittsburgh, PA, USA
e-mail: venkataramanst@upmc.edu

Medical Director, Respiratory Care Services, Children's Hospital of Pittsburgh, 4401 Penn Avenue, Faculty Pavilion 2117, Pittsburgh, PA 15224, USA

B. A. Kuch
Director, Respiratory Care Services and Transport Team & Clinical Research Associate, Department of Pediatric Critical Care Medicine, UPMC Children's Hospital of Pittsburgh, 4401 Penn Ave, Pittsburgh, PA 15224, USA
e-mail: bradley.kuch@chp.edu

© Springer Nature Switzerland AG 2022
A. P. Sarnaik et al. (eds.), *Mechanical Ventilation in Neonates and Children*,
https://doi.org/10.1007/978-3-030-83738-9_9

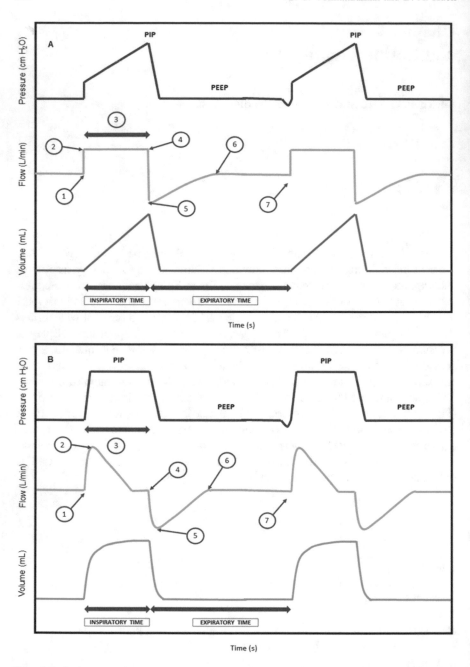

Fig. 9.1 Scalar waveform of volume-controlled time-cycled (**A**) and pressure-controlled time-cycled mandatory ventilation (**B**). This figure shows the graphic display of pressure in the top panel, flow in the middle panel, and volume in the lower panel plotted over time in the x-axis. PIP = Peak inspiratory pressure; PEEP = Positive end-expiratory pressure. The phases of a breath are described in the text

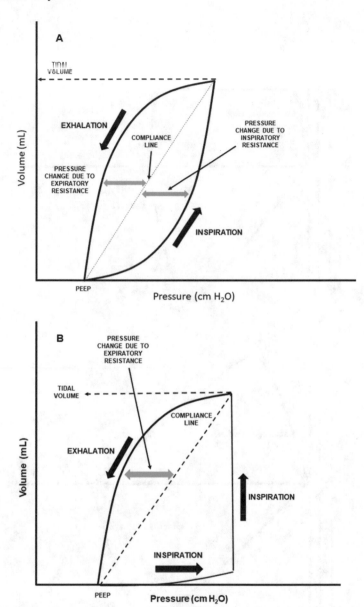

Fig. 9.2 Pressure–volume loop of a volume-controlled mandatory breath (**A**) and a pressure-controlled (**B**) mandatory breath. Figure shows volume on the y-axis and pressure on the x-axis. Inspiration starts at PEEP (positive end-expiratory pressure). The dotted compliance line denotes the static pressure–volume change due to elastance

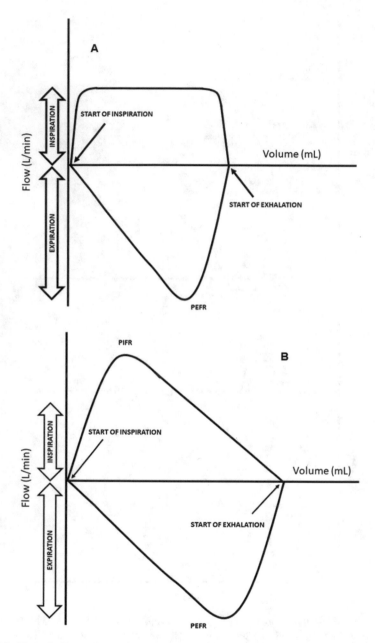

Fig. 9.3 Normal flow-volume loop with volume-controlled (**A**) and pressure-controlled (**B**) breaths. Inspiratory flow-volume curve is above the line and expiratory flow-volume curve is below the line

9.1 Identifying the Phases of a Mechanical Breath

The first step in the clinical application of ventilation graphics is to be able to identify the phases of a mechanical breath, whether it is mandatory or spontaneous. Figure 9.1 shows the scalar waveform of pressure, flow, and volume (on the y-axis) over time (on the x-axis) for both volume-controlled (A) and pressure-controlled mandatory ventilation (B). Points 1 through 7 are shown for the flow-time curve but these points also correspond to the same phases of the breath in the pressure–time and volume-time curves. Points 1 and 7 are the start of inspiration. Point 1, on the pressure–time axis, has no negative deflection and therefore, is a time-triggered mandatory breath. Point 7, on the pressure–time axis, is an example of a patient-triggered mandatory breath due to the negative deflection before the start of the breath. During inspiration, the inspiratory flow reaches a maximum quickly (Point 2). In volume-controlled ventilation, inspiratory flow is maintained constant throughout the inspiratory phase once it reaches the maximum flow (Point 3). With pressure-controlled ventilation (B), inspiratory flow reaches a maximum quickly and then declines. In this example, the inspiratory flow decreases to zero before the end of the inspiratory phase (Point 3). With volume-controlled ventilation, both the volume and pressure increase to their maximum value at the end of the inspiratory time. With pressure-controlled ventilation, tidal volume reaches a maximum when the inspiratory flow decreases to zero while the peak inspiratory pressure (PIP) remains constant throughout the inspiratory phase. Point 4 is the end of inspiration and the initiation of exhalation, referred to as cycling. The cycling mechanism for this breath is time. Inspiratory time is the interval between Points 1 and 4. Point 5 is the peak expiratory flow rate and Point 6 is the end of exhalation. Expiratory time is the interval between Point 4 and the start of the next breath (Point 7).

Figure 9.2 shows pressure plotted versus volume for volume-controlled mandatory (A) and for pressure-controlled (B) mandatory breaths. The dotted line between PEEP and the peak inspiratory pressure is the compliance line, which denotes static pressure–volume characteristics of the respiratory system. The extent to which the inspiratory pressure–volume curve is bowed to the right with volume-controlled ventilation depends on the inspiratory resistance of the respiratory system. When airway resistance increases, the pressure curve bows more to the right indicating greater pressure requirement to overcome the resistance. On the other hand, the inspiratory pressure–volume curve during a pressure-controlled breath reflects the change in pressure in the system and does not represent the changes in lung mechanics. During exhalation with volume-controlled ventilation, the volume of the deflating lung is higher for the same pressure than the inspiratory phase. This difference in volume between inspiration and exhalation and the shape of the pressure–volume curve is called *hysteresis*. The amount of hysteresis will change with changes in lung mechanics that will be described below. The extent to which the curve is bowed to the left is due to the expiratory resistance of the respiratory system with both modes of ventilation.

Figure 9.3 shows a graphic display plotting flow on the y-axis and volume on the x-axis. Ventilator graphics usually display inspiratory phase above the line and the exhalation phase below the line. This figure shows that, with a volume-controlled breath, the inspiratory flow reaches a maximum early in inspiration and remains at that level throughout inspiration. With a pressure-controlled breath, the inspiratory flow reaches a peak level (PIFR) following which the flow declines down to zero. In this example, the flow decreases to zero at the end of inspiration. During exhalation, with both modes, expiratory flow reaches a maximum early during the expiratory phase, the peak expiratory flow rate (PEFR). The rate of decline in flow is smooth and relatively convex downward or straight till the next inspiration. The volume subtended between the start of inspiration and exhalation is the tidal volume. When there is no leak, the volume in the inspiratory phase is equal to the volume during the exhalation phase.

9.2   Identifying the Mode of Ventilation

A mode of ventilation is a specific combination of a breath control variable (volume or pressure), sequence of breaths in a minute (all mandatory, all spontaneous or a combination of both), and any specific built-in targeting scheme (described in Chap. 6). Scalar waveform will show which variable is controlled and the sequence of breaths. A detailed description of the modes is given in Chap. 6.

Figure 9.4 shows scalar waveforms of pressure, flow and volume for both volume-controlled (A) and pressure-controlled (B) mandatory ventilation. With volume-controlled ventilation, the peak inspiratory flow is the same across all breaths. Since the breaths are time-cycled, all breaths are volume-controlled. While the peak inspiratory pressures shown in the figure are the same for all the breaths, a change in respiratory system compliance and resistance will result in a change in pressure while the flow and volume remain the same. All the breaths shown have the same characteristics with no spontaneous breaths occurring. Therefore, this mode is called machine-triggered, continuous mandatory ventilation which is volume-controlled and time-cycled. Figure 9.4B shows that the peak inspiratory flow reaches a maximum early in inspiration and then declines to zero during the inspiratory phase. All the breaths are time-cycled. The peak pressure remains constant in all breaths, making the breaths pressure-controlled. The peak inspiratory pressures shown in the figure are the same for all the breaths. A change in respiratory system compliance and resistance will not result in a change in pressure while the flow and volume will change. All the breaths shown have the same characteristics with no spontaneous breaths occurring. Therefore, this mode is called   machine-triggered,   continuous   mandatory   ventilation   which   is pressure-controlled and time-cycled.

Figure 9.5 shows the scalar waveforms of pressure, flow and volume for assist-control ventilation. In the example shown, panels A and B show assist-control ventilation in the volume-controlled and pressure-controlled modes, respectively. As

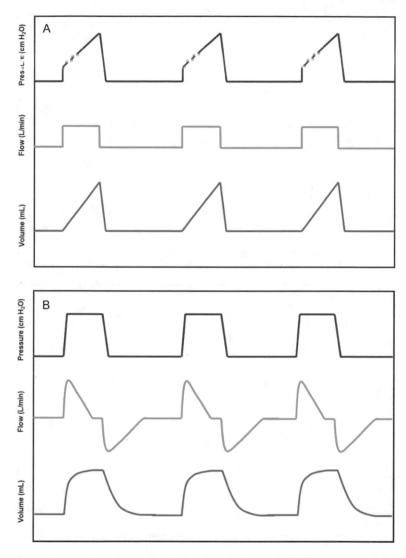

Fig. 9.4 Continuous mandatory ventilation with volume controlled (**A**) and pressure-controlled (**B**) time-cycled ventilation. All the breaths are machine-triggered mechanical breaths and no spontaneous breaths are observed

shown in the figure, every mandatory breath is preceded by a negative deflection in the pressure waveform signaling a spontaneous effort. Since there are no spontaneous breaths between the machine breaths, this is an example of continuous mandatory ventilation that is patient-triggered, also called as Assist-Control Ventilation. Assist-control mode is available in both volume-controlled and pressure-controlled modes in most ventilators.

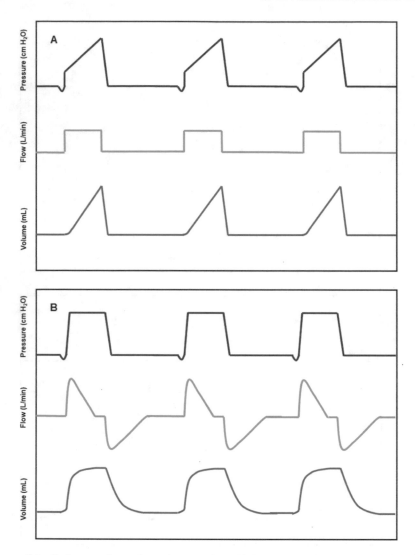

Figure. 9.5. Scalar waveforms for assist-control ventilation. Panel A is volume-controlled and Panel B is pressure-controlled ventilation, respectively. Every mandatory breath is triggered by a patient effort (negative deflection in the pressure curves)

Figure 9.6 shows scalar waveforms of pressure, flow, and volume where all the mechanical breaths are preceded (triggered) by a spontaneous breath. The pressure waveform shows that the pressure reaches a maximum quickly and is maintained till the end of the inspiratory phase. Towards the end of inspiration, the pressure level starts to decline before the start of exhalation. This is in contrast to pressure-controlled mandatory ventilation shown in Figs. 9.4 and 9.5, where the peak inspiratory pressure remains maximal until exhalation starts. All the breaths reach the same peak inspiratory pressure and therefore, these breaths are pressure-controlled. Inspiratory flow reaches a maximum early in inspiration and declines to a predetermined level (usually 25–30% of the peak inspiratory flow) when exhalation begins. All the breaths are spontaneous and the positive pressure breaths are patient-triggered, pressure-controlled during inspiration, and flow-cycled. This is referred to as Pressure-Support Ventilation.

Figure 9.7 shows a graphic display of intermittent mandatory ventilation with volume-controlled (A) and pressure-controlled (B) ventilation. As shown in Fig. 9.7A, the sequence of breaths includes both mandatory breaths as well as spontaneous breaths which occur between the mechanical breaths. All the mandatory breaths are patient-triggered, volume-controlled (A) or pressure-controlled (B) and time-cycled ventilation. The spontaneous breaths that occur in this example do result in inspiratory and expiratory flows and a tidal volume. These spontaneous breaths are not supported by positive pressure. This mode is referred to as Synchronized Intermittent Mandatory Ventilation (SIMV) with volume-controlled (Fig. 9.7A) and pressure-controlled (Fig. 9.7B) ventilation.

Figure 9.8 shows an example of SIMV with pressure-control where the spontaneous breaths that occur between the mandatory breaths are supported by a positive pressure breath. These supported breaths are patient-triggered and flow-cycled breaths. This is referred to as a Pressure Supported Breath. The level of pressure support in this example reaches a peak inspiratory pressure lower than the peak pressure with the SIMV breath and therefore results in a smaller tidal volume. The tidal volume delivered with a pressure supported breath can be adjusted independently of the tidal volume of the SIMV breath. SIMV with pressure support can also be provided with volume-controlled ventilation.

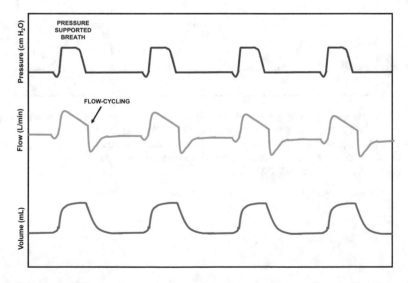

Fig. 9.6 Scalar waveforms of pressure, flow, and volume for Pressure Support Ventilation

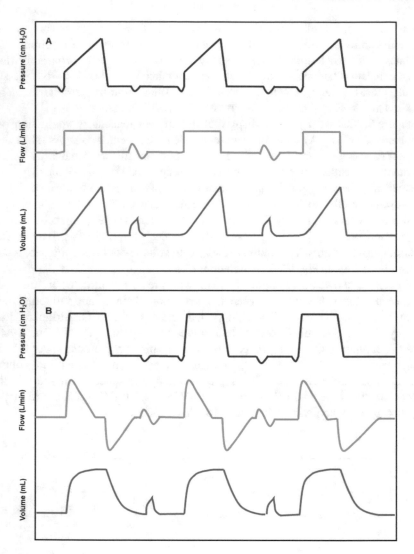

Fig. 9.7 Scalar waveforms of pressure, flow, and volume over time for intermittent mandatory ventilation (IMV). Panel A shows volume-controlled and Panel B shows pressure-controlled ventilation. Spontaneous breaths occur between the mechanical breaths and are not supported by positive pressure. Since every mechanical breath is triggered by a patient effort, this mode of ventilation is Synchronized IMV (SIMV)

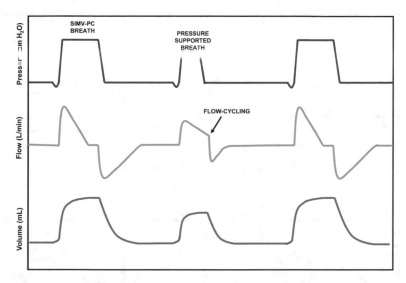

Fig. 9.8 Scalar waveforms of Synchronized Intermittent Mandatory Ventilation (SIMV) with Pressure Support. All SIMV breaths are patient-triggered, pressure-controlled, and time-cycled. Spontaneous breaths also occur between the mechanical breaths which are assisted by Pressure Support

9.3   Recognizing and Measuring Respiratory System Mechanics

9.3.1   Increased Lower Airway resistance

Lower airway resistance is increased in several conditions such as asthma, bronchiolitis, and bronchopulmonary dysplasia. The equation of motion would predict that for volume-controlled ventilation, the total pressure required to inflate the lung with a specific tidal volume will increase according to the pressure required to overcome the resistance (see Chapt. 2). With pressure-controlled ventilation; the tidal volume and flow would be reduced since the total pressure is maintained constant (Chap. 2). This would be evident in the waveforms—both scalar waveforms and the loops. Figure 9.9 shows a volume-controlled time-cycled breath with an inspiratory hold during constant inspiratory flow both in normal lungs (A), in a lung with lower airway disease due to acute bronchospasm (B), and after treatment with a bronchodilator (C). In the normal lungs, the drop in pressure from the peak value (PIP) to the plateau pressure ($P_{plateau}$) is small. Exhalation is complete since the expiratory flows return to zero before the start of the next inspiration. With acute bronchospasm and an increase in airway resistance, PIP increases for the same delivered tidal volume and the drop in pressure from PIP to $P_{plateau}$ increases compared to normal (Fig. 9.9B). During exhalation, the peak expiratory flow rate decreases and the exhalation is incomplete since the expiratory flow does not reach

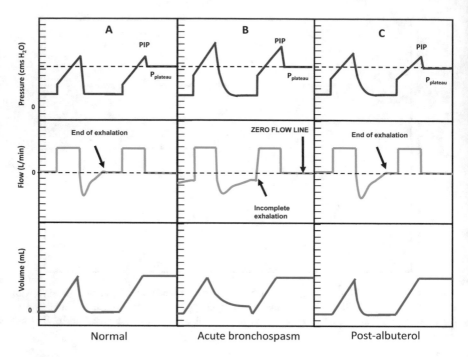

Fig. 9.9 Scalar waveforms of volume-controlled ventilation with normal lungs (**A**), with acute bronchospasm (**B**) and after treatment with albuterol (**C**)

zero before the start of the next inspiration. With albuterol, the magnitude of the drop in pressure from PIP to plateau pressure decreases while the plateau pressure remains the same (Fig. 9.9C). Exhalation is complete with expiratory flow returning to zero. This demonstrates that scalar waveforms can be used to evaluate lower airway obstruction as well as its response to treatment. Measurements of respiratory system mechanics can be estimated either dynamically without any flow interruption or in a static condition with occlusion of flow in the circuit (Chap. 5).

Unlike volume-controlled ventilation, during mechanical ventilation with pressure-controlled mandatory ventilation with acute bronchospasm, the delivered tidal volume decreases while the total pressure remains constant (Fig. 9.10). Acute bronchospasm also results in a reduction in peak inspiratory and peak expiratory flow rates (Fig. 9.10B). Due to increased time constant of the respiratory system, inspiration and expiration terminate before they reach zero flow resulting in reduced tidal volume and air trapping, respectively (Fig. 9.10B). Albuterol restores the scalar waveforms more towards normal as shown in Fig. 9.10C.

Figure 9.11 shows the flow-volume loops with acute bronchospasm with volume control ventilation. The inspiratory flow-volume portion is the same for all the loops as shown in the figure. With normal lungs (blue line), expiratory flow reaches a maximum, the peak expiratory flow rate (PEFR) and returns to zero flow at the end of exhalation. The shape of the expiratory flow-volume curve is smooth and

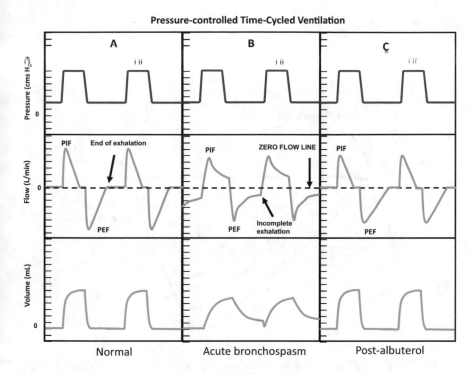

Fig. 9.10 Scalar waveforms for pressure-controlled ventilation with normal lungs (A), with acute bronchospasm (B) and after treatment with albuterol (C)

relatively straight. With acute bronchospasm (red line), PEFR decreases with the expiratory flow not returning to zero flow signaling incomplete exhalation. The shape of the curve after PEFR point is concave to the left and inferiorly. With albuterol (green line), PEFR increases compared to that during acute bronchospasm and in the example shown the flow returns to zero at the end of exhalation. The shape of the expiratory flow-volume curve is slightly concave to the left and inferiorly, signaling prolonged exhalation and residual lower airway obstruction.

Figure 9.12 shows the pressure–volume changes with acute bronchospasm before and after treatment with albuterol. Compared to the normal loops (blue line), the inspiratory limb of the loop with acute bronchospasm (red line) is bowed to the right due to increased respiratory system resistance. Similarly, the expiratory limb is bowed to the left showing increased expiratory resistance. Since exhalation is incomplete the volume does not return to zero. Acute bronchospasm with incomplete emptying results in hyperinflation which decreases the respiratory system compliance. Figure 9.12 shows that the compliance line is shifted to the right with acute bronchospasm. After albuterol (green line), the inspiratory and the expiratory limbs of the loop return closer to the normal loop with a slight decrease in compliance (see compliance line).

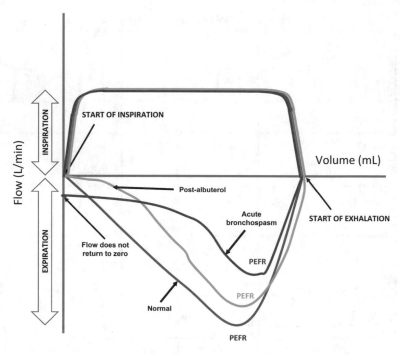

Fig. 9.11 Flow-volume loops with acute bronchospasm and its response to albuterol during volume-controlled ventilation. PEFR = Peak expiratory flow rate

9.3.2 Decreased Respiratory System Compliance

Figure 9.13 shows the scalar waveforms during volume-controlled time-cycled mandatory ventilation with Acute Respiratory Distress Syndrome (ARDS) which results in a decrease in respiratory system compliance. Compared to the normal waveform, PIP and $P_{plateau}$ are both increased by the same magnitude such that the pressure drop from PIP to $P_{plateau}$ remains the same (Fig. 9.13A, B). This is in contrast to increased airway resistance where the PIP increases while $P_{plateau}$ remains the same (Fig. 9.9). During the recovery phase in ARDS, the compliance improves as shown in Fig. 9.13C, where the PIP is lower but the drop from PIP to $P_{plateau}$ remains the same. The change from 9.13B to 9.13C can also been seen in patients who are treated with surfactant with an improvement in respiratory system compliance or with a recruitment maneuver. Lung protective strategy involves not only smaller tidal volumes but also keeping the $P_{plateau}$ less than or equal to 30 cm H_2O. It is, therefore, important to monitor the $P_{plateau}$ during volume-controlled ventilation and make the necessary changes in tidal volume to keep it below 30 cm H_2O. With ARDS, flow-volume loops are not that useful but changes in pressure-volume loops are important to consider as shown below.

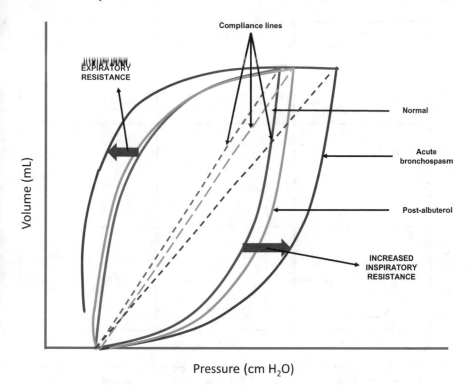

Fig. 9.12 Pressure–volume loop with normal lungs (blue), with acute bronchospasm (red) and after albuterol treatment (green) with volume-controlled ventilation

Figure 9.14 shows the pressure-volume loops with normal lungs (black), with ARDS (red) and during the recovery phase (green) of ARDS. Compared to the normal, for the same tidal volume, the pressure–volume loop is shifted to the right such that PIP is much higher with markedly decreased hysteresis as shown by a narrower loop with ARDS. During the recovery phase of ARDS, as compliance improves, PIP is lower for the same tidal volume and the hysteresis is larger. As shown in Fig. 9.13, PIP-PEEP is larger with ARDS compared to normal for the same tidal volume and as the lung recovers, this difference decreases.

Figure 9.15 shows the scalar waveforms during pressure-controlled, time-cycled mandatory ventilation with normal lungs (black), with ARDS (red) and during the recovery phase of ARDS (green). As shown in Fig. 9.15B, with ARDS, the tidal volume decreases while PIP remains the same. Peak inspiratory (PIFR) and expiratory (PEFR) flow rates are both decreased with ARDS. The flow decreases to zero much earlier than the end of inspiration as well as before the end of exhalation due to the shorter time constants (Fig. 9.15B). During the recovery phase, tidal volume, PIFR and PEFR increase (Fig. 9.15C). The change from Fig. 9.15B to C would also be seen with administration of surfactant or with recruitment.

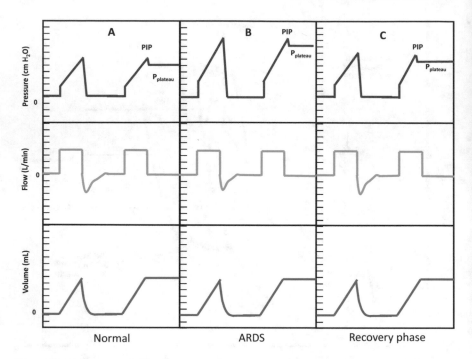

Fig. 9.13 Scalar waveforms during volume-controlled mandatory ventilation with ARDS. ARDS = Acute respiratory distress syndrome, PIP = peak inspiratory pressure, $P_{plateau}$ = Plateau pressure

During pressure-controlled ventilation, changes in lung compliance in pressure-volume loops would be signaled by a decrease in tidal volume since the pressure is controlled during inspiration. ARDS results in a smaller tidal volume compared to normal as shown in Fig. 9.16. During recovery from ARDS, compliance improves and therefore, tidal volume increases for the same PIP.

9.4   Patient-Ventilator Interactions

When a patient is breathing spontaneously during mechanical ventilation, it is important for the respiratory pump of the patient to be synchronous with the ventilator. Patient efforts need to be matched immediately with a level of support appropriate for the patient to provide ventilatory assistance while decreasing the spontaneous work of breathing and avoid wasted effort. The degree to which spontaneous breathing is synchronous with the ventilatory assistance can be evaluated by examining the scalar waveforms.

Figure 9.17 shows some examples of dyssynchronous patient-ventilator interactions. Example A shows a pressure-controlled mandatory breath where a

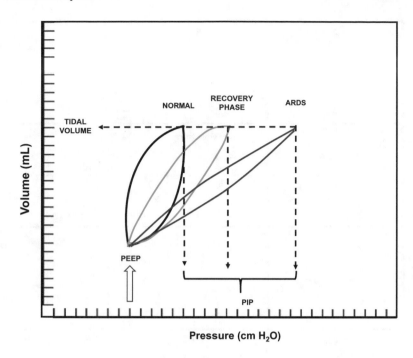

Fig. 9.14 Pressure-volume loops with volume-controlled ventilation showing a normal loop (black), loop with ARDS (red) and a loop during the recovery phase (green)

spontaneous inspiratory effort occurs during the mechanical breath. This results in a negative deflection in both the pressure and flow waveforms. Delivered tidal volume is increased due to the patient effort. Example B shows two spontaneous efforts signaled by the negative pressure deflections below baseline with no flow or tidal volume change. Example C shows a pressure-controlled mandatory breath where an active exhalation effort by the patient occurs. This results in an increase in PIP and the inspiratory flow declines rapidly due to the increase in airway pressure. The total tidal volume delivered is reduced due to the reduction in inspiratory flow.

Figure 9.18 shows some examples of dyssynchronous patient-ventilator interactions during volume-controlled ventilation. Example A shows a volume-controlled mandatory breath where a spontaneous inspiratory effort occurs during the mechanical breath. This results in a negative deflection in both the pressure and flow waveforms. Delivered tidal volume is decreased in this example by the patient effort without additional flow. Example B shows a spontaneous effort signaled by a negative pressure deflection below baseline with no flow or tidal volume change. This represents wasted effort as the triggering mechanism is not activated. Example C shows a volume-controlled mandatory breath where an active exhalation effort by the patient occurs. This results in an increase in PIP and the

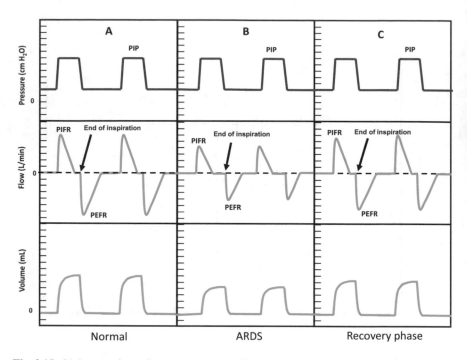

Fig. 9.15 Scalar waveforms for pressure-controlled, mandatory ventilation with normal lungs (**A**), with ARDS (**B**), and during the recovery phase of ARDS (**C**). PIP = Peak inspiratory pressure, ARDS = Acute respiratory distress syndrome, PIFR = Peak inspiratory flow rate, PEFR = Peak expiratory flow rate

inspiratory flow declines rapidly due to the increase in airway pressure. The total tidal volume delivered is reduced due to the reduction in inspiratory flow.

Both active inspiration and exhalation during a mechanical breath can be mini-mized by allowing more spontaneous breathing by reducing the mandatory venti-lator rate. Ineffective triggering is due to the trigger threshold being higher relative to the patient's spontaneous effort. The most common reason for an ineffective trigger is weakness of respiratory muscles resulting in poor effort. Ineffective trigger may require adjustments of the trigger sensitivity as shown in the example (Fig. 9.19).

Figure 9.19 shows scalar waveforms of SIMV with pressure control with pressure support. In panel A, the spontaneous efforts do not result in a pressure-supported breath. Panel B shows the same patient after adjustment of the trigger threshold making it more sensitive. The same patient effort is able to trigger the pressure-supported breath with resolution of the dyssynchrony. With missed efforts, it is important to pay attention to the trigger sensitivity and adjust it accordingly. Care must be taken not to make it too sensitive since that will result in auto-triggering (Table 9.1).

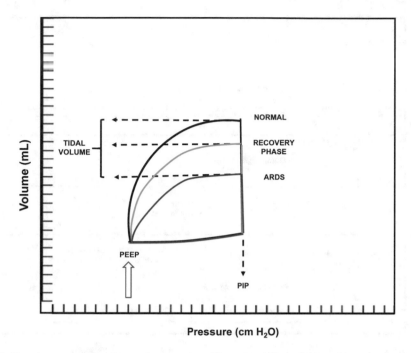

Fig. 9.16 Pressure-volume loops with pressure-controlled ventilation with normal lungs (black), with ARDS (red) and during the recovery phase (green). ARDS = Acute respiratory distress syndrome, PIP = Peak inspiratory pressure, PEEP = Positive end-expiratory pressure

9.5   Trouble-Shooting Suboptimal Ventilator Performance

Both scalar waveforms and loops can be used to trouble-shoot ventilator performance. It is important to distinguish between artifacts in the graphics and "true" indicators of suboptimal ventilator performance. It is common to see pressure overshoot as an artifact, especially when the rate of change in pressure is quite rapid. The electronics in the ventilator cannot distinguish between artifacts and true events and therefore may respond to artifacts as if they are changes in patient's lung mechanics. For example, a pressure overshoot in pressure-controlled ventilation (not shown) might cause the ventilator to decrease the inspiratory flow to decrease PIP. This might result in a reduced delivered tidal volume. One of the most significant contributors to suboptimal ventilator performance is a leak in the system. The leak may be in the circuit, in the patient connection or a leak around the artificial airway. This will result in a substantial amount of tidal volume escaping the circuit. This can be detected both in scalar waveforms as well as the loops as shown below.

The cardinal feature of a leak in the system is decreased tidal volume delivery. Figure 9.20 shows the scalar waveforms with a leak with both volume-controlled (A) and pressure-controlled (B) ventilation. With a leak, PIP, peak expiratory flow

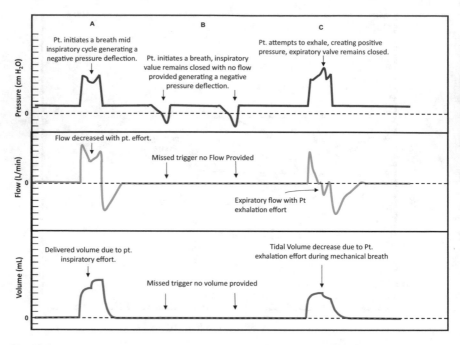

Fig. 9.17 Scalar waveforms showing some examples of dyssynchrony with SIMV with pressure control. A is an example of a spontaneous inspiratory effort occurring during a mandatory breath, B is an example of ineffective trigger, and C is an example of active spontaneous exhalation during a mandatory breath

rate and the exhaled tidal volume are decreased. With pressure-controlled ventilation, the ventilator attempts to maintain PIP by increasing inspiratory flow. This results in a larger machine-delivered tidal volume delivery for the same magnitude of leak with pressure-controlled ventilation compared to volume-controlled ventilation. Therefore, in the presence of a leak around an artificial airway (tracheostomy tube or endotracheal tube), pressure-controlled ventilation might be a better strategy to maintain better tidal volumes.

Flow-volume loops will show that the expiratory flow returns to zero much earlier and the tidal volume exhaled will be smaller than the delivered tidal volume as shown in Fig. 9.21. As described above, the exhaled tidal volume with pressure-controlled ventilation is larger than that with volume-controlled ventilation.

Pressure support ventilation behaves slightly differently depending on the magnitude of leak present in the circuit. Figure 9.22 shows scalar waveforms during pressure support ventilation with a small leak and without a leak. In the presence of a small leak (Panel B), the pressure support level is reached to the same level as that without a leak (Panel A). The flow curve starts to decline much earlier and faster with a leak which is also reflected in a drop in peak inspiratory pressure.

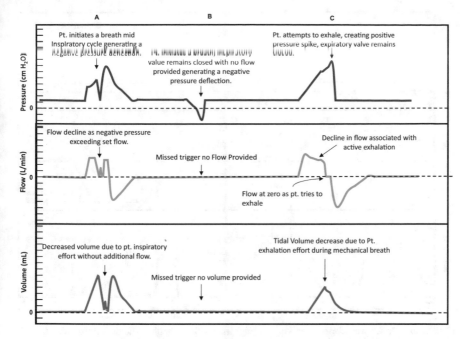

Fig. 9.18 Scalar waveforms showing some examples of dyssynchrony with SIMV with volume control. A is an example of a spontaneous inspiratory effort occurring during a mandatory breath, B is an example of ineffective trigger, and C is an example of active spontaneous exhalation during a mandatory breath

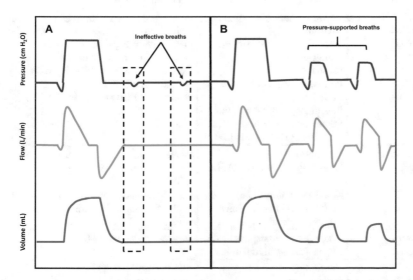

Fig. 9.19 Scalar waveforms showing ineffective triggering in SIMV with PS (**A**) and effective triggering after adjustment of the trigger sensitivity (**B**)

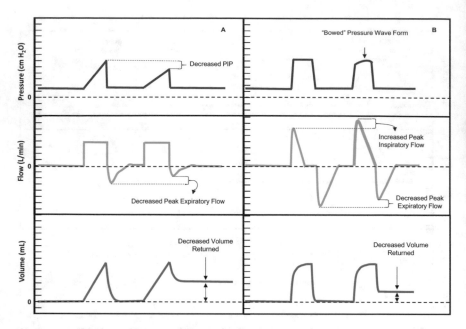

Fig. 9.20 Scalar waveforms showing a significant leak with volume-controlled (**A**) and pressure-controlled (**B**) ventilation

Table 9.1 Types of asynchrony, causative factors and therapeutic approach

Type of asynchrony	Causative factor(s)	Therapeutic approach
Ineffective triggering	**Ventilator:** Inappropriate sensitivity setting or malfunction Prolonged inspiratory time **Patient:** Respiratory Muscle weakness Decreased neural drive Auto-PEEP (Hyperinflation)	Adjust sensitivity (flow is more sensitive than pressure trigger) Decrease inspiratory time Decrease respiratory drive depressants (sedation and NMB) Adjust set PEEP and /or PSV
Double trigging	**Ventilator:** Short inspiratory time relative to neural inspiratory time Low tidal volume in Volume Control ventilation	Increase inspiratory Time or decrease cycling threshold percentage of peak flow (PSV) Consider sedation and/or NMB. Consider modes that allow for variation in tidal volume (i.e., PC)
Reverse triggering	Patient effort in response to a mechanical breath/inflation	Decrease sedation, NMB
Auto-triggering	**Ventilator:** System leak Sensitivity set too sensitive Water in the ventilator circuit	Adjust sensitivity setting Correct leak Remove excessive water from the ventilator circuit

(continued)

Table 9.1 (continued)

Type of asynchrony	Causative factor(s)	Therapeutic approach
	Patient: Cardiac activity resulting in pressure or flow oscillations triggering breaths	Decrease sensitivity setting
Premature cycling	**Ventilator**: Inspiratory time set lower than the patient's inspiratory time **Patient**: Restrictive lung process during use of PSV (?)	VC—decrease inspiratory flow or increase tidal volume PC—increase inspiratory time PSV—decrease cycling threshold percentage or PS
Delayed cycling	**Ventilator**: Inspiratory time set longer then the patient's inspiratory time **Patient**: Obstructive lung process during use of PSV	VC—increase inspiratory flow rate PC—decrease inspiratory time PSV—increase cycling threshold percentage or decrease PS, or decrease rise time
Insufficient flow setting	**Ventilator**: VC—flow rate set to low PC and PSV—inspiratory pressure set to low, rise time to long **Patient**: Increased neural ventilatory drive/demand	VC—increase inspiratory flow rate or switch to PC or PSV (variable flow) Reduce neural drive and metabolic demand: control fever, pain, metabolic acidosis, and anxiety
Excessive flow	**Ventilator**: VC—flow rate set too high PC and PSV—inspiratory pressure set too high, rise time to short	VC—decrease inspiratory flow rate PC or PSV—decrease pressure or increase rise time

Adapted from Alcantara Holanda M, et al. J Bras Pneumol. 2018;(4):321–333

Inspiration terminates earlier as shown by the inspiratory time (I-Time) and the delivered tidal volume is smaller than without a leak.

The effect of a larger leak during pressure support ventilation is shown in Fig. 9.23. Panel A shows the scalar waveforms when there is no leak. When there is a large leak, in this example, the set peak pressure is not reached with initial inspiratory flow. Inspiratory flow continues at this high level to try to achieve the pressure support level. While the lung is inflating, the presence of a leak prevents the peak pressure being reached despite a sustained increase in flow. Termination of inspiration (cycling) also occurs late due to this phenomenon. The delivered tidal volume is decreased due to the leak.

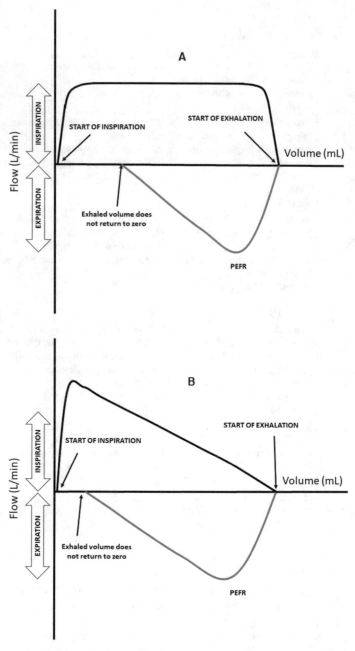

Fig. 9.21 Flow-volume loops with leak for volume-controlled (**a**) and pressure-controlled ventilation (**b**)

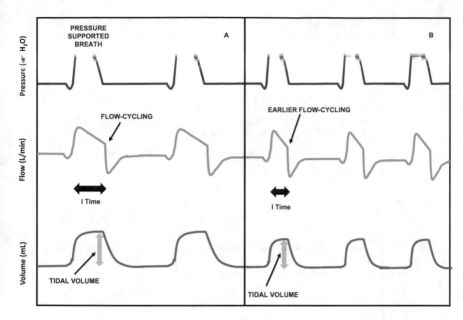

Fig. 9.22 Scalar waveforms during pressure support ventilation with a small leak. Panel A shows waveforms without a leak. Panel B shows waveforms with a small leak. I Time = Inspiratory time

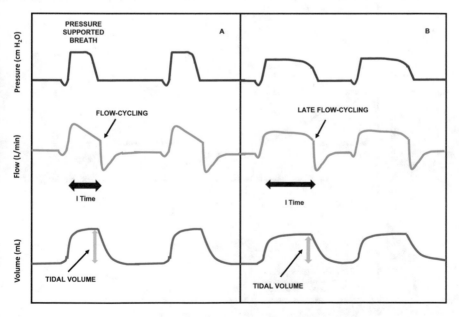

Fig. 9.23 Scalar waveforms during pressure support ventilation with a large leak. Panel A shows waveforms without a leak. Panel B shows waveforms with a largel leak. I Time = Inspiratory time

Leaks around the endotracheal tube can be eliminated by using cuffed tubes with the cuff inflated. There may be leaks due to connections that are not air-tight. Therefore, every connection needs to be checked to verify whether they are

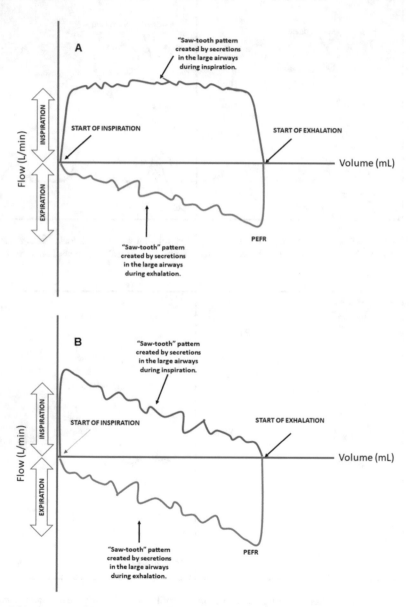

Fig. 9.24 A Flow-Volume loop in Volume control mode **B** Flow-Volume Loop Pressure Control—Saw-tooth pattern created by flow and pressure changes created by secretions in the large airways

adequately tight. Sudden appearance of a leak usually signifies a disconnection in the ventilatory circuit.

The presence of secretions can be identified during mechanical ventilation by the presence of a "saw-tooth" pattern during inspiration and expiration that may be missed during auscultation of the lung fields (Fig. 9.24). The "saw-tooth" pattern is created as air passes over the secretions in the first few airway generations resulting in small flow and pressure changes. When identified, suctioning the patient may improve lung mechanics and decrease the patients' work of breathing.

Suggested Readings

1. Nilsestuen JO, Hargett KD. Using ventilator graphics to identify patient-ventilator asynchrony. Respir Care. 2005;50(2):202–32.
2. Jin P. Mechanical breathing graph waveform monitoring and analysis in the nervous system intensive care unit. J Neurocrit Care. 2018;11(2):63–70.
3. Holanda MA, dos Santos VR, Ferreira JC, Pinheiro BV. Patient-ventilator asynchrony. J Bras Pneumol. 2018;44(4):321–33.
4. Hess DR. Noninvasive ventilation in neuromuscular disease: equipment and application. Respir Care
5. Corrado A, Gorini M, Villella G, De Paola E. Negative pressure ventilation in the treatment of acute respiratory failure: an old noninvasive technique reconsidered. Eur Respir J. 1996;9:1531–44.
6. Corrado A, Gorini M. Negative-pressure ventilation: Is there till a role? Eur Respir J. 2002;20:187–97.
7. Hassinger AB, Breuer RK, Nutty K, et al. Negative-pressure ventilation in pediatric acute respiratory failure. Respir Care. 2017;62(12):1540–9.
8. Sammuels MP, Raine J, Wright T. Continuous negative extrathoracic pressure in the treatment of respiratory failure in infants and young children. BMJ. 1989;299:1253–7.
9. Deshpande SR, Kirshbom PM, Maher KO. Negative pressure ventilation as a therapy for post-operative complications in a patient with single ventricle physiology. Heart Lung Circ. 2011;20:763–5.
10. Shah PS, Ohlsson A, Shah JP. Continuous negative extrathoracic pressure or continuous positive airway pressure compared to conventional ventilation for acute hypoxaemic respiratory failure in children. Cochrane Database systemic rev. 2013 Nov 4;(11)

Chapter 10
Noninvasive Mechanical Ventilation

Bradley A. Kuch, Shekhar T. Venkataraman, and Ashok P. Sarnaik

Noninvasive Ventilation (NIV) is defined as the application of assisted ventilatory support without the use of an invasive airway such as an endotracheal tube or a tracheostomy tube. Continuous airway pressure can be provided without the use of an artificial airway as well and while it does not provide active inspiratory support, it is still included in the discussion of NIV as a non-invasive modality. NIV can be applied via either positive or negative pressure. Positive pressure NIV (NIPPV) is provided by an interface that increases the proximal airway pressure whereas negative pressure NIV (NPV) is provided by creating a negative pressure around the chest wall. In both instances, the transrespiratory pressure, which is the pressure difference between the proximal airway pressure and the alveoli, is raised causing airflow into the lungs. Non-invasive ventilatory support has emerged as an important treatment modality for acute and chronic respiratory failure. Successful implementation of non-invasive adjuncts is related to appropriate patient selection,

B. A. Kuch (✉)
Director, Respiratory Care Services and Transport Team & Clinical Research Associate, Department of Pediatric Critical Care Medicine, UPMC Children's Hospital of Pittsburgh, 4401 Penn Ave, Pittsburgh, PA 15224, USA
e-mail: bradley.kuch@chp.edu

S. T. Venkataraman
Professor, Departments of Critical Care Medicine and Pediatrics, University of Pittsburgh School of Medicine, Pittsburgh, PA, USA
e-mail: venkataramanst@upmc.cdu

Medical Director, Respiratory Care Services, Children's Hospital of Pittsburgh, 4401 Penn Avenue, Faculty Pavilion 2117, Pittsburgh, PA 15224, USA

A. P. Sarnaik
Professor of Pediatrics, Former Pediatrician in Chief and Interim Chairman Children's Hospital of Michigan, Wayne State University School of Medicine, 3901 Beaubien, Detroit, MI 48201, USA
e-mail: asarnaik@med.wayne.edu

© Springer Nature Switzerland AG 2022   185
A. P. Sarnaik et al. (eds.), *Mechanical Ventilation in Neonates and Children*, https://doi.org/10.1007/978-3-030-83738-9_10

firm understanding of the limitations for each interface and device as well as the disease-specific pathology and pathophysiology. Primary benefit of these devices is the reduction in the rates of invasive ventilation and decreased hospital costs.

10.1　Non-Invasive Positive Pressure Ventilation (NIPPV)

NIPPV can be used in the acute (short-term) or sub-acute/chronic (long-term) care setting. Short-term NIPPV is initiated where positive pressure support is needed acutely in a hospital setting for conditions that are usually reversible within a few days (Table 10.1). Long-term NIPPV is indicated in conditions where respiratory failure is likely to be chronic or progressive.

10.1.1　Indications and Contraindications

A patient is considered a candidate for short-term NIPPV if the following criteria are met: (1) the cause of respiratory failure is reversible, (2) gas exchange cannot be maintained without positive pressure, (3) there is no immediate need for intubation and invasive mechanical ventilation, and (4) there are no contraindications to initiating NIPPV (Table 10.1). Short-term NIPPV may also be initiated to facilitate

Table 10.1 Indications and contraindications for short-term NIPPV

	Conditions
A. Indications	1. Potentially reversible condition
	a. Acute hypoxemic respiratory failure (e.g., ARDS)
	b. Acute cardiogenic pulmonary edema
	c. Acute lower airway disease (e.g., asthma, bronchiolitis)
	2. Avoiding intubation
	a. Restrictive chest diseases
	b. Neuromuscular disorders
	c. Post-operative respiratory failure
	d. Post-extubation respiratory failure
	3. Facilitate weaning and extubation
B. Contraindications	1. Need for immediate intubation and invasive mechanical ventilation
	2. Hemodynamically unstable (hypotension, shock)
	3. Poor airway protective reflexes (absent cough and gag)
	4. Recent upper airway and esophageal surgery
	5. Congenital facial malformation
	6. Presence of facial pressure ulcers
	7. Excessive secretions
	8. Lack of cooperation/Agitation
	9. Untreated pneumothorax
	10. Inability for a good mask fit

extubation. In some patients, with certain terminal illnesses such as advanced cancer, NIPPV may be attempted to avoid intubation. If any of the above criteria are not met, the patient may not be a suitable candidate for short term NIV. The need for positive pressure and ventilatory assistance is evidenced by moderate to severe increase in work of breathing, retractions, paradoxical breathing, accessory muscle use, and abnormal gas exchange (ventilatory or oxygenation failure). If the patient requires only positive airway pressure to recruit the lung volume to improve oxygenation, then the patient can be placed on noninvasive continuous positive airway pressure (CPAP) through an appropriate interface. If the patient needs ventilatory assistance based on the clinical signs and symptoms or gas exchange derangements, then the patient is a candidate for NIPPV.

10.1.2 Clinical Application

Once the patient is considered to be a suitable candidate for NIPPV, it is important to choose the correct interface which is appropriately sized. The choice of the interface will depend on the level of support as well as the severity of the distress. If only CPAP is required, then a nasal or oronasal mask may suffice. If ventilatory assistance is required, an oro-nasal or a total face mask would be the most appropriate interface. It might take several attempts before a patient can tolerate the interface. Sometimes, it might be necessary to hold the mask gently in place with without securing it on the head. Once the patient is able to tolerate the interface and the respiratory support provided, it can be secured with the straps provided. Figure 10.1 shows the flowchart for initiation of NIPPV.

Once CPAP/NIPPV has been initiated, patient's response needs to be monitored. The level of CPAP/NIPPV is selected based on the clinical needs. Some patients improve rapidly with the initial settings and may not require further adjustments. If there is not an immediate improvement within 15 min of initiation, the ventilator settings may need to be adjusted further. The patient should be monitored for clinical improvement for the next 2–3 h. The decision-making once CPAP/NIPPV is initiated is described in the flowchart in Fig. 10.2.

Clinical improvement with NIPPV is indicated by: (1) decreased respiratory rate, (2) reduced work of breathing, (3) improvement of dyspnea, (4) an increase in pH, (5) better oxygenation, and (6) decreased arterial carbon dioxide ($PaCO_2$) levels. Additionally, there may be hemodynamic effects such as a reduction in heart rate, improved blood pressures and perfusion. Generally, short-term NIPPV is used continuously until the patient improves or fails.

Fig. 10.1 Flowchart for
initiation of CPAP/NIPPV.
CPAP—Continuous positive
airway pressure;
NIPPV—Noninvasive
positive pressure ventilation

Fig. 10.2 Flowchart of
decision making in the first
2 h after initiation of CPAP/
NIPPV. CPAP—Continuous
positive airway pressure;
NIPPV—Noninvasive
positive pressure ventilation;
*If on CPAP, may need to
escalate to NIPPV

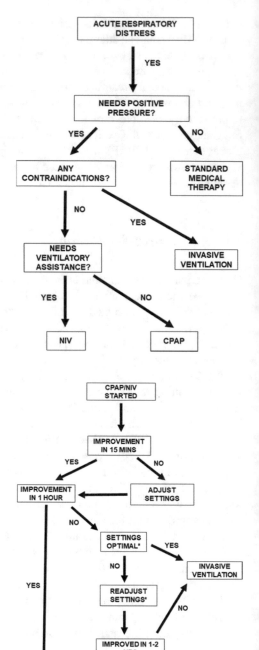

10.1.3   Ventilator Settings

With short term NIPPV, two strategies have been employed. A common approach
is to place the patient on a spontaneous mode with assist which is called pressure
support in ICU-specific ventilators and BiPAP or Bi-Level mode in ventilators
dedicated for NIPPV. The inspiratory pressure is usually set 5–8 cm H_2O above the
expiratory pressure. The inspiratory pressure limit with specific NIPPV ventilators
is called *inspiratory positive airway pressure* (IPAP). The expiratory pressure is
PEEP in ICU-specific ventilators and is called *expiratory positive airway pressure*
(EPAP) in the NIPPV ventilators. Depending on the level of relief of symptoms, the
inspiratory pressure limit can be gradually increased. When the inspiratory pressure
required is > 20 cm H_2O without clinical improvement, then endotracheal intubation and invasive mechanical ventilation should be considered. This is called the
low–high approach—start low and increase to a high level. The second approach is
to start with a high inspiratory pressure (about 20 cm H_2O or higher). The goal of
such an approach is for rapid clinical improvement. Once work of breathing is
reduced and gas exchange has improved, the inspiratory pressure can be decreased
to a lower level which still produces relief of symptoms. This approach is called the
high-low approach—start high and decrease to a lower level. In general, the low–
high approach is better tolerated by the patient, especially smaller children, since
they can adapt to the increasing flow into the nose and face. The flow of gas
associated with the high-low approach is not as well tolerated since the patient is
often uncomfortable with the high flow of gas to the face. On the other hand, work
of breathing may take much longer to be relieved with the low–high approach than
the high-low approach. Within the first 1–2 h, subsequent adjustments may be
necessary depending on the patient response. Expiratory pressure is used routinely
during short-term NIPPV (either EPAP or PEEP). Maximal fraction of inspired
oxygen (FiO_2) with bi-level ventilators is usually about 0.45–0.5. If a higher FiO_2 is
required and endotracheal intubation is not indicated, an ICU-specific ventilator
may be used, with a closed interface system. With this system there is an increased
risk of aspiration.

Care should be taken to prevent excessive skin pressure from the interface with
the use of adequate padding and monitoring how tight the interface is secured. In
some patients, mild sedation may be considered to improve tolerance of the mask.
Sedation of a patient already in respiratory distress needs to be monitored closely to
prevent inadvertent hypoventilation and worsening respiratory failure.
Humidification of the inspired gases is critical to prevent drying of the mucosa and
to avoid patient discomfort.

10.1.4 Optimizing Patient-Ventilator Interaction

Optimal patient-ventilator interaction requires the ventilator to be able to detect the patient's inspiratory efforts as quickly as possible and terminate inspiration (cycling) as close to the beginning of the patient's exhalation as possible. Inspiratory trigger function differs significantly among the ventilators. Factors affecting the inspiratory trigger function include trigger response to the inspiratory flow, leak-induced auto-triggering, and pressure–time and flow-time waveform heterogeneity. Strategies to optimize cycling include setting a suitable threshold for the inspiratory time and adjusting the cycling flow-threshold. Patients with obstructive lung disease tend to do better with high inspiratory flow whereas patients with neuromuscular disease seem to do better with low inspiratory flows. An adjustable back-up rate is available in most modern ventilators used for NIPPV. It is particularly useful when sedation is used to improve patient compliance with NIPPV. Leaks around the interface reduce its effectiveness. Some amount of leak around the interface is expected with NIPPV. Complete elimination of air leak is not desirable as it comes at the expense of a very tight-fitting mask which may lead to patient discomfort and skin breakdown. Ventilators differ in their capacity to compensate for leaks. One of the drawbacks of a large air leak is auto-triggering. In the presence of large system leaks, the ventilator will increase flow provided to compensate for the loss in pressure. The increase in flow decreases the ventilator's ability to sense both the beginning and the termination of the inspiratory cycle. This results in asynchrony, increased work of breathing, and oxygen consumption. In the presence of a system leak, the patient must be assessed for the presence of asynchrony. Humidification is important to prevent mucosal drying. Humidification can be provided using a heated humidifier, heat and moisture exchange, or a pass-over humidifier.

10.1.5 Mechanisms of Improvement

In patients with parenchymal lung disease, the lung has a tendency to collapse due to the high critical closing pressure and closing capacity. Application of CPAP/NIPPV can increase the airway pressures above the critical closing pressure and recruit the lung. Recruitment of the lung increases lung volumes, improves compliance, and decreases venous admixture. CPAP/NIPPV can also decrease the work of breathing by unloading the inspiratory muscles facilitating the inspiratory flow. As an example, in an obstructive disease such as asthma exacerbation, the resistive work of breathing (WOB) is greatly increased (Fig. 10.3).

The equal pressure point (EPP), where airway pressure is equal to intrapleural pressure during expiration, is displaced distally (towards alveoli) with intrapulmonary airway obstruction (Chapter 1). Intrathoracic airway proximal to EPP is therefore subjected to increasing transmural pressure resulting in further narrowing

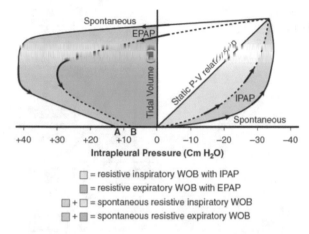

Spontaneous
EPAP
Tidal Volume
Static P-V relation
IPAP
Spontaneous

+40   +30   +20   +10   0   −10   −20   −30   −40
          A B
Intrapleural Pressure (Cm H₂O)

□ = resistive inspiratory WOB with IPAP
▨ = resistive expiratory WOB with EPAP
□ + □ = spontaneous resistive inspiratory WOB
□ + ▨ = spontaneous resistive expiratory WOB

Fig. 10.3 Work of breathing (WOB) in status asthmaticus with and without NIPPV. In the expiratory limb of the respiratory cycle equal pressure point (EPP) is displaced distally causing airways to close at higher lung volume (increased closing capacity), dynamic hyperinflation, and auto-PEEP (Point A). Application of EPAP stents the airways, causes proximal displacement of the EPP, and decreases closing capacity, dynamic hyperinflation, auto-PEEP (Point B), and WOB. In the inspiratory limb, the patient needs to generate less negative pressure to initiate inspiration because of lower auto-PEEP. Inspiratory muscles are further unloaded by IPAP throughout inspiration for the given tidal volume. Both expiratory and inspiratory WOB is thus reduced by application of NPPV. *From Sarnaik AA, Sarnaik AP: Pediatr Crit Care Med 13:484–485, 2012*

and limitation of expiratory airflow. The resistive WOB (pressure x volume) is greatly increased especially during exhalation when airway narrowing is exacerbated. Closure of airways earlier in expiration also results in greater closing capacity, ventilation-perfusion (V/Q) mismatch, auto-PEEP and decreased cardiac output. The dynamic compliance (C_{dyn}) is greatly reduced compared to the static compliance (C_{stat}). The prolonged time constant, results in dynamic hyperinflation and increased end-expiratory-lung-volume (EELV) compared to the expected functional residual capacity based on static pressure volume relationship.

Application of NIPPV addresses many of these pathophysiologic derangements. IPAP is aimed at unloading the inspiratory muscles and therefore decreasing the inspiratory work of breathing. EPAP on the other hand, moves the EPP more proximally (towards the thoracic inlet), stent the airways, decrease transmural pressure and ameliorate airway collapse during exhalation. Delay in airway closure during exhalation will also result in decreased auto-PEEP, dynamic hyperinflation, improved C_{dyn}, and decreased closing capacity with improved V/Q match. Additional advantages of NIPPV in status asthmaticus are improved aerosol delivery to obstructed airways and better distribution of gases such as helium–oxygen mixture.

Clinical decision-making to continue CPAP/NIPPV depends on whether the respiratory failure is resolving, unimproved or worsened (Fig. 10.4). When respiratory failure is resolving, CPAP/NIPPV should be weaned. Depending on the

Fig. 10.4 Flowchart
outlining the clinical
decision-making depending
on the trajectory of respiratory
failure

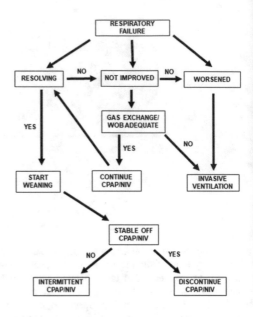

degree of resolution, some patients may require positive pressure support intermittently for a while before they are able to discontinue it completely. When
respiratory failure has not improved or worsened, then invasive ventilation needs to
be considered to provide further respiratory support.

10.1.6 Equipment

Interfaces A properly fitting appliance is essential for the optimal application of
NIPPV. There are currently several devices in use: (1) Adam's circuit and nasal
pillows, (2) Nasal masks, (3) Oro-nasal masks, (4) Total face masks, (5) Helmet or
Head Hood and (6) Mouthpieces. A correctly sized interface minimizes leaks,
improves effectiveness of positive pressure support, and improves comfort.
Current NIPPV delivery devices have the capacity to compensate for significant
leaks. Some devices can compensate for leaks as high as 60 L/min.

Adam's Circuit or Nasal pillows

This device uses a "nasal pillow" which attaches to a manifold and Velcro strap
system (headgear) that is placed over the top of the head. Some patients prefer this
to the nasal mask. "Nasal pillows" are available in various sizes. One advantage
with nasal pillows over the other interfaces is that patients can be fed if the work of
breathing and respiratory rates are normal.

Nasal masks A nasal mask rests between the bridge of the nose and above the
upper lip (Fig. 10.5). As a rule, the smaller the mask, the better the fit. In patients,
who are unable to keep their mouth closed, chin straps may be used to close the

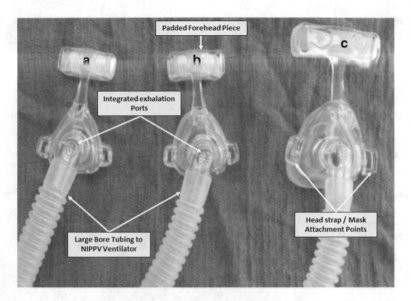

Fig. 10.5 Nasal masks. Three sizes of single-limb nasal masks **a** Newborn **b** Infant **c** Toddler. Integrated exhalation ports create a leak for CO_2 removal. Padded forehead piece maintains a comfortable fixation point on the patient's head, Head strap/mask attachment point holds the bottom portion of the mask to the face. Large bore tubing connects to the ventilator

mouth. Some nasal masks have integrated exhalation ports for exhaled gas to escape and prevent rebreathing of CO_2.

Oro-nasal Masks This is the most common interface used to provide NIPPV in children (Fig. 10.6). The ideal face-mask should be: (1) made of a clear material to allow visual inspection, (2) conforming to the contours of the patient's face, (3) easily moldable from its factory shape, (4) soft and does not apply excess pressure on the skin of the face, and (5) able to maintain its deformed shape (has "memory") when it is removed. The mask should extend from the bridge of the nose to just below the lower lip. The mask is secured using an anchoring system that goes around the head. Oro-nasal masks can be "vented" or "non-vented". Vented masks have integrated hole/holes for exhalation.

Total face mask This mask covers the whole face including the eyes (Fig. 10.7). The advantage of a total face mask is that it does not have to conform to the shape of the face and therefore does not have to be molded to fit every patient. The disadvantage is that it has an increased dead space and therefore, there may be difficulty in eliminating CO_2.

Head hood Also called a "helmet", it has been used successfully in a number of European ICUs. It appears best suited for application of CPAP. Dead space is a major concern and therefore, should be reserved for patients in the ICU.

Mouthpieces These are simple devices to be pursed between the lips for domiciliary mechanical ventilation (Table 10.2).

Fig. 10.6 Oro-nasal mask. Shown is a mask with a leakless elbow swivel used in dual limb ICU-specific ventilators. The type requires an active exhalation value for CO_2 removal. Padded plastic head piece maintains a comfortable fixation point on the patient's head. Velcro mask straps encircle the head and neck, and mask attachment point holds the bottom portion of the mask to the face. This model uses a plastic clasp for easy application and removal

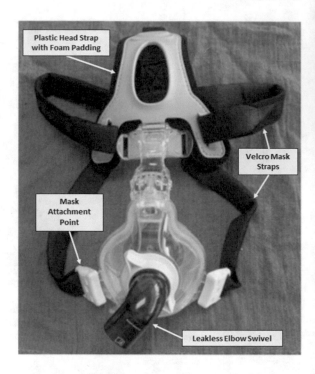

Fig. 10.7 Total face mask. Total face mask with an integrated exhalation elbow swivel for use in single limb continuous flow ventilators allowing for CO_2 removal. The elbow swivel has a one-way valve that closes during inspiration and opens during exhalation. Velcro mask straps encircle the head and neck, and mask attachment point holds the mask to the face. This model uses a plastic clasp for easy application and removal

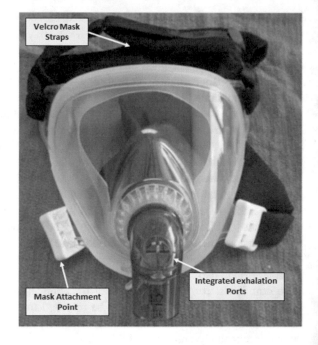

Table 10.2 Advantages and disadvantages of commonly used interfaces

Interface	Feature	Advantages	Disadvantages
Nasal masks	Covers nose not mouth	Possibility of speaking and drinking Allows cough Reduced danger of vomiting Minimum risk of asphyxia	Air leaks if mouth is open Risk of pressure injury Needs patent nasal passages
Full face (or oronasal)	Covers nose and mouth	Few air leaks than nasal masks Cooperation is easier Can be adjusted for comfort	Difficult to fit at times Vomiting (needs NG drainage) Risk of aspiration Claustrophobia Risk of pressure injury Speaking and coughing difficult
Total face mask	Covers eyes, nose, and mouth	Minimum air leaks Little cooperation required Easy fitting and application Surprisingly, less claustrophobia	Vomiting (needs NG drainage) Claustrophobia Speaking difficult Risk of aspiration
Mouthpieces	Placed between lips and held in place	Can be applied as rotating strategy with other interfaces Usually used with sip-ventilation	Salivation Gastric distension Speaking difficulty Possible air leaks

Ventilator devices

The ventilators that are used for NIPPV can be classified into 3 categories: (1) ICU-specific ventilators with a double limb circuit without leak compensation, (2) devices with a single limb circuit with leak compensation, and (3) devices that combine the above 2 categories to include both leak compensation and having a double limb circuit. Category 1 devices can only be used in the hospital. Category 2 and 3 devices can be used both in the hospital and at home. The examples of these devices would be any of the ICU-specific ventilators that can provide pressure support with PEEP (Category 1), Respironics Bi-PAP (Category 2), and the Pulmonetics LTV ventilator (Category 3). The performances of these ventilators vary widely in delivered tidal volumes, air-leak compensation, response to simulated effort, inspiratory trigger, expiratory cycling, rebreathing, response to high ventilatory demands and patient-ventilator synchrony. Category 1 or ICU-specific ventilators operate with high-pressure gas sources with an oxygen blending system. Category 2 and 3 devices can operate without a high-pressure gas source. Bi-level ventilators do not have a blender and therefore, the delivered FiO_2 is unpredictable depending on the oxygen flow rate, ventilator settings, amount of leak, site of O_2 enrichment, and the type of exhalation port. Most common mode of NIPPV is continuous spontaneous ventilation with assist such as bi-level pressure support (referred to as BiPAP) and pressure support ventilation with ICU-specific ventilators. While it is possible to provide volume-controlled or pressure-controlled mandatory breaths for NIPPV, these modes are not as common as the spontaneous modes with assist.

Circuits

Dual-limb and single-limb circuits are the two commonly used circuits with non-invasive ventilation. A dual-limb circuit is usually used with an ICU-specific ventilator to provide NIPPV (Fig. 10.8). The inspiratory limb is separated from the expiratory limb so that there is segregation of inspired and exhaled gases. In modern ventilators, the valves controlling the inspiratory and expiratory limbs are located within the ventilator. The expiratory valve closes during the inspiratory phase and the inspiratory valve closes during the expiratory phase. There is no rebreathing of exhaled CO_2 into the ventilator since the inspiratory valve is closed during exhalation.

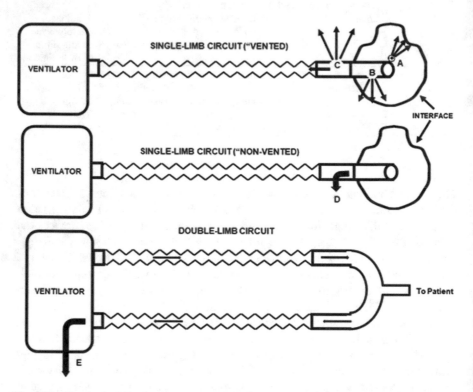

Fig. 10.8 Circuits for NIPPV. The circuit shown at the top is a Single-limb "vented" circuit. The "vent" can be in the interface (**A**), in the connector between the interface and the circuit (**B**), or in the circuit close to the connector (**C**). The circuit shown in the middle is a Single-limb "non-vented" circuit with an active exhalation post (**D**). The circuit shown at the bottom is a Dual-limb circuit where exhalation occurs through the expiratory port of the ventilator (**E**)

Single-limb circuits by definition have only a single hose exiting the ventilator (Fig. 10.8). Single limb circuits that are employed with bi-level ventilators can result in significant CO_2 rebreathing. Included CO_2 needs to vent the circuit without significant rebreathing of CO_2 in the inspired gas. This can be accomplished by either passive or active exhalation mechanisms in the circuit. Exhaled gas can be vented through holes in the interface itself, or the connector between the circuit and the interface or in the circuit close to the patient as shown in Fig. 10.8. Passive exhalation occurs through these "vents" but a portion of the exhaled gas can enter the circuit resulting in some rebreathing of CO_2. With this system, there is a continuous flow through the entire breathing cycle inside the circuits. CO_2 removal (or rebreathing) is affected by EPAP, intentional and nonintentional leaks, and supplemental oxygen entrained in the mask.

The second mechanism by which exhaled gas can exit the circuit without significant rebreathing is to have an active exhalation port which prevents the exhaled gas from the entering the circuit. This can be accomplished by having an exhalation valve similar to a PEEP valve or a valve with a pressure line that is controlled by the ventilator (Fig. 10.9). Rebreathing of CO_2 is lowest when the exhalation port is closest to the patient.

Important points to consider when selecting interfaces and circuits.

When using an ICU-specific ventilator, a non-vented interface is the interface of choice and a vented interface should be avoided since these ventilators do not have adequate leak compensation. When using a single-limb circuit, if there the interface is vented, then the circuit should not have any other ports for exhalation. If the interface is non-vented, then it is important to use a single-limb circuit with a passive or active exhalation port.

10.1.7 Complications and Concerns During Short-Term NIPPV

Aerophagia and gastric distension can occur with NIPPV. Higher the pressures used, the greater the risk of gastric distension. Regurgitation of gastric contents and aspiration into the lungs are major concerns with the use of an oro-nasal, total face masks and a helmet. Close monitoring is needed to prevent aspiration. A nasogastric tube to keep the stomach decompressed is necessary in these acutely ill patients. Pressure sores related to the masks are other major concerns. It should be possible to pass one or two fingers between the headgear and the face. Care should be taken to avoid fitting the interface too tightly. A spacer with a soft padding can reduce the incidence of pressure sores on the face.

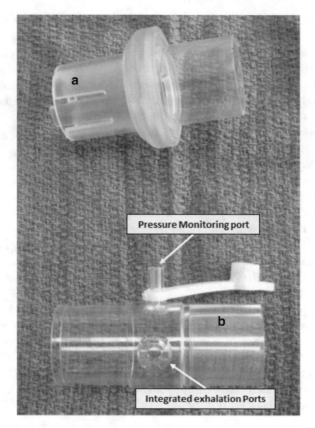

Fig. 10.9 Integrated exhalation valves. Two commercially available integrated exhalation values (e.g., Whisper-valves) **a** Non-disposable—exhalation ring for expired gas evacuation. **b** Disposable—has a pressure monitoring port and an integrated port for exhalation. Both exhalation valves create a leak for CO_2 removal. The rate of escape via the exhalation ports must be greater than the patient's exhaled gas flow

10.2 Negative-Pressure Ventilation

Negative-pressure ventilation (NPV), defined as noninvasive mechanical ventilation where sub-atmospheric pressure is applied to the external chest wall through either a tank/chamber device or chest "shells" causing inspiratory flow into the lungs at timed intervals. The negative pressure applied to the chest wall decreases the pleural and alveolar pressures resulting in chest expansion due to the pressure gradient created between the mouth and the alveoli. This mode of breath delivery provides a more physiologically supported breath by pulling atmospheric gas into the ventilator units, similar to the gas flow created by the diaphragm during inspiration. Usually, exhalation is passive due to the elastic recoil of the lung and chest wall. Some devices are capable of applying positive pressure to the thorax during the expiratory phase to facilitate exhalation in clinically indicated situations.

NPV was first applied via the iron lung to support respiratory failure secondary to the poliovirus epidemic. Popularity of the iron lung waned as a result of its large size, personnel required to support patients, and the detrimental effect on the cardiovascular system. Invasive positive-pressure ventilation alleviated these issues and quickly became the standard of care. Newer NPV devices have addressed the size and venous return issues by developing plastic cuirasses, which create a seal around the thorax—allowing access to the patient, increased patient portability, and providing increase range of motion without loss of ventilation.

10.2.1 Indications

Acute Respiratory Failure: Negative pressure ventilation is used in the pediatric population for treatment of acute respiratory failure such as in bronchiolitis, status asthmaticus, pneumonia, post-cardiothoracic surgery, and extubation support (Table 10.3). The most commonly used mode is CNEP. Evidence regarding the use of NPV in the pediatric population is mostly low-level—consisting of case-reports and single-center retrospective cohort studies. Given the lack of well-designed, controlled trials regarding this indication, use of NPV should be considered secondary or as an adjunct to other support strategies. The risks and benefits should be considered as they relate to other therapeutic options. Upper airway obstruction is a common reason for NPV failure due to upper airway collapse from negative extra-thoracic pressure. The patient should be monitored for paradoxical breathing pattern as this is the hallmark for upper airway collapse in children.

Neuromuscular Disorders: The available evidence suggests NPV provided by a chamber device (i.e. iron lung) can be effective in supporting acute respiratory failure in patient with neuromuscular disease (Table 10.3). However, size, cost and availability of chamber devices create significant barriers regarding its mainstream use within the acute care setting. Currently, only the Porta-lung® chamber is FDA approved in the United States. The device is compatible with older negative-pressure driving systems, such as the Respironics NEV-100 or Emerson 33-CR devices, as well as at the Negavent DA-3 Plus Pegaso V. More commonly

Table 10.3 Indications for NPV	Acute Respiratory Failure
	Post-cardiac surgery
	Chronic respiratory insufficiency
	Neuromuscular disease
	Mask intolerance
	Facial deformity
	Increased pulmonary secretions
	Facial pressure ulcers

used devices are those using a chest cuirass interface that increases access to the patient while adding patient comfort and mobility. These systems allow for addition of adjunctive therapy such as pulmonary hygiene or supplemental oxygen.

Other indications Noninvasive positive pressure ventilation is not effective with the following factors: (1) mask intolerance in infants and younger children, (2) sizing constraints, (3) congenital facial malformation, and (4) the presence of facial pressure ulcers (Table 10.3). Use of NPV may be a viable alternative to provide mechanical ventilation without an artificial airway. Chest cuirass interfaces alleviates the potential for mask intolerance by providing respiratory support without covering the face with a tight-fitting interface. Inability to properly fit a total face or oro-nasal mask in patients with congenital facial deformity results in a failure to deliver consistent pressures and volumes. Improper fit also increases the risk of pressure ulcer across bony prominences. Use of NPV may deliver better respiratory support while decreasing the need for escalation of care.

10.2.2 Contraindications and Side-Effects

Although NPV is indicated in both acute and critical care environments, several important contraindications must be considered when initiating NPV for non-invasive support (Table 10.4).

Children with documented central and/or sleep apnea syndromes should not be considered for NPV support. Absence of a central respiratory drive may result in clinically significant respiratory insufficiency leading to hemodynamic compromise. Negative pressure ventilation also increases the severity of upper airway collapse in obstructive sleep apnea—from negative intrathoracic pressure created by the device. Patients with tracheostomy are potentially less affected by the increase in thoracic negative press as the source of upper airway obstruction is bypassed by the artificial airway. Unconscious or patients with altered mental status are

Table 10.4 Contraindications and side-effects of NPV

Contraindications	Sleep-Apnea Syndrome
	Severe obesity
	Severe kyphoscoliosis
	Claustrophobia
	Rib fractures
	Recent abdominal surgery
	No protective airway reflex
	Extra-thoracic airway obstruction
Side-effects	Extra-thoracic airway collapse
	Back pain or discomfort
	Fatigue or depression
	Esophagitis
	Rib fracture
	Poor tolerance

contraindications, as often there is a loss of protective airway reflexes increasing the risk of aspiration. Some have suggested the use of an oral airway to support patients with upper airway obstruction from structural tissue and posterior displacement of the tongue. Use of an oral airway should only be used as a temporary adjunct until a more definitive airway can be placed. An oral airway should not be used continuously with NPV.

Additional contraindications include the morphology of the chest wall and abdomen. Severe obesity and kyphoscoliosis create an inability for the chest cuirass to fit snuggly are around the chest and abdomen, resulting in situations where neither negative nor positive pressure is achieved inside the cuirass rendering the therapy ineffective. Rib fractures and recent abdominal surgeries are also contraindications as the interface device will create discomfort and potentially result in complications. In these situations, non-invasive positive ventilation may be preferred to increase patient comfort and therapeutic effect.

10.2.3   Equipment for NPV

Design of negative pressure ventilators The basic design of all negative pressure ventilators include a negative pressure generator (pump), large-bore tubing, a pressure monitoring/trigger line (either a nasal cannula or a direct pressure line to the chamber), and a chamber in which sub-atmospheric pressure is created. The chamber may cover the entire body except for the head and neck (tank respirator, isolette, or a body suit) or only the chest and the upper abdomen (cuirass). The tank respirator has both the chamber and the pump in one unit. In all other cases, the two units are separate. The cuirass can be prefabricated or custom-designed to fit the contours of the chest. Custom-designed cuirasses are especially useful in patients with skeletal or spinal deformities. All body suits fit over a hard shell similar to the cuirass placed over the chest and the upper abdomen. Most negative pressure pumps in use today are pressure-cycled which means that when the target inspiratory pressure is reached, inspiration is terminated, and exhalation is started.

Tank/Whole Body Ventilator Modern tank ventilators are either made of aluminum or plastic and have separate rotary pumps. There is a mattress inside the chamber on which the patient's body rests. The head and neck rest on a pad or pillow outside the chamber. Some models have windows and portholes to allow access and to observe the patient as well. One of the advantages of the tank respirator is that they do not need to be designed to fit each patient. It requires only one effective seal at the level of the neck. The disadvantage is that it is difficult to access the patient. Aspiration of material from the pharynx into the trachea and bronchi may occur, especially with swallowing dysfunction.

Inspiration is time-triggered and the pump generates a negative pressure in the chamber. The tidal volume is directly proportional to the peak negative pressure within the chamber and inversely proportional to the patient's respiratory system dynamic compliance. When the negative pressure reaches a peak threshold value, inspiration is terminated and expiratory phase is initiated. The breaths delivered by the tank respirator are all mandatory breaths and pressure-cycled. Ventilator rate and the I:E ratio are selected by adjusting the appropriate controls. Tank ventilators do not allow synchronization of the mandatory breaths to the patient's efforts. This ventilator does not provide any assist to spontaneous breathing like pressure support since all the breaths are mandatory. Supplemental oxygen can be administered through standard oxygen delivery devices such as nasal cannula or a face-mask.

Isolette Ventilator Isolette-type respirator is a negative-pressure ventilator, used in neonates and small infants, consisting of two Plexiglas chambers, one for the body and one for the head. The two chambers are connected by an opening equipped with a neck sleeve. The infant's body is placed on a mattress in the body chamber with the neck placed in the opening between the two chambers. The head is positioned on a head rest. When the neck sleeve is gently closed around the neck to obtain a relatively tight seal with all the openings in both chambers being closed, negative pressure ventilation can be instituted. The depth of ventilation and therefore, the tidal volume, is controlled by the peak inspiratory negative pressure. Ventilator rate and the I:E ratio are selected by adjusting the appropriate controls. Humidified oxygen can be delivered either by nasal cannula or directly into the head chamber. The infant's body temperature can be maintained using servo-control regulation available as part of the isolette. In some ventilators, the mandatory breaths can be synchronized.

Cuirass ventilators Most cuirasses are made of clear plastic with a durable foam seal around the outer edges. The foam creates a seal ensuring that the pressure generated is maintained throughout the respiratory cycle. Located at the top of the cuirass is a large bore opening for the pressure hose to connect. The pressure tubing is large bore so as to accommodate the gas flow that is needed during both inspiration and exhalation. In theory, a cuirass that covers only the chest should be easier to use than a tank ventilator. A properly fit cuirass should cover the chest with an airtight seal and allow the anterior abdominal wall to freely expand during inspiration. In some patients, standard sizes may fit poorly and fail to provide an airtight seal around the chest or allow free movement of the abdomen requiring a cuirass to be custom fit. Development of pressure sores at the points of contact between the cuirass and the patient is a disadvantage that needs to be monitored. Similar to the tank ventilator, the tidal volume achieved with a cuirass is proportional to the peak negative pressure within it.

Jacket ventilation The first effective jacket ventilator was the Tunnicliffe jacket, developed in the 1950s. The design consists of an airtight synthetic garment with an inner framework made of metal or plastic. Most of the models cover the chest and abdomen up to the level just below the hips. Though several sizes are available, they are still too large for the infants and children. They are also not quite effective in patients with skeletal abnormalities. A pump intermittently evacuates the air within the jacket similar to that used in a cuirass ventilator. The developed tidal volumes are usually smaller than that of a tank respirator. The most commonly used are the Tunnicliffe jacket, the Lifecare PulmoWrap, and the Lifecare Numo Garment.

10.2.4   Available Controls

Inspiratory pressure—Inspiratory pressure is the negative extra thoracic pressure applied to the chest wall that generates inspiratory flow into the lungs. Increasing the negative pressure increases the tidal volume which can be measured with a mouth-piece attached to a spirometer. Decreasing the level of negative pressure decreases the level of support, placing more work of breathing on the patient.

Expiratory pressure—Expiratory pressure is the pressure applied to the thorax during exhalation. When it is set to zero cm H_2O, exhalation will be passive due to the elastic recoil of the lung and chest wall. When it is set to be greater than zero cm H_2O, the positive pressure assists the exhalation of the lungs.

Respiratory frequency—These are mandatory breaths that can be set in control, assist control, and assist with plateau modes. Initial rate is usually set at least 2 breaths/min above the patient's current spontaneous respiratory rate. Some devices have synchronization modes, allowing for improved patient tolerance as the device adjusts the rate and shape of breath in response to the patient's pattern and effort.

I/E ratio—While setting the I:E ratios, it is important to pay attention to the actual inspiratory and expiratory times for each breath. Based on the respiratory system time-constants, I:E ratios can be adjusted for optimal lung inflation as well as exhalation.

Plateau pressure—Used in spontaneous mode, the plateau pressure can be used to extend the inspiratory time and maintain the set inspiratory pressure for the additional time. A time is set usually between 1.0 and 2.0 s. The pause allows for longer duration of distending pressure thus increasing mean airway pressure.

Trigger—In most devices, the trigger to initiate a breath is time or pressure. In some devices, just as with synchronized mandatory ventilation (SIMV), a patient effort can trigger the mandatory breath. The trigger to activate such synchronized breaths is pressure which may be sensed in the chest cuirass or a nasal cannula.

10.2.5   Available Modes

There are 2 types of NPV support, which are pressure-controlled ventilation and continuous negative extrathoracic pressure (CNEP). All ventilatory modes in NPV are pressure-controlled—the peak inspiratory pressure is limited or controlled with the tidal volume varying depending on the mechanical properties of the respiratory system. The following summary of the modes available in these ventilators will be described according to Chatburn's classification system with the corresponding proprietary names provided by the manufacturer.

1. Unsynchronized mandatory ventilation—All devices are capable of this mode of ventilation where all the breaths are machine-triggered and machine-cycled using time as the variable for triggering and cycling. The ventilator delivers a set rate with predetermined inspiratory and expiratory pressures and a fixed I:E

ratio. The total number of breaths delivered in this mode of ventilation is the set rate. Patient's spontaneous efforts do not have any impact on the total number of breaths provided by the ventilator and are not used to trigger any of the breaths. This is referred to as the *Control mode* by the Hayek ventilator and as *Timed mode* by the Pegaso V ventilator. The inspiratory pressure limit is set to provide the desired chest expansion. The expiratory pressure can be set to be a negative pressure, ambient pressure (zero) or a positive pressure. When the expiratory pressure is negative, it functions similar to PEEP in maintaining a certain lung volume during the expiratory phase. This mode is also called *Negative Pressure with CNEP*. This is particularly useful in children with parenchymal lung disease with decreased FRC. When the expiratory pressure is set to be positive, the chest is compressed during the expiratory phase providing active exhalation. This is also referred to as *Negative/Positive Pressure Ventilation*. The positive expiratory pressure can facilitate exhalation and CO_2 removal. Conversely, exhalation of the lungs is passive due to chest and lung recoil when the expiratory pressure is set to be zero or negative. When the expiratory pressure is set to be zero, it is also called *Cyclical Negative Pressure ventilation*

2. Synchronized mandatory ventilation—Some devices are capable of providing synchronized mandatory ventilation. The Hayek ventilator can sense patient's breathing efforts both in the cuirass as well as a nasal cannula. The Pegaso V ventilator can sense the patient's efforts using a nasal cannula or a facemask. Just as with the unsynchronized mode, the ventilator needs to have a preset rate, I:E ratio, inspiratory and expiratory pressures. If the patient is apneic or is unable to trigger, then the ventilator will deliver the set number of breaths. If the patient is breathing spontaneously and can trigger a breath, the ventilator will deliver a breath with the preset inspiratory and expiratory pressures with fixed inspiratory and expiratory times. This mode is similar to the Assist-Control mode with positive pressure ventilation. This is referred to as *Synchro-Timed* mode by the Pegaso V ventilator and *Respiratory Triggered* mode by the Hayek ventilator.

3. Synchronized assisted ventilation—Some devices are capable of providing synchronized, assisted ventilation similar to pressure support in positive pressure ventilation. When a patient's effort is sensed, the ventilator delivers a breath with the preset inspiratory and expiratory pressures. The inspiratory and expiratory times that determine the I:E ratio will depend on the patient's own efforts. When the patient makes an expiratory effort, machine inspiration is terminated and exhalation is initiated. During the succeeding exhalation phase, if an inspiratory effort is sensed, a mechanical breath is delivered. Unlike pressure-support ventilation, this mode has a back-up mode which is the unsynchronized mandatory mode with a preset rate, inspiratory and expiratory pressures, and a fixed I:E ratio. The inspiratory and expiratory pressures are the same whether the breath is synchronized and assisted or unsynchronized and mandatory.

Patient-triggered and synchronized pressure control require the use of an interface such as a nasal cannula or a direct trigger line connected to the chamber. The trigger is measured and ranges from 0.6 to 3.0 cm H_2O. The proximal interfaces (i.e., nasal cannula or a mouth-piece near the patient's airway) are more sensitive than the direct cuirass pressure sensing line.

4. CNEP—*CNEP* refers to a spontaneous mode where a constant sub-atmospheric pressure is provided throughout the respiratory cycle. CNEP is like CPAP and is used to support conditions with increased work of breathing associated with small airway disease and V/Q mismatching. Initiation of CNEP usually begin at −7 to −10 cm H_2O and is adjusted as necessary based on gas exchange and work of breathing. Occasionally a more negative setting may be needed. Improvement is identified by better oxygenation and ventilation, a decrease in expiratory muscle use and metabolic acidosis.

5. High frequency oscillator mode—The Hayek ventilator can function as a high frequency ventilator at a frequency between 2 and 15 Hz. The expiratory pressure is set to be a positive pressure of the same magnitude as the negative inspiratory pressure. The total pressure deflection between peak inspiration and peak expiration is called the *Span* similar to the amplitude/power of the high frequency oscillatory ventilators used from invasive ventilation. The high frequency mode is not approved for use as a ventilator in the US.

6. Machine Failure and Alarms Machine failure is indicated by both audio and visual alarms and occur when the device is deemed inoperable. These alarms vary with device. Reasons leading to machine failure include but are not limited to (1) AC power failure, (2) unrecognized hardware failure, (3) pressure sensor fault or failure, (4) faulty pressure valve, (5) software failure, and (6) tank pressure being too low. Both high and low alarms can be set for pressure and rate.

7. Monitoring Clinically, NPV has been associated with improvement in ventilation and oxygenation in a number of clinical situations. Most commonly the modality has been used as an adjunctive support device in conjunction with supplemental oxygen devices. Standard physiologic monitoring should be used to identify clinical improvement or decline during therapy. Clinical evaluation should include a systematic assessment of the upper airway patency, cardiovascular, respiratory, and neurologic status. Respiratory rate and pattern changes are helpful in identifying clinical improvement or worsening. Pulse-oximetry will identify changes in SpO_2, facilitating oxygen titration and identifying need for escalation in therapy. Institutionally accepted oxygen titration guidelines should be used to manage support. Additionally, end-tidal carbon dioxide ($ETCO_2$) monitoring through a commercially available system using a nasal cannula interface may help recognize changing in expired CO_2. Clinicians should be aware of any changes in $ETCO_2$, as it is a key indicator of muscle fatigue or increasing intrapulmonary shutting. If changes in vital sign, SpO_2, or $ETCO_2$ are seen, blood gas measurements should be obtained (Table 10.5).

Table 10.5 Negative pressure generator devices and characteristics of operation

Device	Inspiratory pressure (cm H_2O)	Expiratory pressure (cm H_2O)	CNEP maximum (cm H_2O)	Rate (breaths/min)	I:E Ratio	Modes	Trigger	Alarm
Hayek® United Hayek	−50	10 cm above the inspiratory pressure up to +50	−50	6–150	1:6	C, CNEP	Pressure	Apnea High RR MF
Negavent DA-3 Plus Pegaso V Dima Italia	−5 to −99	−25 to + 99	−25	1–50	1:6	C, A/C, CNEP, A + Plat	Pressure, Flow	P_{max} P_{min} MF

C: Control; A/C: Assist Control; CNEP: continuous negative extrathoracic pressure; A + Plat: Assisted with Plateau pause; P max: Maximum Pressure; P Min: minimum pressure; MF: Machine failure

Additionally, understanding of the operational characteristics (Table 10.5), interface sizing, and device limitations will facilitate the therapeutic effect of NPV. Both the devices are capable using inverse I:E ratios. These are used mainly for secretion clearance purposes and not for ventilatory support.

10.2.6   Secretion Clearance and Cough Assist

High frequency chest wall oscillations using the cuirass ventilators can be used for secretion clearance in patients. It can be used alone or in combination with sigh breaths following which the airway can be cleared of any secretions that are brought up. The sequence of high frequency oscillations followed by the sigh breaths can be programmed into the ventilator. Cuirass ventilators can also be used as cough assist devices with a simulated cough that has a prolonged inspiratory phase with a pressure of -20 to -60 cm H_2O followed by a very short expiratory phase with a positive pressure of the same magnitude as the inspiratory phase.

Suggested Readings

1. Nilsestuen JO, Hargett KD. Using ventilator graphics to identify patient-ventilator asynchrony. Respir Care. 2005;50(2):202–32.
2. Jin P. Mechanical breathing graph waveform monitoring and analysis in the nervous system intensive care unit. J Neurocrit Care. 2018;11(2):63–70.
3. Holanda MA, dos Santos VR, Ferreira JC, Pinheiro BV. Patient-ventilator asynchrony. J Bras Pneumol. 2018;44(4):321–33.
4. Hess DR. Noninvasive ventilation in neuromuscular disease: equipment and application. Respir Care
5. Corrado A, Gorini M, Villella G, De Paola E. Negative pressure ventilation in the treatment of acute respiratory failure: an old noninvasive technique reconsidered. Eur Respir J. 1996;9:1531–44.
6. Corrado A, Gorini M. Negative-pressure ventilation: Is there till a role? Eur Respir J. 2002;20:187–97.
7. Hassinger AB, Breuer RK, Nutty K, et al. Negative-pressure ventilation in pediatric acute respiratory failure. Respir Care. 2017;62(12):1540–9.
8. Sammuels MP, Raine J, Wright T. Continuous negative extrathoracic pressure in the treatment of respiratory failure in infants and young children. BMJ. 1989;299:1253–7.
9. Deshpande SR, Kirshbom PM, Maher KO. Negative pressure ventilation as a therapy for post-operative complications in a patient with single ventricle physiology. Heart Lung Circ. 2011;20:763–5.
10. Shah PS, Ohlsson A, Shah JP. Continuous negative extrathoracic pressure or continuous positive airway pressure compared to conventional ventilation for acute hypoxaemic respiratory failure in children. Cochrane Database systemic rev. 2013 Nov 4;(11)

Chapter 11
Respiratory Care Equipment

Bradley A. Kuch and Shekhar T. Venkataraman

11.1 Oxygen Delivery Devices

Supplemental oxygen administration is the most common therapeutic intervention provided to infants and children presenting with acute or chronic respiratory disease. In order to match the patient's needs with the appropriate device requires an understanding of the patient's pathophysiology and the capabilities of a particular device. The acronym AIM has been suggested as a helpful means to select oxygen delivery device. The AIM mnemonic stands for (A) assessment of patient need, (I) identification of device capability, and (M) matching device/technology with need. Clinical evaluation for the need for supplemental oxygen includes general appearance, responsiveness, pulse-oximetry, and heart rate. Knowing each oxygen delivery device's capabilities and limitations is critical in selecting the right device for the patient's needs. Matching the device capacities with the patient's oxygen needs begins with an evaluation of severity of hypoxemia, patient inspiratory rate, and tolerance of the applied device. Intolerance of the applied device can the stress the patient and increase the work of breathing which may lead to further compromise. Common reasons for ineffective supplemental oxygen therapy include

B. A. Kuch (✉)
Director, Respiratory Care Services and Transport Team & Clinical Research Associate, Department of Pediatric Critical Care Medicine, UPMC Children's Hospital of Pittsburgh, 4401 Penn Ave, Pittsburgh, PA 15224, USA
e-mail: bradley.kuch@chp.edu

S. T. Venkataraman
Professor, Departments of Critical Care Medicine and Pediatrics, University of Pittsburgh School of Medicine, Pittsburgh, PA, USA

Medical Director, Respiratory Care Services, Children's Hospital of Pittsburgh, 4401 Penn Avenue, Faculty Pavilion 2117, Pittsburgh, PA 15224, USA

© Springer Nature Switzerland AG 2022
A. P. Sarnaik et al. (eds.), *Mechanical Ventilation in Neonates and Children*,
https://doi.org/10.1007/978-3-030-83738-9_11

improper fit, inadequate flow rates and educational gaps in understanding technical capabilities and published consensus guidelines.

Blenders and Low Flow Meters

Air-oxygen blenders allow for mixing medical grade air and oxygen to any concentration from 21 to 100% oxygen. The output from the blender may be delivered to a variety of respiratory care devices. Oxygen blenders allow the clinician to set a specific concentration of oxygen supplied to the oxygen device, most frequently a nasal cannula in neonates and small infants. Both the flow rate and the blender concentration can be adjusted to deliver the required FiO_2. It is important to understand that air-oxygen blenders cannot be used reliably to deliver other gases such as helium–oxygen mixture since there is considerable difference in gas density which will not only affect the flow through the blender but also the FiO_2 of the gas output from the blender. Table 11.1 gives a suggested guideline for managing and weaning FiO_2 when air-oxygen blenders are used with flow meters.

Blow-by Oxygen Delivery

Blow-by oxygen method of supplemental oxygen delivery is the simplest and easiest to tolerate. This method is provided in several different ways, which include a high-flow oxygen source connected to large bore or small caliber oxygen tubing with or without a face tent/simple face mask placed in close proximity and directed towards the patient's face. It is most commonly used in the delivery-room for oxygen supplementation during infant stabilization, during the initial evaluation, and during the initial patient presentation with respiratory distress. Blow-by oxygen is the least consistent means to provide a known FiO_2 and for this reason it is only recommended for brief oxygen support until a more definitive device can be applied. But, in patients who don't tolerate more bulky devices or who may have

Table 11.1 Guidelines for managing FiO_2	1. Set blender FiO_2 at 100% and flow at the lowest level (often begin at 1 LPM; rarely >2 LPM) to provide an acceptable SpO_2 (92–94%)
	2. If SpO_2 is >95%, decrease flow rate in small increments that maintains an acceptable SpO_2 level (92–94%)
	3. Continue to wean flow rate (still on 1.0 FiO_2) until the lowest graduated mark on the flow meter
	4. Begin decreasing the oxygen concentration on the blender. Commonly changes of 5% are acceptable, however larger or small titrations maybe indicated
	5. Once patient is stable, the nasal cannula can be removed
	Of note Some clinicians lower oxygen concentrations first instead of the flow rate. However, decreasing the flow rates first will maximize the stability of oxygen concentration over time and decrease the magnitude of FiO_2 changes during weaning. For this reason, weaning flow followed by oxygen concentration is recommended

undergone facial surgery or suffered trauma to the face, head, or neck, blow-by oxygen may be the only reliable method to provide supplemental oxygen. Blow-by oxygen therapy delivers relatively low concentrations of oxygen.

Oxygen Hood or Tent

An oxygen hood or tent is a plastic enclosure surrounding the patient's head or the whole body that provides continuous flow of humidified air-oxygen mixture. The source gas can be delivered by either an air entrainment device or more commonly from an air-oxygen blender. Oxygen hoods are used for neonates and small infants and surround the head and upper torso. One benefit of this device is direct access to the patient's chest and body for ongoing assessment. With adequate enclosure seal, an oxygen hood can provide a delivered FiO_2 from 0.22 to 0.8 with a range of 7–10 L/min. Oxygen tent covers the child's entire body and the range of flow rates used is between 15 and 30 L/min. Due to its size, it is difficult to maintain FiO_2 higher than 0.5 and may not be appropriate for patients who need a higher FiO_2. With these devices, exhaled CO_2 is removed by providing an adequate amount of fresh gas into the device. If the gas flow into the device is inadequate, there is a risk of CO_2 rebreathing. There is a risk of hypothermia if the gas is not adequately heated. Widespread use of nasal cannulas, both for low flow and high flow oxygen delivery, has resulted in these devices being less preferable, especially in infants and small children.

Low-flow Nasal Cannula (Low-flow)

Low-flow nasal cannula is one of the most frequently used oxygen devices in infants and children. Low flow oxygen is delivered via 2 prongs situated in the patient's nares. The proximal end of the cannula is connected to 100% oxygen gas source flow meter or an air-oxygen blender allowing for adjustment of source gas FiO_2. Use of a blender provides more control over the delivered oxygen concentration in smaller patients where device flow rates equal or exceed the patient's inspiratory flow demand. It has been reported that delivered FiO_2 to the neonate via a nasal cannula ranges from 0.22 to 0.95 at a set maximum flow of 2 L/min (Fig. 11.1).

Actual FiO_2 delivered via a nasal cannula is associated with several important factors such as the set flow rate and its proportion to the patient's inspiratory flow demand. Other determinants of FiO_2 include room-air entrainment and the device's inability to meet an acceptable proportion of the patient's inspiratory demand in times of increase minute ventilation needs. This will result in a decreased FiO_2 that may require switching to another means to deliver adequate oxygen delivery. Conversely, patients with decreased minute ventilation as a result of sedation, or being post-ictal following a seizure will have increased FiO_2, as flow will fill the anatomic dead space increasing the FiO_2 delivered. Because anatomic dead space is less in the neonate and infant, low flow nasal cannula will provide greater FiO_2 than in adult population. Oxygen delivered with this method may also be passively humidified to increase patient comfort. Prolonged use or high flow rates without adequate humidification may lead to tissue irritation by drying the mucosa and

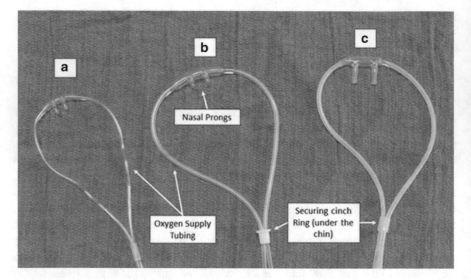

Fig. 11.1 Low Flow nasal cannulas **a** Neonatal **b** Pediatric and **c** Adult Cannula. Nasal prongs fit securely in the nose, tube is draped gently over the ears, and the cinch ring goes under the chin softly hold the tubing over the ears

contribute to patient discomfort. Heating and humidifying the gas source can decrease irritation by adequate humidification and increase patient tolerance.

Heated Humidified High-Flow Nasal Cannula

Definition and Equipment

Heated Humidified High-Flow Nasal Cannula (HHHFNC or shortened to HFNC), is defined as the delivery of heated and humidified oxygen at a flow rate of 0.5–2 L/kg/min through a specially designed nasal delivery system. During normal breathing, the normal peak inspiratory flow rate is about 0.5–1 L/kg/min. The usual starting flow for HFNC can range between 0.5 and 2 L/kg/min. Flow greater than 2 L/kg/min may increase expiratory resistance and decrease the efficacy of HFNC therapy. The FiO_2 of HFNC can range from 0.21 to 1.0. The gas is heated and humidified to increase patient comfort, decrease drying of airway mucosa and facilitate airway clearance (Table 11.2).

HFNC system consist of several primary components, which include:

1. Medical-grade gas source—depending on the configuration, system will require access to air and oxygen to power gas blenders for delivery of varying FiO_2. Commercially available systems have integrated gas-blending systems, removing the need for multiple gas sources.
2. Heated humidifier—conditions gas to a relative humidity of approximately 100% at temperature of 34 and 37 °C, improving patient tolerance, decreasing insensible losses, and improving mucociliary clearance. Additionally, heated

Table 11.2 High-Flow nasal cannula delivery systems and flow generator types

HFNC devices	Manufacturer	Gas generator type
Vapotherm System system	Fisher Paykel Auckland New Zealand	1. Air/oxygen blender with heated humidification system 2. May have an integrated pressure relief valve
Precision Flow®	Vapotherm, Exeter UK	1. Air/oxygen blender with heated humidification system 2. May have an integrated pressure relief valve
Comfort-Flow®	Teleflex Medical, Durham, NC, USA	1. Air/oxygen blender with heated humidification system 2. May have an integrated pressure relief valve 3. Turbine driving with humidifier
Airvo2® with Opitflow®	Fisher Paykel, Auckland, New Zealand	Oxygen only gas source
CPAP/ Conventional Ventilator	Multiple Platforms—ensure the ventilator has non-invasive mode available with select alarm configuration(s)	1. Flow generated by the ventilator, maybe variable 2. Requires non-invasive mode 3. Pressure alarms available

and humidified gas decreases resistance in the nasal cavity, which is an important consideration as it accounts for 50% of the total resistance of the respiratory system.

3. Heated circuit—systems should have an integrated heated circuit to increase temperature control, decrease circuit rain-out, and increase humidity of the inspired gas. These circuit monitor temperature at the chamber and at the distal end of the circuit, which helps the clinician ensure adequate humidity and temperature management. Heated circuit increase patient comfort at high liter flows, increasing device tolerance.

4. High-flow nasal cannula—by definition, high-flow nasal cannula interfaces are non-occlusive, with proper sizing occluding 50% of the circumference of the nares. The leak limits the risk of auto-PEEP/gas-trapping and facilitates CO_2 elimination through an open system during nose breathing with a closed mouth.

5. Oxygen analyzer—commercially available systems have integrated oxygen analyzers to ensure accurate FiO_2 delivery, which adds a margin of safety, facilitates oxygen weaning, and documentation. If an institutionally developed system has been created using a blender, heated humidification device, and

heated circuit, an oxygen analyzer should be placed in-line for accurate FiO_2 measurement.
6. Pressure relief valve—provides a mechanism to relieve pressure at a set level within the circuit to decrease the risk of over-pressurization in the event too large a cannula is used or an obstruction occurs within the system. These are often supplied with the manufacturer supplied circuit systems. These valves should be used as indicated to limit risk to the patient.

The mechanisms by which HFNC may improve the work of breathing and oxygenation are:

1. Decreased inspiratory work of breathing by providing a flow of gas that matches or exceeds the peak inspiratory flow of the patient
2. Decreased dead space

   a. Approximately a third of the exhaled tidal volume is rebreathed during normal respiration
   b. This terminal portion of the exhaled tidal volume contains carbon dioxide which constitutes about 5–6% of this space
   c. HFNC washes out this gas with fresh oxygen-rich gas

3. Maintenance of a higher FiO_2 in the pharyngeal space due to decreased entrainment of atmospheric air
4. With a tight fit in the nares and with the mouth closed, HFNC can generate positive pressure in the airways and produce CPAP. However, the level of positive airway pressure generated in the alveoli is variable and would depend on the ability of the patient to keep the mouth closed, and the tightness of the fit of the nasal cannulas.

Indications and Contraindications

Administration of supplemental oxygen via HFNC is most commonly indicated in children with mild to moderate hypoxemia unresponsive to low-flow oxygen delivery devices. High-flow nasal cannula has also been found to be effective in treating infants and children with underlying lung disorders that require enhanced oxygenation with possibly reducing the work of breathing.

Bronchiolitis Most of the evidence supporting the use of HFNC in the pediatric population is in bronchiolitis. In a large multi-center randomized, controlled trial in infants less than 12 months of age with bronchiolitis, those treated with HFNC received less escalation of care. Additionally, those infants who failed standard therapy, 61% had a response to high-flow rescue therapy. There was no difference in hospital length of stay or duration of oxygen support. High-flow nasal cannula therapy has also been associated with decreased rates of intubation in infants admitted to the PICU with bronchiolitis. A single center retrospective review demonstrated a 68% decrease in intubation in infants less than 24 months of age admitted to the PICU with bronchiolitis after introduction of HFNC into practice.

The authors also reported a reduction in PICU length of stay from 6 to 4 days post introduction of HFNC. These results need to be validated in prospective studies.

Successful use of HFNC in infants with bronchiolitis begins with an early assessment and identification of severity of respiratory distress and therapeutic need. Respiratory Distress Score and oxygen requirement are useful in determining the level of support needed. Infants with mild to moderate respiratory distress and an FiO_2 requirement greater than 0.60 may benefit from HFNC. Severe respiratory distress and higher FiO_2 requirements should be considered for either non-invasive or invasive positive pressure ventilation. Initiation of HFNC should begin at a rate of 0.5–2 L/kg/min and an FiO_2 of 1.0, with FiO_2 decreased to maintain acceptable SpO_2.

Asthma Use of HFNC for asthmatic patients has potential physiologic benefits, which include reduced work of breathing due to auto-PEEP, and potential amelioration of bronchoconstriction by delivering heated and humidified gas. Recently it has been reported that early initiation of HFNC is superior when compared to conventional oxygen therapy in moderate-to-severe asthma exacerbations. It is recommended that use of HFNC in this patient population is based on clinical indications which incorporate clinical respiratory distress scoring. Low flow delivery systems may be adequate to support less severe exacerbations and the application of HFNC may result in an increased resource utilization, length of stay, and costs. Furthermore, use of HFNC may mask the need for more intensive support such as a need for non-invasive positive pressure ventilation. Delivery of nebulized bronchodilator therapy has been suggested via HFNC, however much controversy remains as the delivered dose varies from only 0.5% to 25% of the administered dose. Consideration should be given in the method of aerosol delivery in children supported via HFNC, as an exceedingly low dose is delivered to the lung, with increased nasal disposition, which may result in local toxicity.

Interfacility Transport Interfacility transport is a dynamic low-resource environment, often complicated by patient severity of illness and lack of confirmed diagnosis. Evidence demonstrating the association of the use of HFNC with decreased rate of intubation and escalation of care in both the emergency department and intensive care units, has led to its use in the interfacility transport setting. Benefits associated with HFNC in this environment include the administration of variable level of CPAP, reduced work of breathing through flow-related reduction in anatomic dead space, and patient comfort. A few operational concerns need be addressed in using high-flow therapy in the transport setting. The primary issue is related to a continuous power source for the heater-humidifier. Loss of power will result in a rapid loss of heat delivered humidity and temperature.

Other Potential Uses The success of HFNC with bronchiolitis has increased its potential applications in pneumonia, after cardiothoracic surgery, as well as after extubation.

Contraindications, Risks and Complications

Contraindications for HFNC include suspected or confirmed pneumothorax, severe upper airway obstruction and decreased respiratory drive. Use of HFNC comes with several risks. Most significant concern is the inability to measure the exact level of positive pressure produced. Level of potential PEEP generated by the therapy varies from patient to patient and is affected by patient size, air flow, open-mouth, and the percent occlusion of the nares. These variables allow for inconsistent end-expiratory pressure and may result in gastric distention and/or lung over expansion. Most pediatric lung disease is heterogeneous—producing areas of increased compliance and other areas with decreased compliance. Inconsistent positive end expiratory pressure from a non-occlusive interface results in non-uniform pressure distribution with areas of atelectasis and over-expansion. This may lead to escalation in care such as increased FiO_2 requirement due to V/Q mismatching. A complication rate of 0.9/100 HFNC treatment days has been reported. Of these complications, 4% of the total cohort had either development of new pneumothoraces or chest tube-related air leaks following the initiation of HFNC therapy. A secondary concern is the concentration of oxygen that can be delivered. At high flow rates, it is quite easy to deliver a $FiO_2 > 0.60$, which may mask progressing hypoxic respiratory failure and introduce lung tissue to toxic levels of oxygen. Supplemental oxygen concentration should be weaned to maintain adequate SpO_2. If high levels of oxygen are required to maintain a clinically acceptable arterial saturation, occlusive non-invasive positive pressure ventilatory support should be considered as a more stable mean airway pressure will recruit collapsed alveolar units and result in increased FRC. Paradoxical respiration is a sign of upper airway collapse in small children that is better managed by an occlusive airway device such as nasal prongs, nasal masks, or full-face masks.

Simple Face Mask (Low-flow)

Simple Facemask is a lightweight reservoir mask that fits over the patient's nose and mouth with an elastic strap that is secure around the child's head just above the ears (Fig. 11.2). The mask has open ports on each side—allowing for exhalation and for the patient to draw in room-air during inspiration. Rubber flaps maybe placed on one side of the mask, decreasing room air entrainment, increasing FiO_2 delivered. Set flow rates between 6 and 10 L/min deliver a variable FiO_2 between 0.35 and 0.50. The conical shape and reservoir design may accumulate exhaled carbon dioxide (CO_2) if minimal flows are not ensured. A minimum flow of 6 L/min is recommended for older children and adults to ensure flushing of exhaled CO_2. Sound practice includes that all patients receive no less than 6 L/min when receiving supplemental oxygen via a simple face mask.

No data pertaining to newborns or infants have been reported regarding effective FiO_2 delivery via simple facemasks. Several hazards and complications are associated with the use of simple facemasks. Because the mask is strapped to the infant or child's face, phonation, eating including breast- and bottle-feeding increases the risk of aspiration of vomitus. Particular caution should be taken in patients with

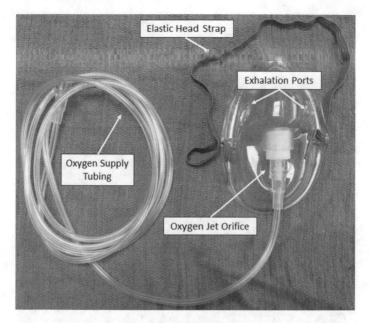

Fig. 11.2 Simple face fask—complete setup with oxygen supply tubing, elastic head strap, and jet orifice. The exhalation ports are open for evacuation of exhaled CO_2. Minimum flow of at least 6L/min must be maintained

altered consciousness and potentially a full-stomach. They should be evaluated for the presence of cough and gag. The elastic strap is also uncomfortable and may cause skin redness and irritation with prolonged use, most notably on the top of the ears.

Air-Entrainment (Venturi) Masks (High-flow)

Air-entrainment or Venturi masks are high-flow masks that provide a fixed concentration of oxygen at a flow rate that meets or exceeds the patient total inspiratory demand. The set flow rate, indicated by the specific device combined with the fixed air-entrainment, exceed the patient respiratory flow demand—ensures that only a fixed amount of room air is entrained. For this reason, these devices are ideal in clinical situations where a reliable concentration of oxygen is indicated. For example, patients with known CO_2 retention whose breathing is dependent on hypoxic drive such as cystic fibrosis, a fixed FiO_2 delivery will decrease the risk of hyperoxia related hypoventilation. Such patients will benefit from an air-entrainment mask. Another clinical situation would be those hypoxic patients with high respiratory rate and tidal volumes, where an air-entrainment mask is capable of meeting the patient's inspiratory flow demand.

The mask fits over the patient's nose and mouth with large ports on each side. The port allows for removal of exhaled gas while providing a means to entrain room air during times of high inspiratory flow demand. The mask commonly has a

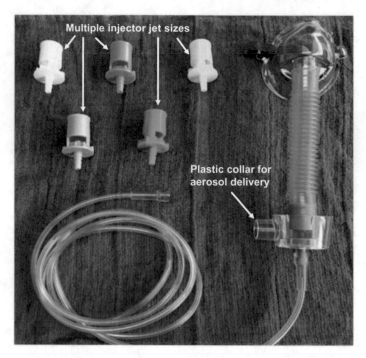

Fig. 11.3 Pediatric Venturi Mask with multiple diluter jet and humidification hood—Carefusion®
Yorba Linda, Ca. USA. Note the plastic collar at the end of the corrugated tubing for aerosol
delivery

50 ml portion of corrugated tubing which acts as a small reservoir. At the end of the
corrugated tubing there is a jet-orifice, which is connected to small-bore tubing.
Some air-entrainment masks come with multiple jet-orifices specifically designed to
deliver the desired FiO_2 (Fig. 11.3), while others have manufacturer provided
adjustable jet orifices. Venturi masks deliver concentrations ranging from 24 to
50%. Each system has oxygen flow requirements indicated to deliver the precise
FiO_2. Increase or decrease in this flow rate will affect delivered oxygen concentration. It must also be noted that backpressure in the system will increase the
delivered oxygen. Back-pressure is commonly caused by blockage of the entrainment ports. Particular attention should be paid to this, as it will limit patient
inspiratory flow and increase FiO_2.

Supplied medical gas is dry and devoid of any humidity. When using an
air-entrainment mask, the high flows needed to meet the patient needs may result in
mucosal drying and airway irritation. The high flows will also result in excessive
backpressure build up if a bubble humidifier is used, resulting in backpressure
pop-off alarm. To address this, some manufacturers supply a humidification hood.
The 22-mm plastic collar (Fig. 11.3) can be attached to a bland-aerosol nebulizer to
provide humidity. Bland Aerosols can either be cool or heated as indicated by the
clinical situation.

As previously mentioned, performance of an air-entrainment mask may be altered by resistance to gas flow occurring distal to the jet–orifice, resulting in less room air entrainment and lower total delivered flow. If the flow in decreased sig. nificantly enough, the patient may only receive room-air. This is the first step in troubleshooting the system when periods of hypoxemia are noted. In addition, at the 50% oxygen setting, total flow delivered is far less than at lower oxygen concentrations. This creates the potential for the patient to receive a lower FiO_2 in times of increased inspiratory flow requirements.

Reservoir Masks

Reservoir masks consist of a mask and plastic reservoir bag with or without a one-way valve to hold oxygen while barring exhaled CO_2 form being rebreathed. Fresh oxygen is supplied to the system via the neck of the mask, directed into the bag reservoir where it can be easily withdrawn during inspiration. The bag increases the total volume of fresh gas supplied for each breath, functionally delivering a higher oxygen concentration. The mask is designed with exhalation ports for exhaled gas elimination. These ports can have plastic valves added to either one or both sides to limit room air entrainment and increase the delivered FiO_2.

Reservoir masks have the capability to provide moderate to high oxygen concentrations. Ensuring these concentrations requires an appropriately sized mask with a tight-fit, which makes these devices less then optimal for long-term use. Reservoir mask are not well-tolerated by infants and small children. They are not recommended for neonates.

Partial Non-rebreather

Partial non–rebreather mask is similar to a simple facemask, but it includes a plastic reservoir bag at the end of the bottom of the mask. It differs from a non-rebreather mask (discussed in detail later) as they do not have a one-way valve to prevent rebreathing of the exhaled breath. The device is designed to conserve oxygen by delivery of 100% oxygen and allowing for partial rebreathing of the exhaled gas, which increases FiO_2 at lower flow-rates. A majority of the exhaled gas is vented through 2 ports, one on each side of the mask. As in all masks, the mask should fit securely on the patient's face with little to no leak. A leak will allow for room-air entrainment decreasing delivered oxygen concentration—a common mistake when utilizing high concentration masks. Oxygen flow should be set at a rate to ensure that the bag remains partially inflated during inspiration. Usually, 6–15 L/min is adequate. In the event the bag deflates totally, more flow is need and the oxygen flow rate should be increased. If inadequate flow is not addressed it may result in CO_2 retention. With a good seal and sufficient flow, a partial-rebreather mask can deliver FiO_2 of up to 0.6. It must be noted as in other oxygen delivery devices, the delivered oxygen concentration will be influenced by the patient's respiratory pattern. Caution should be taken in patients considered to have a full stomach with altered mental status, as the closed design of the mask may increase the risk of aspiration (Fig. 11.4).

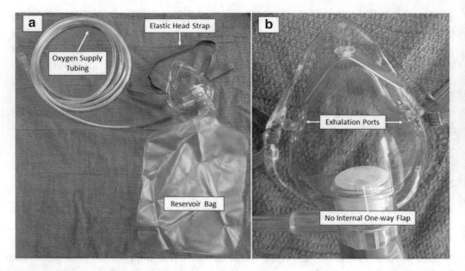

Fig. 11.4 Partial non-breather mask. **a** Complete setup with oxygen supply tubing, elastic head strap, and reservoir bag. **b** Close up of mask with open exhalation ports and no internal one-way flap

Non-rebreather Mask

Non-rebreathing masks are very similar to partial rebreather mask, except they have a one-way valve located between the mask and the reservoir bag to prevent rebreathing of exhaled gas which is directed through the exhalation ports located on either side of the mask. Exhalation ports have one-way rubber/plastic leaflets to prevent room air entrainment. These design characteristics allow for the delivery of higher oxygen concentrations when compared to either a simple facemask or a partial non-rebreathing mask. Like a partial non-rebreathing mask, flow rates should be set at a level high enough to ensure the bag does not completely deflate. If the bag deflates completely, additional flow should be added to meet the patient's inspiratory flow demand. With proper and snug fit, non-rebreather mask can provide oxygen concentrations greater than 90%, and in the best situations close to 100%. Because of its design, these masks can be used to deliver specialty gas mixtures such as Helium–oxygen or sub-atmospheric FiO_2 via a blender set-up. It must be noted that these masks are not intended for long-term use and must be evaluated frequently for pressure breakdown form the strap or non-compliance. Also aspiration risk and CO_2 retention should also be considered when using these mask devices (Fig. 11.5).

Oxymask™ (High and Low-flow)

The Oxymask™ is a high-flow system that incorporates a "Pin and Diffuser" technology, which is designed to concentrate and redirect oxygen flow towards the patient's nose and mouth. The device has an open facemask allowing for room air

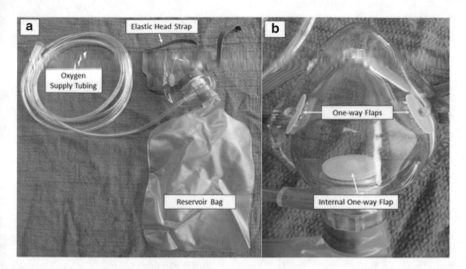

Fig. 11.5 Non-rebreather mask. **a** Complete setup with oxygen supply tubing, one-way flaps preventing room air entrainment and reservoir bag. **b** Close up of mask with internal one-way flap to prevent rebreathing of exhaled gas

entrainment, thus not limiting the patient's inspiratory flow demand while removing the need for valves and reservoirs used in partial- and non-rebreather masks. Oxygen delivery is a function of oxygen flow rate ratio to the patient's inspiratory flow and tidal volume. The device delivers FiO_2 rate form 24 to 90% at flow rates between 1 and >15 L/min. The open mask design allows for carbon dioxide to disperse into the environment during exhalation, removing the risk of CO_2 retention. Additionally, the open mask design decrease the risk of aspiration of vomitus. Other benefits include reduction of setup errors, simplified flow adjustments, decreased oxygen use compared with the traditional oxygen interfaces, and the ability to use one device to manage oxygen delivery across all supplemental oxygen needs (low and high flow delivery systems). Oxymasks come in four sizes, from standard adult to infant appropriate.

An additional option available using the Oxymask™ technology is the OxyMask™ $ETCO_2$, which allows for non-invasive end-tidal carbon dioxide ($ETCO_2$) monitoring. The device allows for low and high flow oxygen delivery with uninterrupted side-stream $ETCO_2$ monitoring. This device delivers FiO_2 ranging from 24 to 65% at 1 to >15 L/min during end-tidal CO_2 monitoring. Oxygen administration and monitoring of $ETCO_2$ are useful during conscious sedation, bronchoscopy, endoscopy, and interventional radiology. The design, oxygen delivery range, and $ETCO_2$ monitoring allow this device the ability to have one oxygen delivery device that supports a wide range of supplemental oxygen needs and flow rates. The OxyMask™$ETCO_2$ version comes in 3 sizes that include standard adult, large adult and pediatric (Table 11.3).

Table 11.3 Comparison of different oxygen delivery systems

Oxygen delivery device	Flow and design	FiO$_2$	Indications	Contraindications
Blow by	Low-flow, Variable FiO$_2$	<0.30	• Low FiO$_2$ requirement • Not tolerating mask • Short-term delivery	• High FiO$_2$ requirement • Lack of SpO$_2$ Monitoring
Oxygen Hood or Tent	Enclosure: High-flow, Fixed FiO$_2$ (hood)/Variable FiO$_2$ (tent)	Hood: 0.25–0.90 Tent: 0.25–0.50	• Small Children • Low- or High FiO$_2$ requirement • Heated Humidity	• Need for on-going access —feeding/ procedures • Sensitivity to sound
Nasal Cannula	Low-flow, Variable FiO$_2$	0.25–0.40	• Low FiO$_2$ requirement • Not tolerating mask • Mobility with oxygen requirement	• Nasal Obstruction • Facial trauma • Choanal Atresia
HFNC	High- or low-flow; variable or fixed FiO$_2$	0.21–1.00	• Low or high FiO$_2$ requirement • Hypoxemia refectory to low-flow oxygen • Oxygen need with increased WOB	• Suspected or confirmed pneumothorax • Severe upper airway obstruction • Absence of Spontaneous ventilation
Simple facemask	Low-flow, Variable FiO$_2$	0.35–0.50	• Moderate FiO$_2$ requirement • Short-term delivery: – Medical transport – Emergency stabilization – Post-anesthesia recovery	Infants or small children requiring low or precise FiO$_2$
Air-Entrainment Masks	Reservoir: High-flow; fixed FiO$_2$	0.24–0.50	• Controlled FiO$_2$ at low to moderate oxygen levels • Increase inspiratory flow demands • Chronic CO$_2$ retention who may hypoventilate with increased oxygen concentrations	• High FiO$_2$ requirement • Lack of SpO$_2$ Monitoring • Does not tolerate mask
Partial rebreather Mask	Reservoir: Low-flow; variable FiO$_2$	0.50–0.60	• Moderate FiO$_2$ requirement • Short-term use during stabilizing efforts	• High FiO$_2$ requirement • Lack of SpO$_2$ Monitoring • Does not tolerate mask

(continued)

Table 11.3 (continued)

Oxygen delivery device	Flow and design	FiO$_2$	Indications	Contraindications
Non rebreather Mask	Reservoir. Low-flow; variable FiO$_2$	0.65–0.95	• High FiO$_2$ requirement • Short-term use during stabilizing efforts	• High FiO$_2$ requirement • Lack of SpO$_2$ Monitoring • Does not tolerate mask
Oxymask™	High- or low-flow; variable or fixed FiO$_2$	0.24–0.90	• High inspiratory flow demand • Low or high FiO$_2$ requirement • Hypoxemia refectory to low-flow oxygen	• Lack of SpO$_2$ Monitoring • Does not tolerate mask

11.2 Humidification Systems

The upper respiratory tract warms, humidifies, and filters the inspired gas. The primary location where this occurs is the nasopharynx, where the highly vascularized moist mucus membrane efficiently conditions inhaled gas because of its large surface area and turbulent flow created by the nasal turbinates. The system is so efficient that in the coolest and dry conditions, the inspired gas reaching the alveolus is fully saturated at body temperature.

Insensible water losses are also a consideration when evaluating airway humidification in children. It is estimated that 30% of insensible losses are from the respiratory tract in children, one and a half times greater than in adults. The remaining 70% loss is from the skin, which is also greater than in adults because of greater body surface to weight ratio. In the clinical setting, adding humidification during artificial respiratory support will decrease insensible water losses from the respiratory tract.

Fundamentals of Humidification

The physical properties of humidification and their role in temperature regulation and mucociliary clearance are essential in supporting respiratory tract homeostasis during both non-invasive and invasive ventilatory support.

Absolute humidity (AH) is the total amount of water vapor that can be contained in a volume of gas, often expressed as mg/L or as partial pressure of water (mmHg). AH increases commensurately with temperature. Clinically, heating the inspired gas in the humidifier provides more humidity to the respiratory tract enhancing mucociliary clearance.

Relative humidity (RH) is the percentage (%) of water vapor contained in a volume of gas relative to its total maximum water carrying capacity. RH may be 100% at low temperatures, as cool or cold gas has a decreased capacity to hold water vapor. For this reason, the relationship of AH with temperature is more important to consider in clinical practice. For example, at a RH of 50%, the column of gas is holding ½ of its maximum possible water vapor it can hold. Clinically, providing only 50% RH will result in water being pulled from the respiratory tract resulting in tissue drying and thickening of secretions. Inadequate humidity may result in mucus plugging and sometimes and airway bleeding.

The temperature at which a gas is 100% saturated with water is the dew point. Clinically, the amount of water vapor in the inspired gas is important as it is responsible for condensation of water in the circuit, often referred to as "rainout". The greater the temperature drop from the heating chamber to the airway, greater the potential for circuit rainout. Heated wire circuits have helped decrease the rainout as the inspiratory gas temperature drop is minimized.

Types and Function of Humidifiers

All patients undergoing mechanical ventilator support via an artificial airway require gas conditioning by either active or passive humidification systems. Passive devices such as heat moisture exchangers (HMEs) are better suited for short-term (≤ 96 h) or during transport. Chronically ventilated patients benefit from HMEs during trips out of the home, as the device provides some filtration while providing acceptable humidification. They are useful in clinical situations where short-term ventilation is needed such as post-operatively. Active humidification is well suited for clinical situations where prolonged ventilation is needed.

Active humidifiers use an external energy source to heat and condition inspiratory gas within a reservoir. Once the water vapor is added to it, the gas travels through the inspiratory limb or oxygen supply line to the patient's airway. Current active devices include a heated-wire in the inspiratory limb of the circuit limiting temperature loss as the column of gas moves away from the heat source toward the airway.

Passover Humidifiers Passover humidifiers add water vapor as inspiratory gas "passes" over a reservoir. This type of humidifier is the simplest and least efficient type of high-flow humidifier. These systems may or may not be heated, and are infrequently used for invasive mechanical ventilator support. These are used for short-term and temporary indications such as use in the emergency department.

Bubble Humidifiers Bubble humidifiers are most commonly used on low-flow oxygen delivery systems such as nasal cannula. Source gas is directed into a tube submerged in a column of water held in a reservoir. The gas exits through a grid at the tube creating bubbles that increases the surface area and adds humidity to the gas. Bubble humidifiers are cost effective for short-term use in non-invasive low-flow systems. However, they do not add enough water vapor for use in invasively supported patients. This is used most commonly in neonates and young infants.

Cascade Humidifiers Cascade humidifiers provide humidity as gas from the ventilator is directed below the water surface contained in the reservoir. The gas bubbles pass through a grid, essentially making the device an efficient bubble humidifier. The incorporated grid creates a foam or froth of small bubbles that absorb water. Cascade humidifiers have a thermostat built into the device to ensure an adequate temperature which is usually set at approximately body temperature (34–37 °C). It is important to note, that cascade humidifiers deliver water vapor, however they may also deliver micro-aerosols to the patient, increasing the risk of bacteria transmitted to the patient if the reservoir is contaminated.

Wick Humidifiers Wick humidifiers are passover humidifiers modified with a "wick" constructed of blotter paper, which is surrounded by a heating element. The base of the wick is submerged in water, which is absorbed. Gas surrounds the heated moist wick, increasing the relative humidity. The large gas/liquid interface adds water vapor without increasing the volume of the reservoir. These types of humidifiers are efficient.

Passive Humidifiers Passive humidifiers use the patient's own temperature and hydration to add humidity, functioning without the electricity or additional water source. They are often referred to as artificial noses since they mimic the action of the nasal cavity by conditioning the inspired gas.

Heat and Moisture Exchangers (HMEs) HMEs contain a condenser element retaining moisture from the exhaled breath returning it back to the less humid inspired gas. Unlike active humidifiers, which are placed in the proximal portion of the inspiratory limb, HMEs are placed at the hub of the endotracheal tube. Limitations of HMEs include the risk of increased airway resistance, increased work of breathing, inadvertent PEEP generation, the need to be removed for aerosol administration, adding dead space and the need to be changed every 48 h.

Several types of HMEs exist, with nomenclature based on device design. Some of the HMEs incorporate layered aluminum with no fibrous component. Aluminum transfers temperature efficiently during exhalation, which allows for condensation to form between the layers. The heat and humidity is then transferred back to the airway during inspiration. Some designs add a fibrous element that aids in moisture retention, and decreases pooling of condensation. These types of HMEs are the least efficient design, though they are most cost effective for short-term use—ideal for operating room setting. Newer HME designs incorporate media that are more efficient in providing both heat and humidity. These include hydrophobic, hygroscopic, and combined designs.

Contraindications: Contraindications to the use of HMEs include thick copious secretions, large leak such that exhaled tidal volume is <70% of delivered tidal volume, use of low tidal volume lung protective strategies, hypothermia (body temperature <32 °C), high minute ventilation, and the need for in-line drug aerosols.

11.3 Respiratory Care Therapeutics

Aerosolized drug administration is perhaps the most widely used therapy in the treatment of infants and children with respiratory diseases. Drug aerosols are used for a variety of diseases from reactive airway disease to lung infections. The unique challenge in drug aerosol therapy in patients with respiratory illnesses is to identify the most effective and practical method of delivery to ensure optimal therapeutic effect without compromising the safety of the patient. The therapeutic index of the drug when administered as an aerosol is enhanced since it is delivered directly to the site of action. Optimal dosing will depend upon the size of the patient, delivery devices used, the procedure used to deliver the medication, and the type of drug used.

Compared to adults, delivery of aerosolized particles to the distal airways in infants and children is poor. Small airway caliber with greater airway resistance, high respiratory rate with a short inspiratory time, increased chest wall compliance, ineffective coordination of effort and inconsistent breath-holding maneuvers all contribute to the poor delivery of aerosols in the airways of infants and children. Despite poor aerosol delivery, a clinical response to inhaled medications is often observed. Knowing that a physiologic response to inhaled medications is determined by the amount of drug that reaches the site of action in the respiratory tract, the goal would be to control as many variables responsible that affect its delivery.

Delivery Devices

The generic term nebulizer includes a number of aerosol-generating devices. Each device has both benefits and limitations. The ideal particle size should be at least 1–5 micron for deposition in the distal airways. Currently, four types of delivery systems are available for clinical use that generate medication aerosols. These are the jet nebulizers (small volume and large volume), ultrasonic nebulizers, metered-dose inhalers, and dry-powder inhalers. Nebulizer performance and the efficacy of therapy depend on the type of nebulizer, gas flow rate, nebulizer volume fill, breathing pattern of the patient, and airway geometry.

Small-Volume Nebulizers Small-volume nebulizers generate aerosols by converting a liquid medication into small particles using a compressed gas source. The primary benefit in the pediatric patient population is the desired dose is given over a longer period of time rather than in one to four breaths, as young children often have irregular breathing pattern. There are many technical and patient-related factors that must be considered when using small volume nebulizers for intermittent therapy. The aerosol deposition in the lungs using these nebulizers with a mouthpiece or a face mask is about 8–12% with almost 30% remaining in the nebulizer.

Large volume nebulizers Large volume nebulizers utilize a similar jet nebulization principle found in the small volume nebulizer but with a larger medication basin, and therefore can be used for longer periods. Duration of therapy is dependent upon the output performance and the amount of medication made available in the basin. This type of nebulizer has been developed primarily for continuous aerosol delivery.

Jet Nebulizers (Pneumatically-Driven) Also known as handheld nebulizers, updraft nebulizers, and unit-dose nebulizers, jet nebulizers are small reservoir gas-powered devices that are the most cost-effective means to deliver an aerosolized medication. These nebulizers utilize the "jet-shearing" principle, created by an external gas source forced through a small lumen contained in a medication cup. As the gas expands—localized negative pressure develops pulling the medication up a feeder tube. The liquid enters the gas stream resulting in the formation of droplets, which then enter a baffle. The smaller particles exit the reservoir following the baffling process. Larger particles drop back into the reservoir for re-nebulization. Two limitations of these devices include large amount of drug wastage, and evaporation with recirculation resulting in increased amount of drug necessary for the therapeutic effect.

Mesh Nebulizers Vibrating mesh nebulizers create a fine aerosol by moving a drug solution through a plate or mesh with small holes. The diameter of these holes or apertures determines the particle size. These devices do not use an external gas source, instead the nebulizer is powered by an electrical power source, which can be battery powered for travel. Lack of additional flow provides the benefit of more normal breath delivery and triggering capacity. In addition to these benefits, vibrating mesh nebulizers also have small dead space volume, ranging between 0.1 and 0.5 mL.

Ultrasonic Nebulizers Ultrasonic nebulizer uses a piezoelectric crystal that produces a highly concentrated output of aerosol particles and has historically been used for cough and sputum production. Ultrasonic nebulizer with its highly concentrated output, may perform better than small volume nebulizer in accomplishing greater deposition of medications in children.

Metered-Dose Inhaler The metered-dose inhaler uses a pressurized canister that dispenses a single bolus of aerosolized medication. They are convenient, cost-effective, versatile, and generally have an effective deposition rate of 10–15%. To optimize the delivery of the drug, the patient must be able to coordinate a series of inspiratory maneuvers while activating the canister. Low inspiratory flow rates, inspiratory pause or sustained maximal inflation maneuver facilitates better deposition. Lower flow rates reduce aerosol impaction in the oropharynx and inner walls of the airways while breath-holding improves deposition by gravity. A spacer device can be a valuable attachment if the metered-dose inhaler is used by children. By adding a spacer device to the inhaler, the synchronized effort is less of a concern and drug delivery is maximized. The canister is activated into the spacer and the medication remains suspended in the chamber until the patient inhales. For younger children or infants, a mask is added to the spacer for more efficient delivery (Table 11.4).

Table 11.4 List of commonly inhaled therapeutic agents

Drug	Site of action	Major effect(s)	Adverse effect
Albuterol	Beta-2 receptor	Bronchodilation	Tachycardia Diastolic hypotension
Levalbuterol	Beta-2 receptor	Bronchodilation	Tachycardia Diastolic hypotension (less than albuterol)
Ipratropium bromide	Muscarinic receptor	Bronchodilation	Dry mucosa Thick secretions
Budesonide	Glucocorticoid receptor	Anti-inflammatory	Thrush Hoarseness
Aminoglycosides (tobramycin, amikacin)	Aminoglycoside binding site on ribosome	Antimicrobial	Thrush Growth of resistant organisms
Antiviral (ribavirin, zanamivir)	Interferes with replication of viruses	Antiviral	Bronchospasm Airway plugging
Colisitin	Bacterial cell-membrane	Antimicrobial	Bronchospasm Neuromuscular blockade
Pentamidine	Nuclear metabolism	Prevents *Pneumocystis jiroveci* infection	Nausea, vomiting Abnormal taste
Hypertonic saline	Mucus	Mucolytic	Bronchospasm
Dornase alpha	DNA	Mucolytic	Bronchospasm
N-acetyl cysteine	Mucus	Mucolytic	Bronchospasm

Aerosols Delivered Through Ventilators

Aerosol delivery is not very efficient when delivered through a ventilator. The endotracheal tube is the most significant barrier to effective delivery. Smaller the inner diameter of the tube, the less efficient is aerosol delivery. In addition to the endotracheal tube, several other factors impact the delivery of aerosols by mechanical ventilators. The nebulizer is most effective when placed near the inspiratory portion of the ventilator circuit which serves as a spacer chamber, similar to the spacer used for metered dose inhalers. The aerosolized particles remain suspended in the inspiratory limb awaiting to be delivered with the ensuing ventilator breath. Aerosols must be generated during the expiratory phase of the ventilator cycle to fill the inspiratory limb. Therefore, a synchronized nebulizer mode is essential where a portion of the preset inspiratory gas is diverted to power the nebulizer. One of the concerns of using aerosols with ventilators is the potential for collection of the particles in the expiratory filter increasing the expiratory resistance or complete blockage of the expiratory port. Filters must be monitored and changed frequently to avoid obstruction or added resistance. In such a circumstances, airway pressures and tidal volumes delivered to the patient should be measured at the hub of the endotracheal tube. An alternative to nebulizers is a metered-dose inhaler, especially with the use of a spacer. Variables affecting aerosol delivery during mechanical ventilation include the nebulizer power source, nebulizer characteristics, ventilator settings, temperature and humidity, location of the aerosol device, and the size of the artificial airway. It is important to consider whether a particular device would be tolerated well by the patient. The aerosol output characteristics are also equally important to consider when selecting an aerosol device.

11.4   Specialty Gases

Altering Inspired Oxygen and Carbon Dioxide Concentration

With certain types of congenital heart disease with single ventricle physiology such as hypoplastic left heart syndrome, it is critical to control pulmonary blood flow and prevent pulmonary over-circulation and systemic hypoperfusion. This can be accomplished by increasing pulmonary vascular resistance and reducing pulmonary blood flow while increasing blood flow to the systemic circulation. One approach is to decrease the FiO_2 to less than 0.21 with a blending of room air with nitrogen which causes hypoxic pulmonary vasoconstriction. The exact FiO_2 delivered must be monitored to avoid administering excessively low inspired oxygen and causing severe hypoxemia. The other approach, especially in patients undergoing mechanical ventilation, both preoperatively and postoperatively, is to increase the inspired carbon dioxide concentration ($FiCO_2$). Increased $FiCO_2$ also increases pulmonary vascular resistance. During mechanical ventilation, increased $FiCO_2$ allows one to hyperventilate, recruit the lungs, and prevent atelectasis without producing hypocarbia. One of the difficulties with a boost in $FiCO_2$ is increased spontaneous ventilatory drive due to an increased $PaCO_2$. This increases the work of breathing and with marginal cardiac reserve, may impose an undue strain on the heart. Therefore, neuromuscular blockade and total ventilatory support may be necessary with increased $FiCO_2$ to avoid an increased workload on the heart.

Helium–Oxygen Mixture

Based on the physics of airflow and the properties of helium oxygen mixture (Heliox), certain outcomes can be predicted with its use: (1) Heliox will results in a higher flow when transairway pressures are held constant, (2) Heliox will result in a lower airway pressure when the airflow is constant, (3) Density-dependent flow meters will underestimate flow, (4) Heliox can decrease the degree of air-trapping and hyperinflation associated with lower airway obstruction, (5) Heliox can decrease the work of breathing, and (6) Heliox can result in better deposition of aerosols administered with it. Helium is usually administered in at least 30% to 40% oxygen. However, for helium to be effective, it should constitute at least 50–60% of the inspired gas. Heliox therapy is therefore not helpful in patients requiring greater than 0.5 FiO_2. Oxygenation should be monitored during administration of helium–oxygen mixture to avoid hypoxemia, especially in neonates.

Inhaled Nitric Oxide

Inhaled nitric oxide produces selective pulmonary vasodilation. Indications for inhaled nitric oxide include diaphragmatic hernia, pulmonary hypertension after repair of congenital heart disease, primary pulmonary hypertension, and isolated right heart failure. Not all patients respond to inhaled nitric oxide. It is prudent to test whether a patient will respond to inhaled nitric oxide. A 2-h trial of inhaled nitric oxide with 20–40 ppm is administered to infants and children with hypoxemic respiratory failure. A good response is defined as improvement in PaO_2/FiO_2 ratio of greater than 100%. A partial response is defined as an improvement in PaO_2/FiO_2 ratio between 50 and 100%. If the response is less than 50%, the patient is considered a non-responder. Inhaled nitric oxide is then continued in only those patients who show a partial or good response. Nitric oxide binds to hemoglobin to produce methemoglobin. Therefore methemoglobin levels should be monitored during the administration of nitric oxide. In addition, nitric oxide combines with oxygen to form nitrogen dioxide. Nitrogen dioxide is known to cause lung injury. Therefore the concentration of nitrogen dioxide should be monitored in the inspired gas to keep it below 1–2 ppm. To minimize complications, the inhaled nitric oxide therapy should be continued at the lowest possible concentrations that are still effective in producing the desired therapeutic effects.

Suggested Readings

1. McKienan C, Chua LC, Visintainer PF, Allen H. High flow nasal cannula therapy in infants with bronchiolitis. J Pediatr. 2010;156(4):634–8.
2. Milesi C, Pierre AF, Deho A, et al. A multicenter randomized controlled trial of a 3-l/kg/min versus 2-l/kg/min high-flow nasal canula flow rate in young infants with severe viral bronchiolitis (TRAMONTANE 2). Intensive Care Med. 2018;44(11):1870–1870.
3. Wing R, James C, Maranda LS, Armsby CC. Use of high-flow nasal cannula in the emergency department reduces the need for intubation in pediatric acute respiratory insufficiency. Pediatr Emerg Care. 2012;28(11):1117–23.
4. Franklin D, Babl FE, Schlapbsch LJ, et al. A randomized trial of high-flow oxygen therapy in infants with bronchiolitis. N Engl J Med. 2018;378:1121–31.
5. Bhashyam AR, Wolf MT, Marcinkowski AL, Saville A, Thomas K, Carcillo JA, Corcoran TE. Aerosol delivery through nasal cannulas: an in vitro study. J Aerosol Med Pulm Drug Deliv. 2008;21:181–8.
6. Corcoran TE, Sallille A, Adams PS, et al. Deposition studies of aersol delivery by nasal cannula to infants. Pediatr Pulmonol. 2019;54:1319–25.
7. Fontanari P, Burnet H, Zattara-Hartmann MC, Jammes Y. Changes in airway resistance induce by nasal inhalation of cold dry, dry, or moist air in normal individuals. J Appl Physiol. 1996;81:1739–43.

8. Byerly FL, Haithcock JA, Buchnana IB, et al. Use of high flow nasal cannula on a pediatric burn patient with inhalation injury and post-extubation stridor. Burns. 2006;32:121.

9. AL Ashry IIS, Modrykamien AM. Humidification during mechanical ventilation in the adult patient. BioMed Res Int. 2014;Article ID 715101;10 pages.

10. Baudin F, Gagnon S, Crulli, et al. Modalities and complications associated with the use of high-flow nasal cannula: experience in a pediatric ICU. Respir Care. 2016;61(10):1305–10.

11. Sarnaik SM, Saladino RA, Manole M, Pitetti R, Arora G, Kuch BA, Orr RA, Felmet KA. Diastolic hypotension is an unrecognized risk factor for ß-agonist-associated myocardial injury in children with asthma. Pediatr Crit Care Med. 2013;14(6):e273–9.

12. Kalister H. Treating children with asthma, a review of drug therapies. West J Med. 2001;174:415–20.

13. Petersen W, Karup-Pedersen F, Friis B, Howitz P, Nielsen F, Stromquist LH. Sodium cromoglycate as a replacement of inhaled corticosteroids in mild-to-moderate childhood asthma. Allergy. 1996;51:870–87.

14. de Benedictis FM, Tuteri G, Pazzelli P, Berotto A, Bruni L, Vaccaro R. Cromolyn versus nedocromil: duration of action in exercise-induced asthma in children. J Allergy Clin Immunol. 1995;96:510–4.

15. Wisecup S, Eades S, Hashmi SS, Samuels C, Mosquera RA. Diastolic hypotension in pediatric patients with asthma receiving continuous albuterol. J Asthma. 2015;52(7):693–8.

16. Davis MD, Donn SM, Ward RM. Administration of inhaled pulmonary vasodilators to the mechanically ventilated neonatal patient. Pediatr Drugs. 2017;19(3):183–92.

Chapter 12
Long-Term Ventilation and Home Care

Shekhar T. Venkataraman

As survival from PICU with critical illness has increased, many children are being discharged from the hospital who are technology-dependent. Respiratory care, in these children, can range from simple supplemental oxygen to mechanical ventilation, which can range from partial ventilation (e.g., night time ventilation) to 24-h ventilator assistance. Long-term care in a tertiary care center is expensive and it can alternatively be provided in a specialized chronic care center or at home. Home care is psychosocially more acceptable to the families, less expensive, and may provide a better quality of life for technology-dependent children. This chapter will review the definitions of chronic respiratory failure, options for support with chronic respiratory failure and the logistics of discharge of these patients.

12.1 Definitions and Causes

Chronic respiratory failure (CRF) is defined as respiratory failure that persists after the primary process has resolved or it is due to a cause that will remain for the foreseeable future even for the entire life span. CRF may be due to persistent or progressive hypoxemia and/or hypercarbia requiring respiratory support. The conditions that lead to CRF can be classified into those that are likely to improve, remain static, or continue to progress resulting in end-stage respiratory failure. Additionally, there are patients who require care related to obstructive sleep apnea,

S. T. Venkataraman (✉)
Professor, Departments of Critical Care Medicine and Pediatrics, University of Pittsburgh School of Medicine, Pittsburgh, PA, USA
e-mail: venkataramanst@upmc.edu

Medical Director, Respiratory Care Services, Children's Hospital of Pittsburgh, 4401 Penn Avenue, Faculty Pavilion 2117, Pittsburgh, PA 15224, USA

© Springer Nature Switzerland AG 2022
A. P. Sarnaik et al. (eds.), *Mechanical Ventilation in Neonates and Children*,
https://doi.org/10.1007/978-3-030-83738-9_12

Table 12.1 Causes of chronic respiratory failure

Cause of respiratory failure	Diseases
Respiratory pump failure	Static muscle weakness/Loss of function
	Spinal cord injury
	Phrenic nerve injury
	Skeletal/Chest wall deformities
	Scoliosis
	Congenital skeletal malformations
	Progressive muscle weakness
	Neuropathies
	Myopathies
	Mitochondrial disorders
	Spinal muscular atrophy
Respiratory drive	Congenital central hypoventilation syndrome
	Brain/brainstem injury
	Central nervous system tumors
	Degenerative CNS disorders
Structural abnormalities	Airway malformations
	Craniofacial malformations
	Tracheomalacia
	Bronchomalacia
	Acquired airway diseases
	Obstructive sleep apnea
Pulmonary parenchymal and vascular disorders	Chronic lung disease of infancy (bronchopulmonary dysplasia)
	Recurrent aspiration syndromes
	Cystic fibrosis
	Congenital heart disease
	Post-inflammatory or post-infectious
	Lung hypoplasia

and those who require support as part of their palliative care (Table 12.1). Ventilator dependence is defined as the requirement for mechanical ventilation for longer than a month.

Individual patients can have more than one cause for chronic ventilator dependency. For example, patients with neuromuscular weakness can develop kyphoscoliosis which produces restriction to breathing and exacerbation of hypercarbia. Patient with anoxic encephalopathy may not only have an abnormal respiratory drive but also develop recurrent aspiration and obstructive sleep apnea from bulbar dysfunction. The approach to chronic respiratory care will be different depending on the natural course of the underlying disease as well associated complications.

12.2   Pathophysiological Considerations of Chronic Respiratory Failure

Respiratory Pump Disorders—Weakness or Absence of Muscle Function

Neuromuscular Diseases

Most neuromuscular disorders are progressive and result in worsening respiratory function due to several mechanisms and result in multiple morbidities. Included in this category are muscular dystrophies and myopathies. Respiratory muscle weakness progresses to ventilator failure requiring increasing levels of support. Airway clearance is compromised predisposing to recurrent episodes of orotracheal aspiration and recurrent episodes of atelectasis and lower respiratory tract infections. Chest wall and skeletal mechanics are also altered and often lead to kyphoscoliosis and rigidity of the thoracic cage due to ankylosis of costovertebral joints and stiffening of the ligaments and tendons, further compromising gas exchange. Lower airway mucus plugging and increased airway resistance are the consequence of small airway caliber both anatomically and functionally. These imbalances lead to a restrictive respiratory system with reduced vital capacity and total lung capacity. These factors increase the work of breathing which coupled with muscle weakness lead to fatigue and ventilatory failure. Sleep disturbance is common in these patients including obstructive sleep apnea due to bulbar weakness. Mechanical ventilation, especially noninvasive ventilation, has been shown to be beneficial and improve the quality of life in these patients.

Nerve Injury or Illness

Nerves innervating the respiratory muscles may be injured or inflamed and cause either muscle weakness or absence of muscle function. Phrenic nerve injury may occur during childbirth, cardiac surgery and other thoracic surgery. The injury may be unilateral or bilateral resulting in either paresis or total paralysis. Often this injury is irreversible and may necessitate positive pressure support. Spinal cord injury above the level of C3 causes paralysis of the diaphragm as well as the intercostal muscles. Long-term mechanical ventilation through a tracheostomy can prolong life in many of these patients. Amyotrophic lateral sclerosis is a disease that causes the death of neurons controlling voluntary muscles and results in progressive muscle weakness and ventilatory failure similar to neuromuscular disorders. Spinal muscular atrophy is much more common than ALS in children compared to adults.

Respiratory Pump Disorders—Skeletal and Chest Wall Diseases

Distortion of the thoracic cage due to scoliosis causes restrictive respiratory disease and may result from muscle weakness, nerve injury or from congenital malformations. Chronically, the load on the respiratory muscles can result in fatigue and ventilatory failure. Chest wall diseases such as asphyxiating thoracic dystrophy cause restriction to breathing and can be life threatening without mechanical ventilation and reparative surgery.

Respiratory Drive Disorders

Several congenital or acquired central nervous system disorders result in an abnormal respiratory drive characterized by an impaired response to hypercapnia. Congenital central hypoventilation syndrome, Prader Willi syndrome, and rapid-onset obesity with hypothalamic dysfunction, hypoventilation, and autonomic dysregulation (ROHHAD) are some examples of congenital disorders resulting in an abnormal respiratory drive leading to hypercarbia from chronic hypoventilation. Children with Chiari malformation can have a blunted response to hypercapnia and can manifest with both central and obstructive apnea during sleep. Acquired brain stem lesions or injury may also affect respiratory drive resulting in chronic hypoventilation leading to hypercarbia. Progressive and degenerative brain disorders such as Leigh's disease can also affect the neurons involved with respiratory drive and cause hypoventilation.

12.3   Approach to Long-Term/Home Care Ventilation

The benefits of home care include: (1) Cost-efficiency, (2) Quality of life, (3) Psychosocial aspects of the family and the patient, and (4) Family cohesiveness. On the other hand; caregiver stress, concern for inadequate care, neglect are some of the issues of home care which may increase the risk for morbidity. The success of home care depends on the willingness and ability of family caregivers to provide care in the home, and community resources. Alternate sites of chronic ventilation are not available as widely despite the need for such centers.

Options for Respiratory Support in Technology-Dependent Children

There are several options for respiratory support for technology-dependent children. These children may be with or without an artificial airway such as a tracheostomy. Supplemental oxygen may be needed either continuously or intermittently for those patients with parenchymal lung disease with intrapulmonary shunting and venous admixture. When the severity of lung disease and gas exchange abnormalities increase, then positive pressure support may be needed. Table 12.2 lists the type of respiratory support that may be needed in technology-dependent children.

HME is described in Chap. 11. The choice of respiratory support depends upon the severity of lung disease and respiratory failure as well as the desired quality of life.

Goals of Respiratory Support

The goals of long-term respiratory care include: (1) provision of comprehensive, cost-effective respiratory care, (2) enhancement of quality of life, (3) reduction of morbidity, and (4) extend life wherever possible. The setting for post-acute care will depend on the degree of medical stability of the patient and availability of resources outside the pediatric intensive care unit. These include a care site within the hospital, a subacute or long-term facility or home care. The first consideration is the

Table 12.2 Respiratory support in technology-dependent children

Without an artificial airway
1. Supplemental oxygen
i. Intermittent
b. Continuous
2. Noninvasive positive pressure support
a. Continuous positive airway pressure
i. Intermittent
ii. Continuous
b. Spontaneous ventilation with Positive pressure assistance (e.g., BiPAP)
i. Intermittent
ii. Continuous
c. Negative pressure ventilation
i. Intermittent
ii. Continuous
d. Sip-ventilation
i. Intermittent
ii. Continuous

With an artificial airway
1. No supplemental oxygen with or without a heat and moisture exchanger (HME)
2. Supplemental oxygen
a. Intermittent
b. Continuous
3. Continuous positive airway pressure
i. Intermittent
ii. Continuous
4. Spontaneous ventilation with Positive Pressure Assistance
i. Intermittent
ii. Continuous
5. Mandatory ventilation with or without Pressure Support
i. Intermittent
ii. Continuous

medical stability of the patient. The minimum requirements are a stable airway (natural or a tracheostomy), stable clinical status and care demands that can be met by the resources of the care site.

The objectives of long-term mechanical ventilation are dependent on the cause of respiratory failure. In patients with reversible causes of CRF, respiratory support is provided to support and improve gas exchange until there is resolution of respiratory failure. CRF such as bronchopulmonary dysplasia is often associated with poor somatic growth with delayed development. Mechanical ventilation, in these patients, can result in improved somatic growth as well as neurologic development.

Consideration for Mechanical Ventilation

Noninvasive ventilation by positive pressure can be delivered through nasal or oronasal interface. Positive pressure can relieve upper airway obstruction as well as improve minute ventilation and unload inspiratory muscles. If long-term ventilatory assistance is provided in the hospital setting, then either intensive care ventilators or portable home ventilators may be used. Portable ventilators use pistons or turbines to generate the selected volume or pressure, and can do so at lower flow rates. Noninvasive ventilation may be used intermittently, usually at night or when the patient is sleeping. With more severe or progressive disease, NIV may be required continuously. Similar to short-term NIV, for long-term NIV the ventilator settings must relieve patient symptoms.

Long-term NIV has significant physiologic effects depending on the disease process. In general, it improves the quality of life for many patients at home. It also improves night time sleep with less disturbed sleep from respiratory distress. In many patients, chronic sleep apneas and carbon dioxide retention can predispose to the development of systemic and pulmonary hypertension. NIV, by ameliorating these manifestations, decreases the incidence of systemic and pulmonary hypertension. In patients with chronic respiratory failure who are candidates for lung transplantation, NIV can act as an effective bridge toward transplantation. Table 12.3 lists the physiologic effects and outcomes from some of the conditions for which long-term NIV is employed.

Invasive ventilation via tracheostomy is needed for children who require continuous mechanical ventilation. Tracheostomy tube should be of an optimal size, neither too large that may cause injury to the trachea nor too small so as to cause a considerable leak around the tube that can compromise minute ventilation. Intermittent use of speaking valve may facilitate speech development. The presence of a tracheostomy increases the complexity of care including training of caregivers

Table 12.3 Physiologic effects and outcomes of long-tern NIV	*Neuromuscular disorders*
	1. Improves daytime gas exchange
	2. Ameliorates hypoventilation
	3. Decreases intermittent sleep apneas and other sleep-disordered breathing
	4. Improves quality of life
	5. Decreases hospitalization
	6. Increases survival especially when coupled with assisted cough and aggressive secretion clearance
	7. Improves thoracoabdominal coordination during sleep in SMA types 1 and 2
	Cystic fibrosis
	1. Minimizes acute on chronic respiratory failure with exacerbations
	2. Ameliorates sleep disturbance
	3. Serves as a bridge to transplantation
	Obstructive sleep apnea
	1. Reverses or reduces obstructive sleep apnea
	2. Improves sleep-disordered breathing
	3. Provides interim solution while allowing the patient to grow and postpone surgery

on suctioning, cleaning and changing the tracheostomy tube. The presence of a tracheostomy tube increases the risk for infection. Airway complications related to the presence of a tracheostomy tube include infection at the stoma site, granuloma formation, tracheal stenosis, and fistula formation. CPAP provided through a tracheostomy can unload respiratory muscles and enhance minute ventilation by relieving upper airway obstruction. BiPAP devices provide positive pressure assistance to spontaneous breaths and may be required in patients with chronic hypercarbia. When mandatory ventilatory assistance is required, the goal of therapy is to relieve distress and allow the patient to breathe comfortably. Care should be taken not to over-ventilate the patient, especially those with neuromuscular disorders to avoid causing respiratory muscle atrophy from disuse.

Ventilator settings must relieve patient symptoms. The approach that is generally recommended for long-term NIV is the low–high approach which consists of starting at fairly low level of support that is gradually increased until desired effect is observed. A back-up rate sufficiently high to control breathing nocturnally can rest the respiratory muscles and prevent apnea, especially in patients with neuromuscular disease. There has been an increase in the continuous use of NIV, especially in patients with neuromuscular disorders. This has resulted in prolonging survival and improving quality of life in these patients.

Transitioning from an ICU-Specific Ventilator to a Portable Home Ventilator

One of the key steps before discharge from the ICU for patients on long-term positive pressure support is to transition to a home ventilator (HV). The patient must be medically stable with the current ventilator settings. If any specialty gases such as nitric oxide or Heliox have been used, they need to be weaned off. The patient must be gaining weight and able to tolerate therapies without significant changes in gas exchange or work of breathing. Airway must be stable, whether it is the natural airway or a tracheostomy. There are no strict guidelines for ventilator settings or pressures to make the transition. Some HVs may not be able to provide the ventilator settings needed for the patient. In that case, either an alternative HV should be tried or the patient needs to be transitioned when the ventilator settings are lowered and tolerated. The ventilator settings in the HV may need to be adjusted further after the transition to ensure that the patient is breathing comfortably with adequate gas exchange. When the patient is able to tolerate HV for at least 2 weeks without any changes made to the ventilator settings, the patient is considered ready for discharge.

An ideal HV should: (1) Be light-weight and portable, (2) Have a long internal battery life, (3) Able to provide continuous flow, (4) Able to compensate for leaks, (5) Have multiple modes of ventilation available, and (6) Easy to trouble-shoot. Most of the current HVs are portable and approved for children weighing 5 kg or greater. Portability and a long internal battery life allow the patients to leave their homes and travel either for appointments or family gatherings. A long battery life may be life-saving in areas where power outages are common. The actual battery life may be different from the manufacturer's estimations since those are based on providing a low level of ventilator support in adults. Battery life is inversely proportional to level of support needed for the patient. Higher ventilator pressures and rates will decrease the battery life. The type of support provided by HV is listed in Table 12.2.

Monitoring of Patients with Long-Term NIV

Monitoring patients who are on long-term NIV requires an assessment of their respiratory function. Pulse oximeters are useful in detecting hypoxemia especially during sleep. End-tidal CO_2 monitors are only used in the clinic or hospital. Treatment of sleep-disordered breathing improves the quality of life and may prolong survival. Polysomnography may be required to document sleep-disorders but is more expensive than nocturnal pulse oximetry. If a patient has bulbar weakness or severe obesity, there may be obstruction of the upper airway or obstructive sleep apnea in addition to sleep hypoventilation. Both problems are treated with nocturnal ventilation.

12.4   Logistics of Home Care

Home care requires a team approach with interaction between several health care personnel, viz., a primary physician, home care nurses, respiratory therapists, social workers, sometimes the State Health Agency, and the family and the patient. First, the patient must be ready for home care. In children who have a tracheostomy, a mature stoma is essential. Inspired oxygen requirement should not be greater than 35%. PaO_2 should be greater than 60–70 torr with a $PaCO_2$ less than 60 torr with a normal arterial pH at relatively low ventilator settings. The family must demonstrate not only a desire to provide home care but also a minimal ability to provide various aspects of home care. Health care personnel must be available in the local community to assist the family in providing care. The home must have adequate facilities to maintain and operate all necessary equipment and supplies. Contingency plans must be made for emergencies. The location of the home has major implications for home care. The home must be easily accessible by standard transportation. A home care provider should be available on a 24-h basis to respond to emergencies. The home must have adequate space to accommodate all the caretakers and the required equipment. A thorough knowledge of the limitations of various devices is essential for the respiratory care personnel coordinating home care. Parents who are motivated to providing home care for their children are willing to take on the cumbersome responsibility of carrying all the necessary equipment from place to place just to have the benefit of having the child at home. When a technology-dependent child is being discharged home, two adults must be willing and able to learn and assume all aspects of the child's daily care, including dosages and indications for all medications being used, feedings, airway clearance and respiratory assessment, ventilator assessment and troubleshooting, and equipment care. If the child is to receive mechanical ventilation through a tracheostomy, the family caregivers must also learn how to suction the artificial airway and perform routine and emergency tracheostomy tube changes. In addition, there must be adequate financial support from third-party payers to provide the equipment and supplies necessary to care for the child at home. The residence in which the child will be cared for must have adequate space for the child, equipment, and visiting health care providers. The home must have running water, heat, electricity, and a working telephone. Entrances must be accessible for patients confined to a wheelchair.

The discharge plan must also include the amount of skilled nursing care the family will require. All families of children who cannot correct an airway or ventilator problem or call for help should be offered skilled nursing care for at least a portion of the day to allow caregivers to sleep with reassurance that the child's welfare is not at risk. Funding for these services, which are the most expensive component of the home care of technology-dependent children, should be guaranteed by third-party payers with periodic reassessments established to determine ongoing needs. While there are no uniform criteria for establishing the number of nursing hours provided, it should be determined by the medical needs of the child, the capabilities of the family, and other demands on family members such as work requirements, care of other children in the home etc. To allow caregivers time off from continuous medical care and monitoring of the child, funded respite care should also be built into the discharge plan as it has been repeatedly identified as an essential component of the home care plan to help relieve stress and caregiver burnout.

Suggested Readings

1. McKienan C, Chua LC, Visintainer PF, allen H. High flow Nasal Cannula therapy in infants with bronchiolitis. J Pediatr. 2010 Apr; 156(4):634–8
2. Milesi C, Pierre AF, Deho A, et al. A multicenter randomized controlled trial of a 3-l/kg/min versus 2-l/kg/min high-flow nasal canula flow rate in young infants with severe viral bronchiolitis (TRAMONTANE 2). Intensive Care Med. 2018 Nov; 44(11):1870
3. Wing R, James C, Maranda LS, Armsby CC. Use of high-flow nasal cannula in the emergency department reduces the need for intubation in pediatric acute respiratory insufficiency. Pediatr Emerg Care. 2012 Nov;28(11):1117−23
4. Franklin D, Babl FE, Schlapbsch LJ, et al. A randomized trial of high-flow oxygen therapy in infants with bronchiolitis. N Engl J Med. 2018;378:1121–31.
5. Bhashyam AR, Wolf MT, Marcinkowski AL, Saville A, Thomas K, Carcillo JA, Corcoran TE. Aerosol delivery through nasal cannulas: an in vitro study. J Aerosol Med Pulm Drug Deliv. 2008;21:181–8.
6. Corcoran TE, Sallille A, Adams PS, et al. Deposition studies of aersol delivery by nasal cannula to infants. Pediatr Pulmonol. 2019;54:1319–25.
7. Fontanari P, Burnet H, Zattara-Hartmann MC, Jammes Y. Changes in airway resistance induce by nasal inhalation of cold dry, dry, or moist air in normal individuals. J Appl Physiol. 1996;81:1739–43.
8. Byerly FL, Haithcock JA, Buchnana IB, et al. Use of high flow nasal cannula on a pediatric burn patient with inhalation injury and post-extubation stridor. Burns. 2006;32:121.

9. AL Ashry HS, Modrykamien AM. Humidification during Mechanical Ventilation in the Adult Patient. BioMed Res Internat. 2014; (715434):12

10. Baudin F, Gagnon S, Crulli, et al. Modalities and complications associated with the use of high-flow nasal cannula: experience in a pediatric ICU. Respir care 2016;61(10):1305–10

11. Sarnaik SM, Saladino RA, Manole M, Pitetti R, Arora G, Kuch BA, Orr RA, Felmet KA. Diastolic hypotension is an unrecognized risk factor for ß-agonist-associated myocardial injury in children with asthma. Pediatr Crit Care Med. 2013 Jul;14(6):e273–9.

12. Kalister H. Treating children with asthma, a review of drug therapies. West J Med. 2001;174:415–20.

13. Petersen W, Karup-Pedersen F, Friis B, Howitz P, Nielsen F, Stromquist LH. Sodium cromoglycate as a replacement of inhaled corticosteroids in mild-to-moderate childhood asthma. Allergy. 1996;51:870–87.

14. de Benedictis FM, Tuteri G, Pazzelli P, Berotto A, Bruni L, Vaccaro R. Cromolyn versus nedocromil: duration of action in exercise-induced asthma in children. J Allergy Clin Immunol. 1995;96:510–4.

15. Wisecup S, Eades S, Hashmi SS, Samuels C, Mosquera RA. Diastolic hypotension in Pediatric Patients with Asthma Receiving Continuous Albuterol. J Asthma. 2015 Sep; 52 (7):693–8

16. Davis MD, Donn SM, Ward RM. Administration of inhaled pulmonary vasodilators to the mechanically ventilated neonatal patient. Pediatr Drugs. 2017;19(3):183–92.

Chapter 13
Case-Based Analysis of Respiratory Failure

Ashok P. Sarnaik and Shekhar T. Venkataraman

As described so far, respiratory failure and respiratory distress have varied etiologies and each case has to be analyzed, diagnosed, investigated and managed individually. While certain broad principles are common to groups of disorders, each patient has his own unique features in presenting symptoms and signs, clinical course, and response to treatment. We present a systematic approach to the analysis of symptomatology, clinical manifestations and pathophysiologic considerations in the diagnosis and management of respiratory failure of varied etiology.

13.1 Breathing Control Disorders

Case 1

A 14-year-old boy presented to the emergency room with somnolence, lethargy, and difficulty in arousing. For the past month, he had been complaining of tiredness, neck pain, and early morning headaches. He was afebrile with shallow respirations of 10/min, heart rate of 88/min and blood pressure of 160/100 mmHg. Pulse oximetry showed SpO_2 of 90%. Pupils were 4 mm and reacted briskly to light. No evidence of

A. P. Sarnaik (✉)
Professor of Pediatrics, Former Pediatrician in Chief and Interim Chairman Children's Hospital of Michigan, Wayne State University School of Medicine, 3901 Beaubien, Detroit, MI 48201, USA
e-mail: asarnaik@med.wayne.edu

S. T. Venkataraman
Professor, Departments of Critical Care Medicine and Pediatrics, University of Pittsburgh School of Medicine, Pittsburgh, PA, USA

Medical Director, Respiratory Care Services, Children's Hospital of Pittsburgh, 4401 Penn Avenue, Faculty Pavilion 2117, Pittsburgh, PA 15224, USA

© Springer Nature Switzerland AG 2022
A. P. Sarnaik et al. (eds.), *Mechanical Ventilation in Neonates and Children*, https://doi.org/10.1007/978-3-030-83738-9_13

trauma was noted. He responded to external stimulation and answered simple questions but went back to sleep. The rest of the physical examination including that of chest and abdomen was normal. Arterial blood gas in room air revealed pH 7.21, PCO_2 70 torr and PO_2 62 torr. Supplemental O_2 via a face mask was applied. Fifteen minutes later, he was found to be unarousable with barely discernible respiratory effort. SpO_2 was 100%. An arterial blood gas showed pH 7.0, PCO_2 100 torr and PO_2 120 torr. Rapid sequence intubation was performed, and volume-controlled ventilation was instituted with respiratory rate 18/min, tidal volume (V_T) 500 ml, inspiratory time (T_i) 1 s and PEEP of 4 cm H_2O. Chest radiograph revealed normal lungs and heart and endotracheal tube at mid-tracheal level.

Clinical Analysis

The patient has severe respiratory failure however, he shows no signs of respiratory distress, has no abnormal physical findings except for weak respiratory effort. His chest radiograph also shows no abnormal lungs or heart findings. Gas exchange shows severe hypoventilation without significant oxygenation deficit suggesting that this is an abnormality of alveolar ventilation with sparing of alveolar capillary apparatus. Central (above the carina) airway obstruction at the level of pharynx, larynx or trachea could explain alveolar hypoventilation. However, lack of respiratory effort to overcome airway obstruction severe enough to cause this level of respiratory failure, makes this group of disorders unlikely. This leaves us with two possibilities: a) ineffective neuro-musculoskeletal function or b) abnormal central control of respiration. Patients with neuropathies (Guillain Barre syndrome, cervical spinal cord injuries etc.), myopathies (muscular dystrophies, botulism etc.) and skeletal abnormalities have diminished capacity to mount effective effort to combat hypercarbia. However, such patients are conscious and responsive. Somnolence and lack of arousal observed in this patient make this possibility also unlikely. That leaves us with the abnormal central control of respiration as the most likely possibility.

By far the most common cause of decreased central chemoreceptor responsiveness is exposure to CNS sedatives such as drugs of abuse or therapeutic administration. Other forms of toxic, infectious, traumatic, and metabolic encephalopathies could also lead to decreased central chemoreceptor responsiveness. The observation that this patient developed further depression of respiration after administration of supplemental O_2 suggests that his control of respiration was much more dependent on hypoxia sensing peripheral chemoreceptors rather than CO_2 sensing central chemoreceptors. Such a situation occurs in brainstem lesions as well as chronic CO_2 retention where central chemoreceptors are blunted or downregulated. Once peripheral chemoreceptor stimulation was abolished in this patient by supplemental oxygen and a rise in PaO_2, the respiratory drive was diminished resulting in CO_2 narcosis due to ineffective central chemoreceptors.

Subsequent Course

After mechanical ventilation and decreasing $PaCO_2$ to normal levels, and as the effect of pre-intubation drugs subsided, the patient awoke and was interactive. He was extubated and a nasal cannula delivering supplemental O_2 was applied. Several hours later he became somnolent again with development of respiratory acidosis requiring reintubation. The clinicians recognized that this was a disorder of central control of respiration and that the patient was mainly dependent on the hypoxic stimulation of peripheral chemoreceptors for spontaneous respiration. Abolishing hypoxic stimulation with supplemental O_2 was blunting his ventilatory drive resulting in hypercarbia and CO_2 narcosis. Brain and brain stem magnetic resonance imaging (MRI) was performed revealing Type I Chiari malformation. Patient underwent sub occipital craniotomy and decompression of the posterior fossa relieving the pressure on his brainstem. Responsiveness of central chemoreceptors to CO_2 was restored and the patient was discharged home with full recovery.

Important Points

1. Pure alveolar hypoventilation results from central airway obstruction, depressed respiratory center, and ineffective neuromuscular function. Clinical manifestations provide clues to diagnosis.
2. Central chemoreceptors are responsive to acute changes in PCO_2 by decreasing the CSF pH. Peripheral chemoreceptors are primarily responsive to hypoxia, but also to hypercarbia to some extent.
3. Response time to peripheral chemoreceptor stimulation is much more rapid than that of central chemoreceptor stimulation.
4. The magnitude of response to acutely elevated PCO_2 is much greater via stimulation of central chemoreceptors compared to peripheral chemoreceptors
5. Peripheral chemoreceptor stimulation persists over a long time, even for a life-time. Central chemoreceptors however get acclimatized over time with blunting of response to elevated $PaCO_2$. In such situations, removal of peripheral chemoreceptor stimulation by O_2 administration could result in serious hypoventilation and CO_2 narcosis.

13.2   Heart Failure

Case 2

A three-month-old infant boy with Down's syndrome and atrioventricular (AV) canal was brought to the emergency department for increasing respiratory difficulty, grunting and retractions for 12 h. Temperature is 38.4 °C, respirations of 36/min, heart rate of 140/min and blood pressure of 90/45 mmHg. Precordial heave is noted. Chest auscultation revealed grade IV holosystolic murmur along the left sternal border. Expiratory wheezing and grunting were heard. SpO_2 was 90%. Chest radiograph showed cardiomegaly, with prominent central vascular markings and air trapping. High flow nasal cannula was applied with 40% O_2. Thirty minutes later, the infant was noted to be diaphoretic with respiratory rate of 60/min, heart rate of 160/min, blood pressure of 88/58 mmHg and SpO_2 of 100%. Pulses were

Fig. 13.1 Chest radiograph of a three-month-old male infant shows moderate cardiomegaly, pulmonary atrial and venous congestion, and hyperinflation of lungs

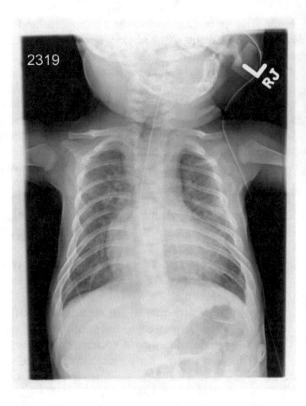

noted to be thready; peripheries were cool with delayed capillary refill. Repeat chest radiograph (Fig. 13.1) showed worsening of cardiomegaly and pulmonary edema.

Clinical Analysis

This infant has a large left-to-right shunt. The systemic arterial blood flow (Q_s) is diverted to the pulmonary arterial flow (Q_p) at both atrial and ventricular level. Such is the case with large ventricular septal defect, atrial septal defect, patent ductus arteriosus and aortopulmonary window. In a normal heart, without any communication between right-sided and left-sided circulations, Q_p is equal to Q_s. In left-to-right shunts, Q_p is greater than Q_s because of lower pulmonary vascular resistance (PVR) compared to the systemic vascular resistance (SVR) The extent to which Q_p exceeds Q_s depends on the size of the shunt and the respective resistances in systemic and pulmonary circulations. The PVR remains fairly high in the neonatal period limiting the left-to-right shunt. As the infant grows, the PVR steadily declines until at the age of 3–6 months, when it reaches the adult value of being 15–20% of SVR. With significantly increased Q_p, the pulmonary blood volume and the interstitial fluid are increased, resulting in decreased lung compliance. Baseline respiratory rates tend to be increased in such situations. The infant probably had respiratory decompensation with an intercurrent viral infection and presented with respiratory distress. Supplemental O_2 administration resulted in a further decrease in PVR increasing the left-to-right shunt, increased $Q_p:Q_s$ ratio and worsening of pulmonary congestion and edema. While SpO2 increased with greater Q_p, he developed systemic hypoperfusion as flow was diverted to the lung from the rest of the body. Maintaining SpO_2 in low 90's should be sufficient for oxygenation without compromising systemic perfusion. Mechanical support of respiration should be aimed at improving FRC and using a low V_T strategy since we are dealing with a disease of compliance. The amount of FiO_2 delivered should be enough to maintain SpO_2 in the low 90's since higher SpO_2 carries the risk of decreasing PVR and increasing the $Q_p:Q_s$ ratio. Use of optimum PEEP (along with positive pressure breathing) will be very helpful since it will: (a) displace alveolar fluid to the extra-alveolar space allowing for better gas exchange thereby reducing the FiO_2 requirement, (b) improving compliance by decreasing the pulmonary blood volume thereby allowing lower inflation pressure, (c) increasing the right ventricular afterload by alveolar capillary compression and therefore decreasing the left-to-right shunt and (d) decreasing left ventricular afterload by positive intrathoracic pressure during both the isovolumic contraction and the ejection phases of systole. The disadvantages of invasive mechanical ventilation in this situation are primarily related to peri-intubation stress and trauma and the use of the necessary sedatives/paralytic agents. Intubation should be performed in controlled conditions.

Subsequent Course

The infant was intubated after appropriate sedation and pharmacologic paralysis. Pressure-regulated volume control (PRVC) ventilation was instituted to deliver 7 mL/kg V_T with a peak inspiratory pressure (PIP) reaching 25 cm H_2O, inspiratory time of 0.8 s, PEEP of 6 cm H_2O, ventilator rate of 25/min and FiO_2 of 0.3. Furosemide was administered for diuresis. Subsequently, the patient exhibited improved perfusion. Over the next 36 h, mechanical ventilation was weaned off and the patient was successfully extubated.

Important Points

1. O_2 administration may result in pulmonary vasodilation in patients with large left-to-right shunts (e.g. VSD, AV canal) and functionally univentricular lesions (e.g. after Norwood operation). In such situations Qp:Qs may increase to such an extent as to result in pulmonary vascular overload, pulmonary edema and systemic hypoperfusion.
2. Positive pressure ventilation is an effective means of decreasing LV afterload. In patients with poor ventricular contractility (e.g. myocarditis, cardiomyopathy), positive pressure ventilation is an effective strategy to mechanically decrease the LV afterload and improve cardiac output.

13.3 Lower Airway Obstruction

Case 3

A 12-year-old boy presents to the emergency department with exacerbation of his known asthma and increasing difficulty breathing for the last 8 h. He is unable to speak in complete sentences. Vital signs are temperature of 37.8 °C, respirations of 24/min, heart rate of 110/min and blood pressure of 108/72 mmHg with pulsus paradoxus of 40 mmHg. SpO_2 while breathing 40% O_2 via a Venturi mask is 89%. Extremities are cool with dusky nailbeds. Examination reveals marked intercostal and subcostal retractions, prolonged expiratory phase and audible wheezing. Very little response to inhaled albuterol and intravenous steroids is noted. Arterial blood gases show pH of 7.12, PCO_2 of 105 torr and PO_2 of 70 torr on non-rebreather O_2 mask. The patient appears to be tiring and lethargic. Rapid sequence intubation is performed and arrangements are made to transport to the ICU for further management. Chest radiograph shows bilateral hyperinflation, flattened diaphragms, perihilar infiltrates, prominent main pulmonary artery, and a relatively small cardiac silhouette (Fig. 13.2). No air-leak is noted. Patient is being manually ventilated via a bag to ET tube with 100% O_2 at a rate of 30/min and inflation pressure of 50 cm H_2O. Repeat arterial blood gas analysis shows a pH of 6.95, PCO_2 of 130 torr and PO_2 of 104 torr.

Clinical Analysis

This patient has marked intrapulmonary airway obstruction with non-uniform ventilation and severe V/Q mismatch. His respiratory time constant (compliance X

Fig. 13.2 Chest radiograph of a 12-year-old boy with status asthmaticus. Note severe bilateral lung hyperinflation, flattened diaphragm and prominent pulmonary artery. Perihilar infiltrates are seen bilaterally

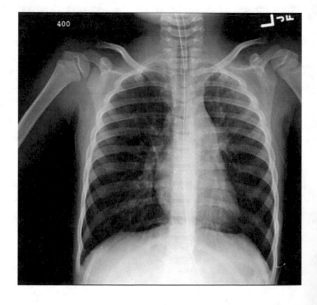

resistance) is markedly prolonged and since the obstruction is intrapulmonary, his equal pressure point (EPP) is displaced far more distally resulting in widespread airway collapse during exhalation. Thus, the expiratory time constant is much more prolonged compared to the inspiratory time constant which is also prolonged. With insufficient time for complete exhalation, there is air-trapping, auto-PEEP, decreased dynamic compliance, impaired venous return and decreased cardiac output. Markedly increased pulsus paradoxus before intubation is indicative of wide swings in intrathoracic pressure during inspiration and exhalation, decreased LV preload and increased LV afterload during inspiration. In order to deliver tidal volume effectively, we need to use sufficient time for both inspiration and exhalation because of his prolonged time constants. This can only be achieved by decreasing the respiratory rate to allow for longer time for each respiratory cycle. Furthermore, exhalation time (T_e) should be more prolonged compared to inspiratory time (T_i) to allow for greater alveolar emptying. This would improve dynamic compliance, decrease auto-PEEP, reduce the risk of barotrauma and increase venous return. Thus, the strategy should be that of a low mandatory rate with a high PIP/or V_T ventilation while monitoring both exhaled V_T and alveolar ventilation. His gas exchange worsened after intubation and manual ventilation. This is most likely because of being ventilated at too high a rate to allow for adequate delivery of V_T and alveolar emptying. On mechanical ventilation, PRVC or pressure controlled ventilation (PCV) would allow for better distribution of delivered volume compared to volume controlled ventilation which will be preferentially distributed to relatively lower resistance areas compared to higher resistance areas with resultant increased inflation pressure and barotrauma. A certain amount of PEEP would help to move EPP more proximally, decrease transmural pressure and reduce airway collapse. Inspiratory and expiratory flows along with auto-PEEP should be monitored by flow-time waveforms. Similarly, exhaled tidal volume should be monitored at different ventilator rates and PIP/V_T combinations to deliver a desired minute ventilation with minimum injury. The threat to life in status asthmaticus is mainly from hypoxia and not from hypercarbia. Hypercarbia and severe acidosis however, may impair cardiac performance, raise intracranial pressure and decrease efficacy of bronchodilators. The emphasis of desired gas exchange should be that of maintaining adequate oxygenation (O_2 saturation $\sim 95\%$) and allowing for permissive hypercapnia as long as pH is ≥ 7.3. Once corticosteroids and bronchodilator therapy decrease airway resistance as reflected in improved gas exchange, increased exhaled V_T and decreased autoPEEP, weaning could be started first by decreasing the PIP, decreasing mandatory breaths and gradually switching to pressure support ventilation.

Subsequent Course

Patient was managed on PCV mode under pharmacologic sedation and paralysis at a rate of 12/min, T_i of 1.2 s, T_e of 3.8 s, inflation pressure of 35 cm H_2O and PEEP of 4 cm H_2O. Clinical examination, ventilatory graphics, exhaled V_T, dynamic compliance and auto-PEEP were monitored. Permissive hypercapnia was allowed. Treatment with steroids and bronchodilators was continued. He also received intravenous magnesium sulphate. Intravenous fluid boluses of 0.9% saline (10 ml/ kg) were administered 3 times with improvement in his perfusion. Over the next 18 h, his dynamic compliance improved along with his gas exchange. Inflation pressure was decreased, pharmacologic paralysis was discontinued, and he was switched to pressure support ventilation while decreasing mandatory breaths. He was extubated 24 h after intubation.

Important Points

1. Diseases with increased resistance have prolonged time constants. Longer time is necessary for both delivering the V_T and alveolar emptying. Expiratory time constant is prolonged more than the inspiratory time constant. Mechanical ventilation should be performed at a relatively low mandatory rate and with higher inflation pressure or V_T.
2. EPP is displaced distally in intrathoracic airway obstruction resulting in widespread airway collapse and auto-PEEP. The consequences of auto-PEEP include decreased dynamic compliance and venous return. Application of extrinsic PEEP and longer T_e will help decrease auto-PEEP.
3. Sustained inflation pressure, either with PCV or PRVC results in better distribution of V_T compared to primarily volume controlled ventilation.
4. Monitoring of flow waveforms and auto-PEEP along with dynamic compliance is very helpful in determining the most effective and least harmful combination of mandatory breaths and inflation pressure (or V_T).
5. The goal of mechanical ventilation should be to maintain adequate oxygenation, reasonable pH and minimize complications.

13.4   Parenchymal Lung Disease

Case 4

A 16-month-old previously healthy girl presents to the emergency department with fever and progressively increasing respiratory difficulty over the past 12 h. Vital signs show a temperature of 39.5 °C, respiratory rate of 50/min, heart rate of 144/ min, blood pressure of 70/36 mmHg and SpO_2 of 75% while breathing room air. Examination shows an anxious, irritable, toxic appearing child, with cool extremities and delayed capillary refill time. Appropriate fluid resuscitation and intravenous antibiotics were given. FiO_2 of 1.0 was administered via a high flow nasal cannula. There was no significant improvement in SpO_2. The decision to institute mechanical ventilatory support was made. The patient was pre-oxygenated with 100% O_2, given sedation and paralytic agents while providing bag and mask ventilation with a PEEP valve set at 10 cm H_2O.

After stabilization, endotracheal (ET) intubation was performed. Bag to ET tube manual ventilation was continued with 100% O_2 and PEEP of 10 cm H_2O, at a rate

Fig. 13.3 A 16-month-old girl with fever and respiratory distress. Radiograph shows bilateral fluffy infiltrates in the lower lobes with extension in middle and upper lobes. Lung volume is decreased

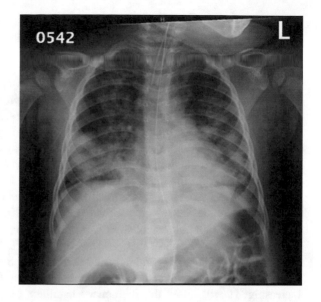

of 30–40/min with an I:E ratio of approximately 1:1. SpO_2 improved to 96% and the patient was transported to the ICU for further management. Chest radiograph showed ET tube at mid-tracheal level, decreased lung volume, and bilateral coarse and dense opacities throughout the lung but more in lower lung fields (Fig. 13.3). Pressure-regulated volume control (PRVC) ventilation was instituted to deliver 7 ml/kg tidal volume at a PIP of 30 cm H_2O, ventilator rate of 30/min, with a T_i of 0.8 s, PEEP of 10 cm H_2O, and an FiO_2 of 1.0.

Clinical Analysis

This child has severe parenchymal pathology with primary involvement of the alveoli. Most likely cause is pneumonia of bacterial origin. She also exhibits signs and symptoms of septic shock which mandates appropriate antibiotics and fluid expansion along with inotropic support. The pathophysiologic consequences of the pulmonary involvement include reduction in FRC and decreased time constants for both inflation and deflation. Decrease in FRC will result mainly in hypoxemia since the pulmonary capillary blood will have less O_2 to pick up during exhalation. Critical opening pressure is increased for the alveoli. Reduction in alveolar pressure during exhalation carries the risk of alveolar collapse (de-recruitment) and alveolar-airway junction stress during inspiration (tidal recruitment), the main cause of volutrauma. Decreased lung compliance with relative sparing of airway resistance implies shortened time constants. The airway pressure and alveolar pressure take relatively shorter time (compared to normal) to equilibrate with each other. The end result is that both inflation and deflation will be completed relatively quickly. The pressure volume relationship with this type of mechanical abnormalities can be represented by an early phase where less volume change occurs for a given pressure ($\Delta V/\Delta P$), followed by a lower inflection point with an increasing $\Delta V/\Delta P$ with another inflection point after which there is decreasing $\Delta V/\Delta P$. Thus, the dynamic compliance is greatest between the two inflection points. The alveolar pressure below the lower inflection point reflects de-recruitment (atelectrauma) and above the upper inflection point represents overdistension (volutrauma). Keeping PEEP below the lower inflection point carries the risk of alveolar de-recruitment and opening them again with an inspiratory pressure—a process sometimes referred to as "tidal recruitment"- exposing the delicate alveolar-terminal airway junctions to shear stress and rupture. PIP beyond the upper inflection point will subject the lungs to unnecessary volutrauma or barotrauma. The challenge to the clinician is to keep the tidal ventilation between these two points, by providing sufficient PEEP to keep alveoli recruited and limiting peak inflation pressure to avoid overdistension. The predominant gas exchange abnormality is hypoxemia. The safest strategies to manage hypoxemia are (a) an adequate PEEP and (b) increasing the inspiratory time (T_i). PEEP will help establish FRC and allow the pulmonary capillary blood to equilibrate with a higher PAO_2. The optimal PEEP can be inferred with improvement in PaO_2/FiO_2 and dynamic compliance. Both these measurements are helpful in keeping the tidal ventilation in between the two inflection points. Increasing Ti will allow the pulmonary capillary blood to equilibrate with the higher PAO_2 during inspiration while still enabling complete exhalation because of the short time constant. Weaning the FiO_2 to maintain sufficient SaO_2 ($\sim 95\%$) will reduce oxytrauma.

Subsequent Course

Patient was managed with PRVC to deliver V_T of 7 ml/kg, rate of 30/min, T_i of 0.8 s, PEEP of 10 cm H_2O and PIP limit of 35 cm H_2O. C_{DYN} was frequently monitored to make appropriate adjustments of PEEP. Pharmacologic sedation and paralysis were introduced to minimize asynchronous ventilation. Blood culture yielded methicillin sensitive *S. aureus*. The patient had a stormy clinical course requiring inotropic support and intravenous fluid expansion. Pulmonary infiltrates worsened with decreasing compliance and PaO_2/FiO_2 ratio, and greater need for oxygen and PEEP. High frequency oscillatory ventilation was employed with MAP of 26 cm H_2O, FiO_2 of 1.0, amplitude pressure of 30 cmH_2O and a frequency of 6 Hz. A steady improvement occurred with an increase in PaO_2/FiO_2 and lung aeration. She was transferred back to PRVC mode of ventilation when her MAP requirement was around 15 cm H_2O. Pharmacologic paralysis was discontinued. FiO_2 was weaned to keep SpO_2 $\sim$ 95%, mandatory rate was decreased to allow for pressure support ventilation. Patient was successfully extubated after a total of 10 days of mechanical ventilation.

Important Points

1. Time constant is decreased in diseases characterized by reduced compliance. This means that the proximal airway pressure and alveolar pressure equilibrate with each other in relatively a short period of time.

2. The major pathophysiologic consequence of alveolar/parenchymal diseases is decreased FRC and hypoxemia.
3. Alveolar recruitment by restoration of FRC with PEEP is a major therapeutic strategy.
4. Ventilation with low PIP/V_T at an appropriate FRC is a proven method of lung protection in pulmonary parenchymal disorders such as ARDS and pneumonia.
5. V_T should be delivered between the lower and upper inflection points. This can be determined by calculation of C_{DYN} at various levels of PEEP.
6. Increase in T_i can lead to improved oxygenation by increasing the time available to pulmonary capillary blood for gas exchange with higher PAO_2 during inspiration.
7. Patient disconnection with PEEP such as during suctioning carries the potential risk of alveolar de-recruitment and hypoxia. Such procedures should be performed while PEEP is being maintained.

13.5   Restrictive Chest Disease

Case 5

A 14-year-old boy with cerebral palsy and severe scoliosis is admitted with fever, tachycardia, hypotension, and poor peripheral perfusion. Clinical evaluation revealed a urinary tract infection with elevated inflammatory markers (white blood cell count, C-reactive protein, and procalcitonin) and combined respiratory and metabolic acidosis. An ABG revealed a pH of 7.06, $PaCO_2$ of 80 mmHg, PaO_2 of 80 mmHg, HCO_3 of 24 meq/L and a Base excess of −8 meq/L with a lactate level of 4 mmol/L. He also presented with a decreased mental status from baseline and respiratory distress with increased work of breathing.

Q. What would be the appropriate response at this time?

1. High-flow nasal cannula
2. Non-invasive ventilation with BiPAP
3. Intubation and invasive mechanical ventilation.

Answer: He definitely has acute on chronic respiratory failure with acidemia. While high flow nasal cannula might reduce his work of breathing and decrease his dead space, it is unlikely to correct his respiratory failure back to baseline. Noninvasive ventilation would not be recommended since he has decreased mental status from baseline. Therefore, the best response would be intubation and invasive mechanical ventilation.

The patient was intubated and placed on invasive mechanical ventilation. His chest x-ray showed the ET tube to be in mid-tracheal position, severe scoliosis, with small lung volumes (not different from prior films when he was well), the right lung being considerably smaller than the left lung, with no infiltrates or effusion. His initial settings were a tidal volume of 8 mL/kg, a rate of 16/min, FiO_2 of 1.0, a PEEP of 5 cm H_2O, with an inspiratory time of 1 s on volume control ventilation. His peak inspiratory pressure was 40 cm H_2O with a plateau pressure of 35 cm H_2O. His ABG an hour after mechanical ventilation was pH of 7.20, $PaCO_2$ of 70 mmHg, PaO_2 of 350 mmHg, HCO_3 of 26 meq/L, and a base excess of −7 meq/L.

Clinical Analysis

The patient has urosepsis with acute on chronic respiratory failure with combined respiratory and metabolic acidosis. His severe scoliosis has produced a restrictive chest disease characterized by low lung volumes, decreased respiratory system compliance despite a normal looking lung on chest x-ray and chronic hypercarbia. There are many aspects of physiology to consider in optimizing mechanical ventilation in patients with restrictive chest disease. First, airway pressures are too high even with a tidal volume of 7 mL/kg on volume control ventilation. It would be preferable to limit the peak alveolar pressure by reducing the tidal volume. While the tidal volume can be reduced in volume control to limit the plateau pressure, the patient also has differential lung volumes due to severe scoliosis. The distribution of ventilation would be uneven and exacerbated by volume control ventilation. With a pressure-controlled time-cycled breath, the peak alveolar pressure would be limited to the same level in all alveoli, albeit with the lung segments having different time constants for inflation. Therefore, the preferred mode of ventilation in this patient would be pressure-controlled time-cycled ventilation. Secondly, by reducing the tidal volume, total minute ventilation would be decreased exacerbating the hypercarbia. Therefore, a much higher rate than 16 would be required to control the hypercarbia. Since he has chronic respiratory failure, his $PaCO_2$ does not have to be reduced to normal levels. Since he has no lung disease, it would not be necessary to increase his PEEP any further. His FiO_2 can be safely decreased to less than 0.5 and weaned from there as tolerated. When his sepsis is under control and he is being weaned, it might be prudent to extubate him to noninvasive mechanical ventilation.

Subsequent Course

He was extubated to noninvasive mechanical ventilation. Since this critical illness made him weaker, he needed noninvasive ventilatory assistance to maintain his gas exchange. He was weaned to intermittent BiPAP support and discharged on intermittent BiPAP support without any supplemental oxygen. About a month later, he was able to wean off the intermittent BiPAP.

Important Points

1. The choice of respiratory support must be tailored to the patient's condition. Invasive mechanical ventilation would be the choice for management for respiratory failure when there is altered mental status with inability to protect the airways from aspiration of secretions

2. Restrictive chest disease in this patient is due to several factors including sco-
    liosis, ankylosis of costovertebral joints as well as sternocostal joints. With the
    result, the chest does not expand normally. Even with a lung protective strategy
    with a tidal volume of 6–7 mL/kg, the peak inspiratory and peak alveolar
    pressures reached in the lung may be too high. Therefore, these patients may
    need an even lower tidal volume. However, the ventilator rate has to be
    increased to maintain adequate minute ventilation.
3. With scoliosis, even though the lungs are relatively normal, lung expansion is
    asymmetric between the two lungs due to different time-constants between the
    two lungs. Volume-controlled ventilation, in this circumstance, results in
    uneven distribution of tidal volume and may result in atelectasis in the lung of
    the stiffer chest cavity while causing overexpansion of the compliant thorax.
    Therefore, the preferred mode of ventilation for this clinical situation is
    pressure-controlled time-cycled ventilation with an inspiratory time sufficiently
    long for adequate inflation.
4. In patients with chronic CO_2 retention, it is not necessary for ventilatory support
    to normalize $PaCO_2$. Permissive hypercapnia is the appropriate management
    strategy targeting a $PaCO_2$ closer to his baseline or higher, whichever is nec-
    essary to provide the most lung protection.
5. It might take longer for many of such patients to regain baseline respiratory
    function requiring a higher level of support after discharge from the ICU to
    adapt to the altered respiratory function. Home management with BiPAP may be
    necessary for some time before the previous respiratory status is established.

13.6 Respiratory Pump Disorder

Case 6

A 16-year-old male with no past medical history presented with a 1-day history of
progressive lower limb weakness and paresthesia. He felt tired the night before
when he went to bed. Morning of admission, he was able to walk but with support.
There was no back pain, upper limb weakness, diplopia, dysphagia or shortness of
breath or trauma to the spine. A week before his current visit, he had a fever and a
cold which lasted about 3 days. Upon initial examination, he was alert, conscious
and not in respiratory distress. His presenting vital signs were as follows: blood
pressure of 120/68 mmHg, heart rate of 85 beats per minute (bpm), temperature of
37 °C, SpO_2 of 96% on room air. His lower limb examination revealed a muscle
power of 1/5, absent tendon reflexes at the patellae and ankles and bilateral plantar
flexion response to plantar reflex. He is now unable to walk even with support. Rest
of the neurologic examination is unremarkable. No spinal tenderness is noted. His
complete blood count, renal profile with electrolytes, liver function, cardiac
enzymes, blood gas and random blood sugar tests are within normal limits. His

electrocardiogram is normal. His lumbar puncture shows 5 cells/mm^3, glucose of 75 mg/dL with a serum glucose of 110 mg/dL, protein of 220 mg/dL. Gram stain is negative. MRI of the spine shows surface thickening and contrast enhancement on the conus medullaris and the nerve roots of the cauda equina.

Differential diagnosis would include Guillain–Barre syndrome (GBS), transverse myelitis, or acute demyelinating myelitis. Since there is no sensory loss, transverse myelitis would be ruled out. Additionally, the typical MRI appearance in transverse myelitis is a central T2 hyperintense spinal cord lesion extending over more than two segments, involving more than two-thirds of the cross-sectional area of the cord. Acute demyelinating myelitis would also show lesions in the spinal cord as opposed to the nerve roots. Nerve conduction abnormalities in GBS would include slow or blocked nerve conduction, prolongation of distal latency and f-waves. His clinical course is most consistent with acute motor axonopathy, a variant of GBS.

Q. Where should this patient be admitted and what monitoring is required for this patient?

Answer: He has rapidly progressive weakness within a day. He is likely to develop worsening ascending paralysis. The concern would be the weakness affecting his respiratory muscles. Therefore, he needs to be admitted to the ICU where he can be monitored closely. His monitoring should include respiratory muscle strength assessment. There are 2 tests that are commonly employed to evaluate the respiratory muscle strength. One is the maximal inspiratory pressure that can be generated by the patient. The other is vital capacity. Maximal inspiratory pressure is measured by using the digital vacuum manometer attached to a unidirectional expiratory valve and a face mask or a mouth-piece. Patients will be able exhale through the valve, but inspiration will close the valve and generate a negative pressure. Care must be taken so as not to permit the negative pressure generated by the sucking action of the buccal muscles to influence the measurement. For this, an appropriate mouth piece is required to negate the action of the buccal muscles. Normal maximal inspiratory pressure is about −60 to −80 cm H_2O. Indication for intubation is a maximal inspiratory pressure of −20 cm H_2O or higher (less negative).

Vital capacity measurement also requires a maximal respiratory effort from the patient. Volumes are measured using a spirometer that can be attached to a mouth piece or a face-mask. Patients are encouraged to make a maximal inspiration followed by a maximal exhalation. The exhaled volume from maximal inspiration to exhalation is the vital capacity. Normal vital capacity is 60–80 mL/kg. A vital capacity of 15 mL/kg is an indication for mechanical ventilation.

On admission, the patient's maximal inspiratory pressure was −50 cm H_2O and his vital capacity was 40 mL/kg. Nerve conduction studies confirmed the diagnosis of GBS. He was treated with IVIG. Six hours later, he was complaining of air hunger and dyspnea. His maximal inspiratory pressure was −15 cm H_2O and his vital capacity was 15 mL/kg. His SpO_2 was 95% in room air and a blood gas showed a $PaCO_2$ of 50 mmHg. A decision was made to provide mechanical ventilation.

Q. Would non-invasive mechanical ventilation be appropriate for this patient?

Answer: This patient has rapidly progressive respiratory compromise. Therefore, noninvasive ventilation would not be appropriate for this patient.

Subsequent Course

The patient was intubated and placed on invasive mechanical ventilation. A volume controlled (V_T 10 mL/Kg) SIMV mode at rate of 16/min was used with a pressure support of 10 cm H_2O. He was treated with IVIG for 5 days with improvement in his muscle weakness. While he was being ventilated his maximal inspiratory pressure and vital capacity were measured daily.

Q. What would appropriate levels of maximal inspiratory pressure and vital capacity to consider weaning towards extubation?

Answer: His maximal inspiratory pressure should be at least −20 cm H_2O and vital capacity should be at least 20–30 mL/kg before weaning towards extubation is commenced. If his maximal inspiratory pressure and vital capacity are closer to normal, then he could be weaned and extubated to complete spontaneous breathing without any positive pressure assistance. If his measurements are low but above the threshold stated above, the patient could be extubated to noninvasive mechanical ventilation provided that wakefulness and airway protective reflexes are adequate.

Important Points

1. Rapidly progressive muscle weakness is an indication for ICU care even if the patient at the time of admission does not require any positive pressure support. The more frequent and intensive monitoring available in the ICU will allow the appropriate respiratory support to be provided as soon as necessary for the patient.
2. In a potentially progressive neuropathy, inspiratory muscle strength and capacity needs to be monitored closely and frequently. The decision to intubate would be made more by the index of inspiratory muscle strength and capacity rather than blood gases. Blood gases may be normal before the inspiratory muscle strength reaches the threshold for intubation.
3. Rapidly progressive muscle weakness especially with the ascending involvement of the intercostal muscles is a contraindication for noninvasive ventilation. Noninvasive ventilation, under these circumstances, may delay intubation and can result in an emergent situation with its attendant complications and morbidity.
4. Once the patient is on invasive ventilation, the clinical progress is monitored by serial measurement of inspiratory muscle strength and capacity. When the inspiratory muscle strength has improved sufficiently, the patient should be considered ready to be weaned off mechanical ventilation.

13.7   Abdominal Distension

Case 7

A one-year-old with biliary atresia, s/p Kasai procedure with portal hypertension and ascites is admitted with viral pneumonia. Chest x-ray shows bilateral diffuse patchy infiltrates mainly in the lower lobes. He is intubated and placed on mechanical ventilation. His initial ventilator settings are a tidal volume of 6 mL/kg, PIP of 30 cm H_2O, PEEP of 6 cm H_2O, FiO_2 1.0, rate of 25/min, and an inspiratory time of 0.8 s in pressure-controlled time-cycled ventilation. He is sedated and paralyzed. His first ABG shows: pH 7.36, $PaCO_2$ 50 torr, PaO_2 of 70 torr, HCO_3 25 meq/L, base excess −1 meq/L. His SpO_2 is 95%. His abdomen is distended and tense with an umbilical hernia and a fluid thrill. His chest x-ray shows the ET tube to be in the mid-tracheal position, with bilateral infiltrates (lower lobes > upper lobes), elevated diaphragm, and 7 rib expansion.

Case Discussion

From a respiratory point of view, he has severe ARDS (PaO_2/FiO_2 ratio < 100) with adequate ventilation (mildly hypercarbic). He has decreased lung volume, and his oxygenation is adequate.

Q. What should the next steps be?

1. Repeat a blood gas in an hour before making any change in ventilator settings
2. Accept current settings and gas exchange
3. Start inhaled nitric oxide
4. Increase PEEP to 8 cm H_2O.

Answer: Given the fact that his lung volume is reduced and he has severe oxygenation failure, the appropriate next step is to recruit the lungs and maintain the recruitment. That can be reliably done with an increase in PEEP. Repeating a blood gas in an hour is only postponing the necessary change in ventilator settings since the gas exchange is unlikely to change in an hour. Accepting the current settings in the setting of de-recruited lungs is not an optimal solution. Inhaled nitric oxide is not appropriate as there is no evidence of pulmonary hypertension.

Case Progression

PEEP was increased to 8 cm H_2O. A repeat ABG showed a pH of 7.35, $PaCO_2$ of 52 torr, PaO_2 of 72 torr, HCO_3 of 24 meq/L and a base excess of −2 meq/L. SpO_2 was 95%. Why did this patient not respond to an increase in PEEP? The reasons are either the patient requires a higher level of PEEP or that his lungs are not recruitable. This patient has abdominal distension as well as an increase in intraabdominal pressure. Increased abdominal pressure restricts the amount of lung inflation in the lower lobes close to the diaphragm. When the airway pressure at the bases is less than the intrabdominal pressure, the lung segments exposed to the intrabdominal pressure will collapse. In order to open these lung segments, one must apply a pressure that is equal to or preferably slightly higher than the intrabdominal pressure. There are two ways one can find the appropriate level of PEEP for this patient. One is to measure the intrabdominal pressure and to set the PEEP just a couple of centimeters above the intraabdominal pressure. Intrabdominal pressure can be measured either by measuring the bladder pressure through a urinary catheter or intragastric pressure through a nasogastric tube. The second method is to do a bedside PEEP titration. With this method, PEEP is increased in steps of 2 cm H_2O to observe the delivered and exhaled tidal volumes with a change in PEEP. In a recruitable lung, as PEEP is increased, tidal volume will also increase in pressure-controlled ventilation due to an improvement in lung compliance. The best PEEP would be the level at which the maximum increase in tidal volume was observed. If the lung is not recruitable, then there would either no change in tidal volume or a decrease in tidal volume if the lungs are hyperinflated. In the case of increased abdominal pressure, as PEEP is increased, one may see an abrupt increase in tidal volume when the PEEP level is above the intrabdominal pressure. This patient had both maneuvers performed. His bladder pressure was 12 cm H_2O. During the PEEP trial, with a change in PEEP from 6 to 8 to 10 to 12 cm H_2O, no change in tidal volume was observed which was set at 6 mL/kg. When PEEP was increased from 12 to 14 cm H_2O, tidal volume increased to 9 mL/kg, and further increased to 10 mL/kg when PEEP was increased to 16 cm H_2O but at this level of PEEP, his blood pressure decreased and heart rate increased. His PEEP was set at 14 cm H_2O. His PIP could be reduced to 30 cm H_2O to maintain a tidal volume of 6 mL/kg. His repeat ABG showed a pH of 7.36, $PaCO_2$ of 50 torr, PaO_2 of 245 torr, HCO_3 of 24 meq/L and a BE of −2 meq/L. This case illustrates the concept that the transpulmonary pressure, the alveolar pressure minus the surrounding pressure should be greater than zero for the alveoli to remain open. In patients, with increased abdominal pressure, increasing PEEP can have negative hemodynamic effects. Therefore, the optimal level of PEEP would be the one that results in improvement in lung mechanics and gas exchange while balancing the negative effects on the circulation. Increases in PEEP can however, adversely affect venous return and cardiac output. To counteract this, abdominal pressure should be reduced by paracentesis. Paracentesis can be associated with hypotension due to hypovolemia and may require an appropriate volume infusion. Decreasing abdominal pressure can also increase transpulmonary pressure by decreasing the forces opposing alveolar pressure.

Important Points

1. In order for an alveolus to remain open, the transpulmonary pressure (alveolar pressure minus the pleural pressure) must be positive. If the transpulmonary pressure is less than zero, it will result in atelectasis of the involved alveoli and contribute to intrapulmonary shunting.
2. With abdominal distension, intrabdominal pressure increases. This means that the alveoli exposed to the abdominal pressure near the diaphragm need a higher pressure to overcome the abdominal pressure. During inspiration, the inspiratory pressure may be higher than the abdominal pressure and open the alveoli. But,

during exhalation, if the PEEP level is below the intraabdominal pressure, the alveoli will collapse and contribute to venous admixture.

3. Repeated opening and closing of alveoli will contribute to atelectotrauma. To avoid this, alveoli need to be maintained open both during inspiration and exhalation. Setting the PEEP as described above, so that the transpulmonary pressure is positive throughout the respiratory cycle, is an important component of ventilator management.

4. Moderate to severe intraabdominal pressure increase, especially due to fluid accumulation, may require paracentesis to drain the fluid and decrease the intraabdominal pressure.

5. It is important to remember that both paracentesis and PEEP titration are strategies to increase the transpulmonary pressure and may need to be combined in many patients.

6. Removal of fluid from the abdomen, especially when it is under high pressure, may result in hypotension due to hypovolemia requiring the restoration of circulating blood volume. It would be prudent to administer the fluid before paracentesis is performed to mitigate the decrease in blood pressure.

Correction to: Mechanical Ventilation in Neonates and Children

Ashok P. Sarnaik, Shekhar T. Venkataraman, and Bradley A. Kuch

Correction to:
A. P. Sarnaik et al. (eds.), *Mechanical Ventilation*
in Neonates and Children,
https://doi.org/10.1007/978-3-030-83738-9

The original version of the book was published with images where the labels and text were misaligned and were inadvertently processed as such for the chapters 1, 2, 3 and 7. The erratum chapter has been updated with the changes.

The updated versions of these chapters can be found at
https://doi.org/10.1007/978-3-030-83738-9_1
https://doi.org/10.1007/978-3-030-83738-9_2
https://doi.org/10.1007/978-3-030-83738-9_3
https://doi.org/10.1007/978-3-030-83738-9_7

Index

© Springer Nature Switzerland AG 2022
A. P. Sarnaik et al. (eds.), *Mechanical Ventilation in Neonates and Children*,
https://doi.org/10.1007/978-3-030-83738-9

Printed in the United States
by Baker & Taylor Publisher Services